FIND NEW HELP FOR . . .

- Jet Lag
- Memory Problems
- Sexual Dysfunctions
- Prostate Disorders
- Diabetes
- Heart Disease and more

AMAZING MEDICINES
THE DRUG COMPANIES DON'T WANT YOU TO DISCOVER

AMAZING MEDICINES

THE DRUG COMPANIES DON'T
WANT YOU TO DISCOVER

Revised and Updated

HANS KUGLER, PH.D., AND CHASE REVEL

BERKLEY BOOKS, NEW YORK

NOTE: Every effort has been made to ensure that the information contained in this book is complete and accurate. However, neither the authors nor the publisher are engaged in rendering professional advice or services to the individual reader. The ideas, procedures and suggestions contained in this book are not intended as a substitute for consulting with your physician and obtaining medical supervision as to any activity, procedure or suggestion that might affect your health. Accordingly, individual readers must assume responsibility for their own actions, safety and health and neither the authors nor the publisher shall be liable or responsible for any loss, injury or damage allegedly arising from any information or suggestion in this book.

AMAZING MEDICINES THE DRUG COMPANIES DON'T WANT YOU TO DISCOVER

A Berkley Book / published by arrangement with the authors

PRINTING HISTORY
Laservision, Inc. hardcover edition published in 1995.
Berkley revised and updated edition / June 1999

All rights reserved.
Copyright © 1995 by Chase Revel and University Medical Research,
© 1999 by Laservision, Inc.
Book design by Tiffany Kukec.
Cover design by Erika Fusari.
Cover photograph by Abrams/Lacagnina-Image Bank.
This book may not be reproduced in whole or in part,
by mimeograph or any other means, without permission.
For information address: The Berkley Publishing Group, a division
of Penguin Putnam Inc., 375 Hudson Street, New York, New York 10014.

The Penguin Putnam Inc. World Wide Web site address is
http://www.penguinputnam.com

ISBN: 0-425-16943-X

BERKLEY®
Berkley Books are published by The Berkley Publishing Group,
a division of Penguin Putnam Inc., 375 Hudson Street,
New York, New York 10014.
BERKLEY and the "B" design
are trademarks belonging to Penguin Putnam Inc.

PRINTED IN THE UNITED STATES OF AMERICA

10 9 8 7 6 5 4 3 2 1

Contents

Carefully Tested!

YOU ARE ABOUT to learn some cold hard realities about the drug companies, their "alleged" watchdog—the Federal Drug Administration (FDA), the widespread greed of doctors and, most important, medicines that work for which you don't need a doctor's prescription.

You'll also learn about a few prescription drugs not available in the United States that have proven to be sensational answers to certain problems, and how to get them.

In the field of alternative medicine, you are exposed to a lot of stories about the benefits of certain vitamins, nutritional supplements, herbs, flavonoids and other organic extracts. Unfortunately, most of them are written by vitamin companies or herbalists who are touting their products, often stretching the truth.

Today we live in a scientific world where technology has reached a point that we can test the use of a medicine or nutritional supplement and carefully evaluate its effects in an unbiased way. The accepted method of evaluating a substance by scientists worldwide is called a "double-blind" study. A scientist must eliminate the possibility of bias and the placebo effect. The placebo effect is simply the power of one's mind to achieve what it believes will happen if a certain medicine is taken.

In a double-blind study, the director does not have any contact with the patients being tested. Researchers handle the patients. The director makes up one group of pills (for example) that contain the ingredient being tested combined with an inert substance. He also makes up another batch of pills that look identical but contain only the inert substance. These are placebos.

The researchers are given packets of pills marked for a specific patient. They don't know whether the pills are placebos or the real thing. All patients are told that they are receiving something that should help them, which prevents the placebo effect from skewing the results. Also, it is less likely that the researcher can influence the results.

If the real ingredient shows substantially more positive results than the placebo, and there are enough patients tested, the study will be considered statistically valid. When the results are published in a scientific journal, other scientists around the world try to duplicate the results in other double-blind studies. If they can, then scientists in this field usually believe that the ingredient has value.

In this book, our research team examined 266 research projects conducted by over 500 medical scientists worldwide. We eliminated all claims for nonprescription medicines and supplements where there was no scientific testing done. In most cases, we name the scientists and tell where the results were published so you can investigate further if you wish.

The purpose of this book is to make you aware of natural substances you can use not only to prevent illnesses and diseases, but also ones which cure or alleviate the disorder. A portion of medical scientists believe that we can prevent many illnesses except where they are genetically caused. And every day, genetic researchers are discovering genes that cause certain diseases and ways to manipulate these genes to correct specific problems.

Health care in the future is certain to be mostly preventive maintenance or genetic correction, instead of just trying to control the symptoms as doctors do today. We are finally learning in a big way how to correct the causes, not only the symptoms. Hippocrates would be proud!

AMAZING MEDICINES

THE DRUG COMPANIES DON'T
WANT YOU TO DISCOVER

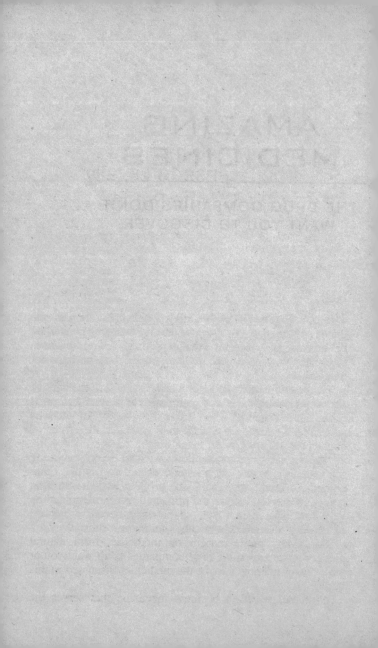

1

The License to Legally Rip Off the Public

THE U.S. PATENT Office describes a patentable item as one that is new, unique, not in existence prior to being created by the inventor and performs a useful purpose. Therefore something that exists in a plant, animal, or the earth or air is not patentable.

For example salicylic acid, which is found in the bark of poplar and willow trees, is commonly known as aspirin. It could not be patented when it was discovered. All vitamins and minerals exist in plants and animals, therefore, of course, can't be patented.

The big drug companies don't want to market anything for which they can't get a patent. The reason is that other companies could also make the product and the ensuing competition would cause the price and profit margins to be very low. That means that all patent-protected drugs are essentially "designer chemicals," not natural substances.

So, a low profit margin on medicines from natural sources is the reason the drug companies don't want you or your doctor to know a lot of the medicines discussed in this book!

Chemical World, a business magazine that serves the

pharmaceutical or drug industry as well as other chemical users, recently reported that "The drug business is one of the most profitable industries in the world."

The reason is that the federal government gives the drug companies a monopoly on a newly patented drug for seventeen years during which they can charge any price for it they wish. No one can copy that drug or create a generic brand for seventeen years.

On the surface that's fair because an inventor's creativity should be protected. However, we're not discussing inventing a Polaroid camera. The Polaroid inventor had seventeen competition-free years to recoup his development costs and be rewarded with the profits from his creativity. But there is a difference between a product such as a camera and a drug.

When the Polaroid camera was first sold it was so expensive that only upper income people could afford it. However, there is a common law in economics that states, "the more people who can afford your product, the more you will sell." Polaroid followed that law and steadily found ways to lower the price of the camera over the years so more people could afford it. This was in spite of the fact that inflation caused labor and material costs to go up an average of 5 percent per year.

Drug companies don't have to deal with this basic law of economics because patients are told by their doctors that they *must* have the drug. Therefore the drug companies charge as much as they think the market can bear. The cost of manufacturing most drugs is minuscule compared to the price charged. The bottle, label and box often cost as much if not more than the ingredients.

When questioned about their prices, the drug companies scream that they spend $50 to $200 million developing and testing a drug before it goes to market. They have to amortize that cost into every bottle sold, they argue.

On the surface that sounds like a legitimate argument except for some interesting questions. One, why are drug companies' net profits the highest of all industries? Two, why is it that European drug manufacturers, who contend with equal or even higher labor costs than the United States, spend an average of only $50 million per drug to develop and test it?

According to the annual statements of the large publicly traded drug companies, last year they spent about $8 billion on research and development of drugs. However, they also spent *over $10 billion on advertising!* Of course, advertising costs are also amortized into the price of each bottle.

This $10 billion expenditure indicates that advertising should be about 50 percent of a drug company's cost for the drug. After they add their profit margin and overhead and pharmacies and hospitals double it again for their profit, a five-dollar cost of advertising becomes twenty dollars to the patient.

But what we don't understand is why they must spend so much on advertising. The public can't buy their drugs without prescriptions. The costs of mailing an announcement and test results to doctors couldn't be more than a couple of dollars each, or about $1 million per drug.

In addition, at most there are less than one hundred "new" drugs brought to market in even the most prolific years. That amounts to $100 million to get the information to doctors in a year. Where do they spend the other $9.9 billion of their advertising expenses?

Well, we've found that a substantial portion of it goes toward persuading doctors to prescribe each drug. How do they do it? We'll give you the details in the next chapter.

The balance of their advertising is directed at the public, apparently to convince people that they have a medical problem that they didn't realize they had. Rarely does one of their "public service" ads mention a specific product, because they would have to mention all the side effects. But if you go to the doctor for that medical problem, you can bet the only drug available is theirs.

Most of the time, their public relations experts deliver stories to newspapers, magazines, TV and radio stations as "public service" or "educational" announcements. The drug companies cleverly avoid mentioning a product name, so the media immediately sends it out to the public as "news." The stories might be better described as "scare the consumer" publicity campaigns.

These scare tactics definitely create a demand for the drugs. In fact, the *Wall Street Journal* quoted Jerry Jackson, the marketing chief for the drug company Merck, as saying, "We had to create a market as well as develop a drug." He was referring to Merck's anticholesterol drug, Lovastatin.

Most people with high cholesterol can control it by changing their diet, but many people would rather take a pill. Two of the highest dollar-grossing prescription drugs are for cholesterol medications.

And it seems the cholesterol story changes every time you pick up the newspaper. First, it was that all cholesterol is bad. Then we had good and bad. The most recent one was that some of the good is bad. Next week we'll probably hear that some of the bad is good. Yet many scientists insist that the doctors are treating a symptom and not a cause.

Another very successful scare campaign focused on high blood pressure. Literally hundreds of thousands of people feared they had a problem and visited their doctor, who promptly gave them a new drug for lowering high blood pressure. Although it may have helped a few people with extremely high blood pressure, mild pressure readings can usually be controlled with diet and lifestyle changes.

There has been an extensive ad campaign recently backed by the drug company Merck to "educate" men on the dangers of prostate disease. Merck manufactures the prostate drug Proscar, but apparently it is not doing very well. Most general practitioners will refer you to a urologist if they suspect that you have a prostate disorder. Much to Merck's dismay, the urologists are not writing many prescriptions for Proscar.

A recent article in *Newsweek* stated, "The problem, it seems, is that urologists would rather do surgery than prescribe a drug that *might cut back on their business*" (our emphasis).

This disturbs us greatly because it has been shown that surgery is practically worthless. Even though Proscar isn't effective in many cases, it would be better for the patients than surgery. But we've found much better natural medicine for prostate problems which we'll detail for you in the chapter 7.

In 1982, a standard package of children's vaccines was priced at $7. Ten years later, that same package averages $130! There's no difference in the contents, and the cost of producing those vaccines hasn't risen much above the cost of inflation—about 5 percent per year. Five percent compounded for ten years would only raise the price to about $10.30. Maybe someone at the drug company put a decimal point in the wrong place!

In Europe, the prices of Americanmade drugs average 50 percent less than they do in the United States. The reason is that European health insurers, which are often the governments, just won't pay any more than that. These drugs are made by the same manufacturers, contain the same ingredients and are produced in the same controlled conditions as those available in the United States.

The government has allowed the drug companies to grab us right where it hurts and wring every nickel out of us. Americans are charged more because health insurance and government Medicare/Medicaid programs pay for 80 percent of our prescription drugs. President Clinton could cut health-care costs almost in half if he forced drug companies to sell their drugs at prices comparable to those in Europe and stopped them from spending $10 billion on advertising and "educating" doctors about their products.

Life is sacred. Why shouldn't good health also be sacred? When you are in pain or your life is threatened, you'll pay anything for relief, and the drug companies know it. Is that fair and democratic? Is good health so much less sacred that the government should allow scheming profiteers to gouge us every step of the way to death?

Dr. Charles Moertel, a cautious cancer reseacher at the Mayo Clinic, discovered that levamisole, a deworming drug used for sheep, could reduce the reoccurance of colon cancer in humans. Under an $11 million federal grant, Dr. Moertal tested the drug on thirteen hundred colon cancer patients and proved that levamisole reduced reoccurance by

41 percent and the overall death rate by 33 percent. The government gave Johnson & Johnson approval to market it (brand name, Ergamisol).

Shortly thereafter, Mrs. Annie Rhymes of Rockport, Illinois was operated on for colon cancer. Her doctor prescribed levamisole (Ergamisol) after her release from the hospital. She was dumbstruck when her pharmacist said it would cost $200 for a month's prescription—especially since she knew that the same drug for sheep sold locally for $6.39.

Sandoz Pharmaceuticals found a simple way to double its profits: water down the medicine by 50 percent, put it in the same size bottle and charge the same price! According to *U.S. News & World Report*, attorney generals in thirty-four states accused Sandoz of doing exactly that with their Triaminic Cold And Cough Medicine For Children. And they had the gall to call it "new, improved."

Sandoz has since agreed to drop the "improved" from its label and give customers refunds or coupons for an additional bottle. (Send the label or other proof of purchase to: Sandoz Consumer, Box 476, East Hanover, NJ 07936. Indicate whether you want cash or a coupon.)

The Orphan Drug Act was enacted by Congress in 1983 to encourage drug companies to develop remedies for people who have rare diseases. The act states that any pharmaceutical company developing an orphan drug for treatment of conditions affecting less than 200,000 people gets a tax credit for up to 50 percent off the development and marketing costs, plus a seven-year monopoly on the drug if it is not patentable.

The act was a great concept, but it has been totally abused by drug companies with our government's approval. For example, take Taxol, the new drug for ovarian cancer that was processed from the bark of the yew tree. Our government-funded National Cancer Institute (NCI) spent $30 million developing and proving that Taxol works. The research was then "given" to Squibb Company to complete the FDA-required testing and to market it.

Even though Squibb had very little expense in bringing Taxol to cancer patients, the charge for it ranges from

$4,000 to $6,000 per year for each patient, according to the *New York Times*. If that isn't patient exploitation, we don't know what is.

Officials of Ralph Nader's Center For Study of Responsive Law says that NCI paid another drug company only 12 percent of Squibb's wholesale price to make the initial supplies of Taxol for testing. Unfortunately the Orphan Drug Act does not control what the drug companies charge!

New studies by NCI show that Taxol also works on six other malignancies, including lung and breast cancer, which together afflict over 160,000 people yearly. It is also being tested on eighteen other cancers with high hopes. Taxol will be a bonanza for Squibb even without the benefits of the Orphan Drug Act—yet the FDA is leaving it under the act.

Another orphan drug Ceredase, used in the treatment of Gaucher's Disease, costs some patients, Medicare or health insurance companies over $300,000 a year per patient.

AZT, the AIDS drug, was also developed by government scientists with your tax dollars. Burroughs-Welcome was given the exclusive right to manufacture and sell it under the Orphan Act and began charging patients $10,000 a year each. Only after intense pressure by political activists has the price dropped to $6,400.

Drug companies also use the trick of slicing up the market for a drug to qualify for the Orphan Act. The slang for this trick in the industry is "slicing the salami." Here's how it is done. Let's assume a company creates a drug for asthma but applies under the act as a treatment for the rare steriod-dependent asthma. Less than two hundred thousand people have this rare disease so it qualifies. The drug company has a drug protected by the act but will probably sell it to all 10 million asthma sufferers.

According to the *Wall Street Journal*, Biogen, Inc., developed the drug "r-IFN-beta." They applied and received Orphan privileges as a treatment for metastic renal cell carcinoma. Three months later, the same drug company applied and received Orphan Act privileges for using it to treat cutaneous malignant melanoma. And then after two weeks, the company applied for and received Orphan Act status for treating cutaneous T-cell melanoma. But that wasn't enough. Shortly thereafter, the FDA approved Biogen's Orphan application for treating some AIDS-related conditions.

Biogen has a market of nearly a million patients for a drug that it split into five applications; yet the FDA looks the other way. This is a case of severe abuse of the act, and taxpayers are footing the bill.

When the act was first written in 1983, it required drug companies to show that the potential market for the drug under consideration was too small to be profitable. In 1984, due to the tremendous power and money of the drug-company lobbyists, the act was quietly amended, leaving out that requirement. Not only do we have rapacious drug companies, but our elected politicians are their coconspirators!

2

United States Senate Hearing on Drug Company Fraud and Bribery

THE SCARE PUBLICITY campaigns by drug companies are a more recent scheme to market drugs. The old standby method is to "encourage" or bribe doctors into prescribing certain drugs. There are about a dozen major drug companies and many smaller ones that make generics, so the practice can be quite lucrative for doctors. Much of this chapter has been excerpted from the transcript of a Senate hearing before the Senate Committee On Labor And Human Resources chaired by Senator Edward Kennedy. The primary testimony is by Sidney Wolfe, M.D., director of the Public Citizens Health Research Group, a nonprofit watchdog of the drug industry.

Dr. Wolfe obtained many of his leads for the information he gave at the hearing from a Doctor Bribing Hotline where doctors, doctors' office personnel, drug company employees and others report unethical and illegal behavior of the drug companies. The most outrageous case of bribery that Dr. Wolfe found was executed by a company called Physicians Computer Network (PCN). According to the information uncovered by Dr. Wolfe, this company was fully funded and run by the ten largest drug companies.

PCN gave doctors an elaborate "practice management" software and hardware package that computerizes details of every patient case, the diagnosis of their ills and the drugs prescribed, in addition to billing and other bookkeeping chores. There were two conditions necessary to receive this equipment: one, allow PCN to hook it to a phone modem so they could access the information any time (except for name and address of the patient); and two, the doctor must watch thirty-two ads each month that appear on this computer system and answer one clinically-oriented question per ad. That's not much in exchange for a $35,000 system—about thirty-two minutes of the doctor's time per month.

First, they get incredibly accurate and valuable marketing information about patients which they could *not* get elsewhere which they use to fuel their own product marketing and to convince other doctors to prescribe their drugs.

Second, they get to view the doctors' prescribing habits. That information is passed on to each drug company's "detail person." These are actually sales people who call on doctors, giving them free samples and promoting certain drugs. Obviously, the sales person will corner the doctor, asking why he or she is prescribing a competitor's drug.

Third, and most important, the drug companies have a captive audience with the thirty-two ads that the doctor must watch in order to answer a question about each. A psychologist told us that this is a highly clever and effective way to advertise because the doctor must concentrate on each ad to answer the question. By doing that, the information will probably stay in the doctor's memory. When those symptoms appear in a patient, the doctor is very likely to prescribe the drug he saw on the computer ad.

This information has been turned over to the Human Health Services (HHS) inspector general for further investigation.

In another incident reported by Wolfe, sales people from the drug company Roche contacted doctors, asking them to participate in a "clinical study" for their synthetic variant of penicillin called Rocephin. The salesperson virtually dictated a letter to the doctor's secretary that was to be sent by the doctor to Roche requesting money for the "study." Roche responded by immediately sending the doctor a letter of acceptance with a check for $600 stating that another $600 would be sent when the study was finished.

All the doctor had to do was record the age, diagnosis, antibiotic sensitivity, dose and duration of therapy using Rocephin of twenty hospitalized patients. It may seem like a lot to do, but it required only four minutes per patient. That's eighty minutes of work for which the doctor received $1,200—equivalent to $900 per hour.

The wholesale prices of drugs are listed in a book for pharmacists called the Redbook. From Redbook prices, Dr. Wolfe calculated that two grams of Rocephin given to twenty patients for ten days would result in gross wholesale revenues of $11,400. Certainly $1,200 in promotional costs to generate $11,400 in sales is quite a bargain.

But it is no bargain for the patients, Medicare and the health insurance companies. The hospital will double the wholesale price and bill the patients for $22,800. That's about $15,000 higher than the cost of generic penicillin. Rocephin is just a synthetic version of penicillin. Roche is hiding behind its very thin veil of "alleged research." What will happen? Well, our guess is that now that it has been reported to HHS, and they've started an investigation, Roche will probably drop the program and start a different one.

Dr. Wolfe also discovered a program created by the drug company Wyeth-Ayerst to protect the sales of Inderal, a hypertension drug which had just run out its seventeen years of patent protection. In a cooperative deal with American Airlines, Wyeth offered doctors one thousand frequent flier miles for every prescription of Inderal written. All the doctor had to do was fill out a simple form which required a few words about the patient's condition and about which drug Inderal replaced.

The doctor had to write *only fifty* prescriptions to be rewarded with a free ticket *anywhere* in the United States. It's possible that some doctors write that many hypertension drug prescriptions in a week! American Airlines would not reveal how many doctors had flown at Wyeth's expense, but an American Airlines spokesman did say, "It was a very successful program from our standpoint."

A few thousand passengers probably wouldn't be significant, so we bet that literally tens of thousands of doctors participated in the program. Obviously the drug companies know that there are a lot of doctors who will grab this kind of offer—otherwise they wouldn't keep using these programs.

Massachusetts is the only state that has a law against doctor bribery by drug companies, but it applies *only* when Medicaid paid for the drug. That leaves individuals and health insurance companies out in the cold. In 1989, Massachusetts launched a criminal investigation of Wyeth-Ayerst which later culminated in the following statement: "The pharmaceutical company, Wyeth-Ayerst, which promoted the use of a new heart drug by offering Massachusetts physicians free airline tickets, diagnostic equipment and medical books, will pay the Commonwealth of Massachusetts $195,000 and cease its promotional program as part of an agreement reached today with Attorney General James M. Shannon."

"This office is increasingly concerned with marketing practices of pharmaceutical companies which provide gifts and other incentives designed to influence physicians in prescribing drugs—a practice that violates the state's Medicaid False Claims Act," Shannon said. "It is important that medical decisions be made solely in the best interest of the patient and not on the basis of inducements offered by drug companies."

There is also a federal law that prohibits bribery, but only where Medicare or Medicaid payments are involved. Even the federal government doesn't think the rest of us are important. HHS claimed they were investigating this case, but no publicly announced results were found. We wonder why!

According to a report by the inspector general's office of HHS, Connaught Laboratories was caught by HHS giving doctors "points" redeemable in merchandise for every vaccine package that they prescribed. The merchandise included VCRs, video cameras, computers, software, TVs, medical equipment and medical education programs. HHS Inspector General Richard Kusserow wrote, "This program functions like the supermarket green stamp programs of the past."

Connaught was neither indicted nor sued. They claimed no Medicare or Medicaid funds were involved but agreed to discontinue the program. They received not even a slap on the wrist. It's amazing what the drug companies can get away with.

Dr. Ken Arndt, a dermatology professor at Harvard, received a letter from Sandoz regarding the use of Sandimmune, an immune suppression drug. The FDA had approved it *only* for preventing organ rejection in people receiving kidney transplants. The purpose of the letter was to get Dr. Arndt to read a two-page report on the use of Sandimmune to treat psoriasis. He was promised one hundred dollars if he would answer questions afterwards.

Dr. Ardnt was outraged by this, as it appeared to be a blatant campaign to get doctors to prescribe the drug for an *unapproved* purpose. Dr. Ardnt pointed out that a recent article in the British Journal of Dermatology stated that 46 percent of the people being treated with this drug for psoriasis had to discontinue its use because of serious side effects. There are no reports of Sandoz being reprimanded for this behavior. Why is the federal government looking the other way?

Regularly doctors are being paid one hundred to two hundred dollars plus a gourmet dinner with expensive wines at exclusive, pricey hotels to listen to lectures on the benefits of new drugs. The drug companies get around any bribery complaints by calling the payments "honorariums" or "consulting fees." An article in the drug promotion magazine *Medical Marketing And Media* said the increasingly widespread practice of promotional dinners means that 175,000 to 180,000 doctors will attend such dinners this year.

A promotional dinner expert commenting on the ultimate

measure of success of these events (increased prescription sales) said, "Every promotional dinner doesn't result in a marked increase in the sales curve. They fail 15 to 20 percent of the time."

Well, in the general marketing world an 80 to 85 percent success ratio is considered unbelievably successful. If a salesperson could sell eight out of ten prospects approached, he or she would be considered the greatest salesperson in the world. If you are ever in a position to observe or obtain knowledge of other bribery by drug companies, please report it to the Public Citizen Hotline, 202–872–0320. Ask for Dr. Sidney Wolfe. Let's keep up the pressure on this. Maybe something will happen.

A Harvard study reported that over 10,000 people died in one year in New York City hospitals due to doctors' mistakes or malpractice. By extrapolating that figure nationwide, we estimate that 186,000 people die across the country from doctors misprescribing drugs or practicing medicine poorly. Doctors even have a fancy word for it. They say, "The person died of 'iatrogenic' causes!"

Perhaps many of those people died because doctors prescribed the wrong drugs under the influence of drug companies' promotional campaigns. If a judge gets caught accepting a bribe, usually he or she will get prison time and the total loss of reputation and career. While the judge's decision will cost him or her money and maybe result in a prison sentence, rarely does it result in death.

Yet, if a drug company bribes a doctor, and he or she kills someone with the wrong prescription, nothing happens to either the doctor or the drug company, except for the remote possibility that a loved one will press a malpractice suit. Isn't it time we did something about this awful situation?

Sometimes the doctor can't be blamed for misprescribing drugs. For example, the FDA approved the drug Dipentum for use only in adults to help them maintain remission of ulcerative colitis. According to a report in the *Wall Street Journal* Kabi Pharmacia, Inc., the manufacturer, sent its representatives to doctors claiming children could use it, that it was the best choice for all stages of active ulcerative colitis, and that it was superior to Sulvasalazine, the generic drug prescribed for this disease.

Apparently none of these claims were proven or accepted by the FDA. The *Wall Street Journal* reported that a consent decree signed by Kabi and filed in federal court demanded the company stop making unproven claims to doctors and spend $300,000 to advertise that Dipentum's only use was the one originally approved by the FDA. Apparently this happens all the time. FDA Commissioner Dr. David Kessler said, "As a physician, I think we would be burying our heads in sand to assume that this is an isolated instance. The company's goal was to increase sales *at the expense of patient care*" (our emphasis).

Pfizer has set up a $500 million fund for problems from its now-discontinued artificial heart valves: they have a tendency to crack inside the body, killing the person, according to a story in *Time* magazine.

The biggest story is about Dow Corning Wright, a company accused of failing to report that its silicone gel breast implants were associated with severe side effects such as rheumatoid arthritis and lupus. Between one and two million women have implants made by Dow and other manufacturers.

Dr. Norman Anderson, one of the FDA's advisory panel members, said that he was amazed when he read dozens of documents from a breast-implant liability suit. Apparently seventeen Dow internal memos dating back to the mid-1970s revealed numerous problems with the implants. Dow had previously assured the FDA that they had disclosed all relevent details about the implants. However, Dr. Anderson concluded that the memos leave "little doubt of Dow's misrepresentation of the facts." The FDA declared a moratorium on sales of the implants while it studies the problem.

Yes, "studies" the problem. From our perspective, this was a criminal act. We've seen people go to jail for a lot less. It's about time that the government started putting some drug company executives in jail. That might stop some of this rampant corruption.

The drug company Bolar allegedly forged documents in

seeking FDA approval of Dyazide, its generic high-blood-pressure pill. The pill was found to be defective. Bolar was fined $10 million and its pills pulled from the market. Bolar's top executive, Robert Shulman, went to jail.

Generic drug manufacturers must prove to the FDA that an individual generic drug performs the same as the formerly patent-protected drug. The research director of Vitane Pharmaceuticals ordered a proven brand-name drug to be substituted for their generic version of the drug in the required equivalency tests. He also forged the initials of employees on test batches and raised the size of the test batches in reports to the FDA, according to a story in the *Washington Post*. The company sold more than $11 million of the drug triamterene hydrochlorothiazide, before the government recalled it. Twenty executives of the company have been convicted or pleaded guilty to charges of fraud, racketeering and obstruction of justice. The company was fined $2 million and is now in bankruptcy.

Generic drug companies are usually very small in comparison to the top ten companies. Vitane would be a grain of sand next to a boulder compared to one of the top ten. Why is it that the FDA viciously attacks the little companies and not the big ones? We suspect the big ones have too much political power.

Vitane was the tenth drug company to plead guilty to fraud and misrepresentation in the last three years. U.S. District Judge John Hargrove said, "There is virtually no testing of some products . . . and they are thrown out into the market."

During the investigation of those ten companies, detectives discovered that five key employees of the FDA had taken bribes from the drug companies to speed up the approval of their applications for new drugs.

Last year allegations arose regarding research grants given by drug companies to prominent scientists. It seems the grants were conditioned on the scientists writing positive papers on new drugs about to be marketed—and those papers being published in a major medical journal. The grants ranged as high as $50,000 and involved several scientists and drug companies. Sources claim papers were actually published; which, of course, influenced perhaps hundreds of thousands of doctors to prescribe the drugs. No intense investigation was done because both the scientists and the drug companies denied any collusion. We think the investigators were pretty naive to expect either party to admit to something so devastating to careers of the scientists and the profits of the companies involved.

When drug companies test a new drug, they don't have to submit the raw data to the FDA. The FDA relies on the companies' own analyses and conclusions. Often it takes ten years from creation through testing until a drug comes to the market. Drug companies claim the cost ranges from $50 million to $250 million per drug. Let's say your drug company has spent $200 million, and it later discovers some problems with the drug. A $200 million investment is a mighty big incentive to downplay the problems. *Time* magazine quoted Robert Temple, chief of the FDA's Office of Drug Evaluation, as saying: "They definitely have rose-colored glasses!"

The FDA makes big promises of changes in the system. FDA chief Robert Kessler told the press, "The honor system is out the window. . . . " That sounds great, but Washington observers say that the FDA has neither the staff nor subpoena powers to discover problems before it is too late.

Just how a profit-driven system can be expected to operate on honor and trust is beyond us. Yet every sick person's life depends on it!

In England, the British Parliment has proposed the Medicines Information Bill. This bill, if passed, would provide the public with a full report on the safety trials of each drug. British drug companies, several of which are owned by American drug companies, are fighting it vehemently with the most suspicious defense. They claim it would eliminate healthy competition between drug companies. Maybe that's exactly what we need—less competition and more human concern!

Occasionally with a prescription drug you get a leaflet in the package that describes possible side effects of the drug.

If you have a powerful magnifying glass, you can possibly read the tiny, cramped together four-point type (that's a fraction of the size of the type on this page), but understanding the language requires a doctoral degree in biology, chemistry or medicine. Dorothy Smith, president of the Consumer Health Information Service, says, "Ninety-seven percent of the material on drugs written for patients cannot be understood by the average consumer."

People over the age of sixty are affected more than anyone because they take 59 percent of all the prescriptions. Vision gets poorer the older they get and many have less than a high school education. Why are the drug companies hiding the truth about drugs? Is it so bad that no one would risk taking the drug? Or is it that they are not concerned about the patient's well being? It's pretty obvious to us that they simply don't care and want to hide any problems.

Most doctors are not aware that drug dosage should often be lowered for elderly people. About 70 percent of doctors treating Medicare patients flunked an exam concerning their knowledge of prescribing to older adults. Also, certain combinations of drugs are dangerous—such as taking Warfarin, a blood-thinning agent, while taking aspirin. It can lead to fatal bleeding in some elderly people.

The average elderly person takes four prescription drugs and two nonprescription substances regularly. Often they experience side effects caused by the combination, but usually write it off as just another affliction of old age.

Drug companies are not required to make any tests specifically on elderly people to determine if the dosage should be modified. The big pussycat FDA folks said they issued a guideline in March 1993 that *strongly urges* drug manufacturers to evaluate the effects on elderly people and print the information on an enclosure to go with the drug. Well, whoop-dee-do! Why doesn't the FDA just whip them with a wet noodle? It would have about the same effect. We thought federal regulatory agencies made rules and regulations, not strongly worded urges!

Many drugs block vital nutrient uptake, according to a USDA-financed study at the Human Nutrition Research

Center on Aging at Tufts University. The more drugs you take and the longer you take them the greater the risk of nutritional side effects. Deficiency in a nutrient can cause other illnesses which may force you to go to the doctor again. Very few doctors have any education in nutrition, so they'll try to find another prescription drug in their kit for your problem. That's like pouring gasoline on an out-of-control fire!

Dr. Earl Mindell's *The Vitamin Bible* lists sixty-four prescription and nonprescription drugs or medicines that rob your body of vital nutrients. For instance: aspirin removes vitamin C, B and folic acid; cortisone and prednisone remove zinc; laxatives and antacids deplete vitamins A, D, E and K; and diuretics destroy potassium. Dr. Mindell's book is available in most bookstores and is a worthy addition to any home library.

According to the government's General Accounting Office (GAO), a study found that more than half of the prescription drugs approved by the FDA between 1976 and 1985 caused serious side effects. They were either pulled from the market or relabeled with warnings. An FDA spokesman claimed the study was "alarmist and inaccurate"! The GAO accountants just compiled hard statistics and were less likely to lie than the FDA, which was protecting its territory.

Many of the side effects of these drugs resulted in hospitalizations, permanent disability and death, according to the GAO report. A Public Citizen Health Research Group newsletter reported that 22 percent of older patients given three or more prescriptions upon release from hospitals had prescription errors that were potentially serious or life-threatening.

With an estimated 186,000 people dying every year from iatrogenic causes (complications in treatment), it is believed that a substantial portion were drug-induced. According to published studies and the Public Citizen Research Group (PCRG), 119 out of 364 drugs most commonly prescribed for the elderly should not be used because safer alternatives are available and effective. Every year 659,000 older adults have to be hospitalized due to side effects of the drug. Close to another 9 million suffer at home from these adverse drug reactions.

■ Twenty-nine Drugs May Give You Parkinson's Disease!

This will shock you but it is true! Imagine taking a drug, and having it cause the terrible, dehabilitating Parkinson's disease. Well, over 61,000 people experienced that last year! There are actually twenty-nine drugs on the market that can cause Parkinson's.

There are another 65 that can cause you to go crazy— dementia! PCHR says there are also: 86 drugs that cause depression; 105 that cause hallucinations; 46 that can make you fall and probably break bones; 22 that can cause auto accidents; 119 that cause sexual problems; 88 that cause constipation; and 18 that will keep you from sleeping well!

There's a book that may give you some protection. PCHR, a nonprofit association, has published a book, *Worst Pills/Best Pills II* by Dr. Sidney Wolfe. It offers the plain truth in understandable English about 346 drugs most commonly prescribed to older adults. It includes seventy of the newest, most promoted ones such as Prozac, Mevacor, Cipro, Pepcid and BuSPAR. Dr. Wolfe and other experts warn about 119 of these drugs which they feel you shouldn't use, and give advice on safe, effective alternatives.

Write to:
Public Citizen
2000 P. Street NW, Dept. AM
Washington, DC 20036

3

FDA's Gestapo Tactics Against Vitamins

SEVERAL YEARS AGO on the suggestion of the FDA, state health inspectors in Texas raided health food and vitamin stores throughout the state and confiscated thousands of products. Shoppers were astounded as the inspectors took vitamin C, aloe vera products and herbal teas from the shelves.

Worse yet, in Kent, Washington, sixteen bullet-proof-vested FDA agents brandishing guns burst into the Tahoma Clinic commanding the employees to "freeze." The agents took all of Dr. Jonathon Wright's medical equipment (worth over $100,000), patients' records and his inventory of vitamins. They also arrested him.

The FDA claimed Dr. Wright was making illegal drugs and injecting them into patients. The "illegal drugs" were vitamins. Alex Straus, director of Citizens for Health, said, "For God's sake, we're talking about vitamin C and B_{12} shots!"

■ Patient Films Attack

Fortunately a patient in the waiting room had his video camera with him and recorded the whole fiasco. It was broadcast on news programs nationally. The biggest newspaper in the area, the *Seattle Post*, warned in an editorial, "If there is any plausible excuse for the gestapo-like tactics used in the raid of Dr. Wright's clinic, it better be forthcoming and fast!"

■ FDA Says Mixing Vitamins Is Illegal

The FDA says its actions were "grounded in hard science and law." Since when is mixing vitamins illegal? You can buy multivitamins everywhere! Also when was a law enacted that says doctors *cannot* inject vitamin B_{12} and other vitamins? Most doctors give B_{12} shots!

A year later, the FDA did not prosecute or impose criminal penalties as a result of any of its raids. Yet they have not returned Dr. Wright's equipment, records or inventory— essentially putting the man out of business! We called the Texas state health inspector's office, and no one seemed to know whether they had returned the health food store's merchandise.

What we're even more appalled at is the way government cops (city, county, state and federal) seem to love to pretend to be Rambo or SWAT teams. Is it something about dressing up in their "shoot-'em-up" outfits? Why does a big powerful government agency need to use sixteen burly cops in bulletproof vests with guns drawn to serve a search warrant on a little doctor and three employees?

■ FDA Treated Them Like Columbian Drug Lords

Neither the doctor nor any of his employees had arrest records. None of them even had a gun registered in their names. If a single government cop comes to most law-abiding people's homes or businesses with a search warrant, do they pull out guns and try to shoot the cop? No! It's simply a case of cops and government out of control.

Fortunately the FDA gestapo team drew tremendous heat from the public. Within twenty-four hours, over two thousand letters were sent to the president and hundreds more went to the FDA. Numerous nonprofit citizens' groups were formed to assault Congress with their displeasure and rage. Why is it that a government agency that is supposed to protect our health allows big drug companies to get away with all kinds of fraud and chicanery, yet sticks guns in the faces of people taking and selling vitamins?

4

The Number-One Reason for Becoming a Doctor—Money

A SURVEY OF MEDICAL students revealed that 83 percent wanted to become doctors because of the big money they would earn! Did you really think people would go through years of tough medical school studies *just* to help sick people?

The average medical doctor in the United States earns in excess of $300,000 annually if they have their own practice. The top 20 percent earn over $1 million. Those that have other doctors working for them (and heart surgeons) often earn over $3 million per year.

It's easy to see how heart surgeons make so much money when you look at the cost of open-heart or bypass surgery. The price of that procedure ranges from $30,000 to $50,000. For a half day's work, the chief surgeon will take home $15,000 to $25,000. The balance goes to the anesthesiologist, assisting surgeon and the hospital.

If the doctor averages just three such procedures a week, he or she will gross $3.9 million for the year with a month vacation. We would say that that kind of money is a pretty good incentive to go to medical school.

Many doctors make patients wait anywhere from thirty

minutes to three hours before they see them—and then with
no apology. In the business world, no one would make you
wait for more than thirty minutes for a scheduled appointment. And if it were more than fifteen minutes, you'd get a
very serious apology for being made to wait. If you went
into any retail business to spend money and were made to
wait for more than a few minutes, you'd almost certainly
walk out and go to a competitive store where your business
would be appreciated.

Doctors found out long ago that they could get away with
it because people are resistant to changing doctors. No matter how inconsiderate the doctor is of the patients' time, they
still go back! The doctors also found that about 5 percent of
patients either cancel their appointments at the last minute
or don't show up. Therefore, doctors overbook patients to
take up the slack.

Everyone gets delayed once in a while for unexpected
reasons, and doctors are no different. But have you ever
walked into a doctor's office in a major city at the exact time
of your appointment and been immediately taken in to see
the doctor? We took a survey of our office staff, and *everyone* said that they have to wait every time they go to their
doctor's office. The only exception was dentists: many people said that they usually don't have to wait very long for
them.

So, if a doctor usually runs late every day, why doesn't he
or she book fewer appointments? Obviously doctors have no
concern that you have to waste your valuable time sitting
there reading old magazines. What they are really concerned
about is jamming as many patients into their schedule as
possible in order to make as much money as they can.

With many HMOs restricting the prices doctors can
charge, overbooked schedules have become the norm. Some
doctors see as many as twelve patients per hour. With an
average doctor's visit in most major cities running about
$60, that's $720 per hour. In eight hours they have grossed
$5,760, less rent, utilities and office help. If the doctor does
that five days a week, forty-eight weeks a year, he or she will
take home about $1.2 million annually.

If all the working adults in this country only go to their doctor once per year during normal working hours, and they wait an average of one hour, that's 183 million work hours that Americans lose if on an hourly wage—or businesses lose on salaried employees. Even estimating an hourly salary of only ten dollars, doctors cost us almost $2 billion in lost wages.

According to the drug promotion magazine *Medical Marketing and Media*, 175,000 to 180,000 doctors accepted the one hundred to two hundred dollars plus fine wine and gourmet food to listen to a pitch on a new drug—a clearly unethical practice.

There are no figures available on how many participated in drug-company inducements to write certain prescriptions, such as the frequent flier miles, points for merchandise, free computers, phony research study programs, et cetera.

There's a general attitude among the people in this country that it is all right to rip off insurance companies whenever given the chance. Doctors are probably no different. And there are no figures available on how many doctors overbill insurance companies and charge them for unnecessary lab tests, X rays and other procedures.

Out of the 552,000 members of the American Medical Association (AMA), we're betting the same 83 percent who went into doctoring for money are unethical in some aspect of their practice.

- **A Clever and Profitable Reaction to Malpractice Insurance Rate Increases**

In the 1970s, insurance companies experienced a big surge in malpractice claims, and in turn dramatically increased insurance rates they charged doctors. The outcry was enormous. Every time you turned on the TV or picked up a paper, doctors were claiming the increase would put them out of business.

Of course, doctors are not dummies. They went to their attorneys to find out how they could avoid malpractice claims. Not surprising, doctors with few or no claims were paying the lowest insurance rates. There was a simple way to avoid claims, attorneys reasoned. Give the patients numerous lab tests, X rays and other tests even remotely related to a given problem. That way doctors would certainly be covered when something unusual popped up that could cause a claim.

Also, the attorneys and insurance companies made up a form for each patient to sign. That form, which goes under many different titles, essentially takes away the patient's rights to a jury trial and forces all malpractice claims into the hands of an arbitrator. Arbitrators rarely ever give high awards, especially million-dollar ones, even where malpractice is clearly proven.

The attorneys also suggested that since the doctors would be conducting such a high volume of medical tests, that they could support their own laboratories and medical testing equipment. In doing so the doctors could double or triple their income.

Up until the 1950s, the AMA considered it unethical for a doctor to own or have even an interest in laboratories, pharmacies, hospitals, clinics or drug companies (if they deal directly with patients). It was called "double dipping," because the doctor would be making a profit from something he was prescribing. The AMA apparently felt that a greedy doctor could easily abuse that system with unnecessary tests, prescriptions and hospitalizations.

However, in the fifties, the AMA doctors voted out the old system and allowed themselves to own all sorts of businesses that had customers or patients who could be generated from their practices. The idea caught on slowly, probably because most doctors had been brought up with a more idealistic and ethical attitude toward medicine. But during the malpractice scare of the seventies, lawyers convinced many doctors that it was the thing to do. Of course, realizing they could double or triple their income was no small incentive either.

According to a survey by the *Health Alert Newsletter*, doctors in Miami own 93 percent of all diagnostic MRI centers. However, in Baltimore, for some unknown reason, very few are owned by doctors. Would you want to take a guess

doctors prescribed more $800 MRI scans? You're
The Miami doctors ordered scans twice as often as
in Baltimore!

The University of Arizona conducted a study of 65,000
patients. They found that doctors who had MRI equipment
in their offices conducted four times as many scans as doctors who referred patients elsewhere. Over 40 percent of
doctors own labs or treatment facilities. A study of a portion
of those doctors showed that the doctors' labs did *twice as
many tests per patient* as independent labs—double dipping
to the extreme.

But the independents aren't sacrosanct. In California,
National Health Laboratories, Inc. was caught in a fraudu-
lent lab-tests claims scheme. They agreed to return *$111
million* to Medicare/Medicaid, according to a story published in *Playboy* magazine.

- ## Seminar for Bill Padding

There are seminars that doctors pay to attend where they
learn "creative billing." They are taught tricks of padding
bills to get even more money out of your health insurance
company. A story about this phenomenon appeared in the
November 25, 1991, issue of *Time* magazine.

Who pays for these padded bills and superfluous tests
that are making doctors even more wealthy? Either you or
your doctor pays higher insurance premiums. If employers
pay more, then they must raise the price of their products or
services to cover these additional costs. So even if you don't
pay for health insurance directly, you pay for it with the
higher prices of consumer goods. Do doctors really deserve
the tremendous amounts of money they get?

- ## Overprescribing Drugs

The *Washington Post* reported that Lurlyne Tompkins,
age seventy-eight, took nine drugs every day: four pain medications, a thyroid drug, an ulcer drug, a diabetes drug, a
high-blood pressure drug and a drug for vascular problems.
Her son discovered that often she didn't know whether it
was day or night. He took her and her basket of drugs to the

Geriatric Assessment Center at Johns Hopkins Medical Institute. They found Mrs. Tompkins was taking several drugs she did not need and reduced the dosages of the ones she needed. Amy Goldstein, staff writer for the *Washington Post*, wrote, "Mrs. Tompkin's case is not rare . . . (it's) a common phenomena among elderly people."

Elderly people often have several doctors. Almost 40 percent of those over sixty-five take five prescription drugs daily. Another 19 percent take at least seven drugs, according to a study done by the National Council on Patient Information and Education.

Mixing drugs can cause all sorts of problems—many of which are unpredictable. The common reactions are diminished mental ability, dizziness, memory loss and bladder problems. Combining a high blood pressure drug with Valium can cause severe mental problems. Arthritis drugs often react with coffee or alcohol to damage the stomach. Diuretics combined with heart medications multiply the effect of each drug, and sometimes dangerously. Even aspirin taken with blood-thinning drugs can cause internal bleeding. Eyedrops for glaucoma can cancel the benefits of diabetes and asthma medications.

Clearly it is the doctor's responsibility to ask patients what drugs they are already taking. However, you can't depend on them to ask or to know what is dangerous to mix. Always tell the doctor what you are taking, including nonprescription medicines. Ask him or her what side effects you can expect. Also it would be wise to own a copy of the *Physicians Desk Reference (PDR)* which you can get or order in most bookstores. The PDR explains the side effects of each drug and is available in hardback or paperback. The *Pill Guide*, also available in bookstores, covers the most popular drugs, and it is less expensive than the PDR.

If you experience any new and/or negative feelings while taking medication, call your doctor immediately. Your life might depend on it. And take only the recommended dosages. A federal report stated that over eighty thousand people last year went to emergency rooms because of prescription-drug overdoses. Often the drugs involved were

...ers. such as Valium. Xanax and sedatives. Many ...will prescribe a tranquilizer to any patient that asks. ...octor in New Mexico was responsible for 28 percent of *all* Valium prescribed to Medicare patients in the state.

Nine states have recognized the problem and have instituted a special three-part prescription form. One copy is kept by the doctor. one goes to the pharmacy. and the third part goes to the state health agency. That way the states can track the doctors (like the one in New Mexico) responsible for overprescribing drugs.

As a result of this program in New York. California. Illinois and Texas. prescriptions for dangerous tranquilizers and sedatives have dropped 35 to 50 percent. The state of New York found that the reduction in just one class of sedative drugs saved their Medicaid program $24 million the first year. according to a story in the *New York Times*.

Why don't all the other states have this prescription-control system? Because of strong opposition from the fat-cat drug-company lobbyists who contribute heavily to political campaign chests. The drug companies should be concerned. They stand to lose up to 50 percent of their sales of tranquilizers. sedatives and amphetamines which needlessly addict millions of people. We're talking about several *billion* dollars of lost sales.

- **Over 80 Percent of Medical Procedures Don't Work!**

The federal government has a department called the U.S. Office of Technology Assessment. which studies and analyzes the technological progress of various industries. According to their report on the medical field. over 80 percent of conventional medical procedures don't work and have little scientific basis. Research shows that *many people just heal despite what doctors do to them*.

For example. three separate studies have shown that people don't live any longer after having bypass surgery. The heart surgeons don't like you having this knowledge. As a group they gross $28 million *a day* doing bypass surgery, according to the *Wellness Letter*. Per capita. Americans have twice as many bypass surgeries as Canadians and five times as many as people in France. Yet 20 percent more people in the United States die of heart disease than in Canada per capita.

When anyone suggests that we do away with competition in the health services field, the drug companies and hospitals scream that prices will go up if there's no competition. What they know is that doing away with competition that is, converting our system to a form of socialized medicine, means the advent of price controls.

The state of Arizona formerly controlled the number of hospitals that could do open-heart surgery. During Reagan's "cut the regulations" campaign, the Arizona authorities got the idea that if more hospitals did open-heart surgery, the price would drop. They were wrong. Seven new hospitals in Phoenix joined the four existing facilities that offered open-heart surgery. Within only one year the price rose over 50 percent, and *35 percent more patients died!* Apparently, doctors with less experience made the major contribution to the death rate.

A Harvard study of heart patients found that 84 percent of those who were told by their doctors that they needed bypass surgery *were found not to need it*. The *Wellness Letter* reported that 17,500 patients die every year from this procedure itself. This clearly shows the awful greed of many doctors, and their complete disregard for human life! If the Harvard study is accurate, and we don't doubt it is, then 84 percent, or 14,875 people who were operated on last year might still be alive today!

The "science" of angioplasty, carotid endarterectomy and cancer chemotherapy is just "hope and a big medical bill." Cancer scientists admit that the success rate of chemotherapy is low for many types of cancer, but heart doctors are not so forthcoming about their hot new techniques.

Cardiac catherization is another popular procedure with which heart doctors pad their income. The cost is $4,000 to $5,000 but scientists say that out of the tens of thousands done each year, few are necessary. Several uncomplicated and *inexpensive* stress tests will provide the same information about the patient. However, cardiac specialists love catherization, and so do the hospitals. Their share of the charge results in over 70 percent profit!

When a person is in a hospital, his or her doctor has the power to call in as many specialists as the doctor chooses. Often this goes way beyond the patient's needs. A resident doctor at a major hospital says it is not unusual to see as many as five specialists on a case that is so simple *none was needed*. The resident Dr. Jones (not his real name), said, "What they are doing is repaying favors. You fill my pocket, and I'll fill yours! And the insurance companies or Medicare have to pay for their 'consulting'."

At the same hospital, a young intern fresh out of medical school told us that the administrator had billing clerks checking patients' records to find the ones whose insurance would pay for "physical rehabilitation." The reason? The hospital had just opened a new physical rehabilitation ward! Who cares about patients' needs? They are in this to make money!

An analysis of Ford Motor Company's expenses reveals that the company spends about *$1,300 per car produced just to pay for health insurance*. No wonder Japan can produce better cars for less money! Every product you buy that is made in the United States is effected the same way Ford cars are. So you are paying to fatten the coffers of drug companies, hospitals and doctors; not only through the higher costs of products you buy, but also with the tax money that is spent on Medicare/Medicaid!

Our health system is so complicated by doctors padding bills and doing unnecessary procedures that insurance companies require *ten times the normal amount of employees* just to analyze claims. For example, it takes as many claims administrators to authorize claims coming from doctors and hospitals at Blue Cross for 2.6 million policyholders as it does for *the entire Canadian Health Insurance Program*, which covers over 26 million people! It is no wonder that hospitals are as bad as doctors when it comes to padding insurance claims. Most hospitals are owned by a group of doctors, or they have a substantial interest therein.

The average three-hundred-bed hospital in the United

States has 36.4 billing employees. Yet in Canada, one billing clerk can handle the entire hospital! Why the big difference? Several insurance company administrators told us that practically every claim from hospitals is loaded with inaccuracies and charges for unnecessary tests and procedures. Because of those problems, claims administrators must spend inordinate amounts of time on the phone with hospital billing clerks demanding explanations and documentation.

One way you can help is by demanding that someone go over every item on your bill and explain it to you when you check out of the hospital. Also try to keep track of every item that they deliver to your room or you—even Kleenex, because you'll be charged (exorbitantly) for it. The unfortunate part is that when you are sick in the hospital (and often doped up), you are neither in the mood nor the condition to pay attention to those details. It appears that that is obvious to hospital administrators, and they take advantage of the situation!

Unfortunately our society has given doctors tremendous prestige and we have naive faith in them because we presume that they control life and death. That credibility has apparently carried over to the drug companies and hospitals. However, as we have shown, today the name of the game is money, and most doctors, drug companies and hospitals are out to get as much of it as they can.

They are totally out of control. The health costs in this country are of a higher percentage of the gross national product than that of any other country in the world. The responsible parties are the doctors, drug companies and hospitals. The Clintons started out with the aim of giving every single person in this country health insurance—a noble cause. Apparently they don't see that it will just make the doctors, drug companies and hospitals richer while the taxpayers foot the bill. We believe there are several ways to control these insidious profiteers and probably cut our health-care costs by 75 percent!

Socialized medicine has certainly controlled and cut the costs dramatically in England and Canada. But this country's government employees are already way too numerous. Socializing medicine would add tremendous numbers of government employees, and bureaucracies tend to grow rapidly.

Almost a century ago, the leaders of this country began realizing that the utility companies (water, electricity) needed to be controlled because they had monopolies and could charge whatever they wanted. You can't get your electricity from another company today, because there is only one company. Laws were created that prevented utilities from raising their prices without first proving to the government that their operating costs have increased. Also, the government regulated how much profit they could make, a very low percentage compared to what drug companies make.

Today, the company that sends gas into your home by pipeline is a utility (the oil companies aren't). Your local telephone (not long distance), some local bus companies and your cable TV company are all under the utility laws.

The doctors and drug companies have a monopoly! They don't advertise their prices. Do you get on the phone and call doctors around town to see who has the best price? With the drug companies, you don't have a choice of what you pay for the prescriptions because the doctor dictates what you take. If that isn't a monopolistic situation, Websters better change the definition in the dictionary!

And doctors have abused their monopoly. We are already paying much more than we can afford. Pity the poor person living on a few hundred dollars of Social Security payments each month. If they pay for the average four prescriptions, and have to pay 20 percent of their prescription costs under Medicare, they probably are doing without some other necessities such as good food!

Here are some very workable answers to the problem:

1. Put all drug companies under the same laws as utilities, controlling their prices and profits.
2. Enact laws banning drug companies from advertising prescription drugs to the public and distributing phony

"public service" announcements and press releases, and enforce those laws with criminal penalties.

3. Restrict drug companies' advertising to doctors and hospitals to a package of test results on each drug once per year. In the case of generics, restrict them to a simple announcement of the availability of the substitute drug.

4. Make them eliminate their drug sales force, which they call "detail persons."

5. Enact laws making it illegal to offer any inducement to doctors for prescribing drugs with criminal penalties.

6. Require drug companies to cross-test any drug against any other drug that possibly might be taken at the same time.

7. Make it mandatory that the potential side effects and dangers of other drugs taken at the same time be written in eighth-grade English and Spanish, printed in twelve-point type and distributed with every prescription and refill.

8. Pay royalties to any government-funded research center that creates a new drug that the drug company manufactures and sells.

The only realistic argument that we anticipate from by the drug companies is that the lack of advertising and salespeople will eliminate competition. It most certainly will. But if a drug company patents a new drug, they have seventeen years of competition-free sales anyway. And besides, we're discussing health, life and death. "Competition" doesn't seem very fitting for such sacred subjects.

All states have utility commissions that audit and control the utilities' prices and profits. So it would be easy to put doctors under similar control. The following are the changes we see that are necessary to control doctors:

1. Under the utility laws, control the net profit of a doctor relative to the number of patients handled and the amount of schooling they needed to reach their specialty.

2. Set a national standard price for all medical procedures, modifying it relative to regional cost differences. Allow increases tied to annual inflation figures.

3. Make it reasonably possible for doctors to attain an income in the upper 20 percent level. However, entrepreneurial doctors who employ other doctors or have more than one office should be rewarded for their extra effort and investment.

4. Make the three-part prescription form mandatory in every state with monthly analyses of each doctor's prescription-writing habits. Any doctors who overprescribe dangerous drugs will be prosecuted and their licenses revoked.

5. Require any doctors, who as a course of their business, prescribe drugs, tests or hospitalizations to sell their interests in any drug company, hospital, laboratory or any other profit center outside their normal practice. Make it illegal to have such interests, which are similar to insider trading.

6. Put all medical laboratories, hospitals, clinics and testing centers that deal with prescribing doctors under the utility laws.

7. Require all doctors who deal with patients to take a college course on nutrition before their license is renewed. According to a recent study by the American Journal of Nutrition, the nation's doctors are not only ignorant about nutrition, but their arrogance thwarts the education of patients on the subject. Most doctors, when asked about vitamins or other nutrients, will say, "Just eat good foods. You don't need any vitamins or minerals."

The doctors apparently don't understand that today most vegetables, fruits and grains are grown in nutrient-depleted soils with chemical fertilizers. These chemical fertilizers don't replace many minerals needed by humans. Nor do they acknowledge that food processing eliminates many vitamins.

8. Require doctors to complete a college course on preventive medicine, and demand that they discuss prevention measures with each patient. Have the federal
health agencies create printed handouts for the majority of health disorders.

If we put our shoulders together and push our congress-
people to the wall, maybe we can solve this situation. We'll
be sending a copy of this book to every congressional repre-
sentative and senator shortly. However, the greatest impact
will be your letters and calls to them.

One of the nation's largest insurance companies has
made a giant step forward in promoting preventive medicine. Mutual of Omaha announced that it would conduct a
pilot program with people suffering from coronary artery
disease who are candidates for bypass or other heart surgery.
The company will pay $3,500 per patient for a program
developed by Dr. Dean Ornish, the director of the Preventive
Medicine Research Company of Sausalito, California. The
program will be conducted at six locations around the country and last for two years.

Several hundred heart patients will eat a vegetarian diet
low in fat and cholesterol, exercise moderately, be taught
meditation techniques to relieve stress and attend support
group meetings. Terry Calek, senior vice president of public
affairs at Mutual of Omaha, said, "What Ornish's program
has done has proven that this is a viable alternative to costly
bypass surgery and drug treatment."

Blue Shield and Blue Cross are also considering similar
plans. Several HMOs began the trend by counseling patients
on various recurring illnesses during the last year.

According to statistics, heart and blood vessel diseases
kill more Americans than *all other diseases combined*! Dr.
Ornish says, "I believe that 95 percent of those problems
could be prevented or even reversed!"

Literally thousands of scientists and doctors throughout
the world believe that Ornish's techniques apply to most illnesses and diseases that are not of genetic origin. Part of

what you will learn in the following chapters will be about successful tests conducted under rigid scientific standards that prove you can prevent many illnesses. You'll also learn, of course, about many other medicines for which you don't need a prescription. You should actively look for a doctor who understands the science of nutrition and preventive medicine. Consult with him or her before trying any of the suggestions in this book.

5

■ ■ ■

Poor Memory and Depression May Be Caused by Poor Digestion

FROM THIS CHAPTER title, you might think that medical scientists have rocks in their heads, but they don't. The technological breakthroughs in the past two decades have given medical researchers some amazing tools and techniques for seeing into the most complex organ in the body—the brain. More has been learned about the brain in the last twenty years than in the previous one hundred years.

For example, any food, nutrient or drug can be tagged with a radioactive isotope and then followed as the stomach processes it and sends it to its ultimate destinations. Molecular biologists, using three-dimensional computer displays and advanced chemical analysis, can illustrate exactly what happens to a vitamin or drug when it reaches the brain or any other organ.

If you were a medical scientist and your memory began to fade, wouldn't memory research be particularly interesting to you? For that reason, brain research has attracted the best and most experienced scientists, and consequently, new discoveries have come along fast and furiously.

One of the most significant findings shows that *how we think has to do with what we eat!* Like most people, you've probably had days when you were mentally slow; what we call "our dumb days." The cause may be what you *didn't eat* that day.

■ Diet Caused Animals to Forget

Tests with animals have shown that when certain nutrients were withheld from their diets, the animals forgot tricks they had learned or could not find their way out of a maze which they had easily transversed many times before their diet was changed.

In animals and humans, the problem is compounded by the natural aging process. Our bodies start a slow deterioration beginning between the ages of twenty-five and thirty. By the time we reach the age of fifty, we begin to notice the changes because the mechanical efficiency of every organ has dropped.

After fifty, the decline accelerates. The first organ that makes us painfully aware that we're getting older is the stomach as we experience heartburn, acid indigestion and constipation more often. Even the most robust eaters, who formerly could eat anything without problems, begin to avoid certain foods to prevent potential discomfort.

Most twenty-year-olds can eat voluminous amounts of foods of all kinds without the slightest problem. The reason is that their stomachs are operating very efficiently. Indigestion is the result of a deteriorated digestion system.

It's not the discomfort of digestive problems that the scientists are concerned with; it's the loss of important nutrients. No matter whether you have digestion problems or not, many scientists believe that by the age of sixty, your body is absorbing an estimated one-third less nutrients from food than a twenty-year-old.

So what does that have to do with your memory? A lot, according to scientists. They have found that your brain needs a daily supply of fifteen different nutrients in order to operate efficiently. A shortage of any one of those nutrients can effect your memory and mental ability.

Literally dozens of clinical tests have shown that the majority of people over sixty who enter hospitals have a deficiency of one or more nutrients. Poor eating habits and insufficient absorption of nutrients by the stomach are two causes, but there is another, more important one—*lack of nutrients in our food!*

Before World War II, farmers used manure to fertilize crops, but after that era, chemical fertilizers became the vogue. Manure replaced all the nutrients in the soil, but chemical fertilizers contain only nitrogen, potassium and phosphorus. Enzymes in the soil can only make a limited variety of nutrients from those three chemicals.

In the fifties, tremendous numbers of livestock (cattle, hogs, sheep, chicken and turkeys) began getting diseases never seen before to any extent in animals, such as heart disease, cancer and arthritis. In most cases, veterinary scientists traced the cause to specific nutritional deficiencies.

To give you an example, when turkey ranching became automated (i.e. they were grown in cages and never touched the ground) several hundred thousand died due to cerebral hemorrhages—strokes. It was a tragedy that financially wiped out many turkey ranchers. Scientists finally traced the cause to a lack of nutritional copper in the turkeys' diets. Today, with copper supplementation, turkeys rarely get strokes.

■ You Can't Take a Chicken to the Doctor!

Farming and ranching is strictly business, and the owners don't spend money unless it is a necessity. Let's face it: one doesn't take a chicken worth two dollars or even a lamb worth fifty dollars to a doctor. Today, all livestock producers supplement their animals' diets with a variety of vitamins, minerals and other nutrients—*out of necessity!*

Before 1960, most people ate a lot of fresh fruit and vegetables; however, the sixties gave birth to fast-food franchises and factory-processed, ready-to-eat foods. Today, it is estimated that over 60 percent of the population lives on ready-to-eat foods, rarely ever touching fresh fruits and vegetables.

A study by the National Food Review Board showed that freezing and recooking food destroys up to 93 percent of the nutrients in some foods. All the important enzymes are destroyed at temperatures above 129 degrees Fahrenheit which is way below normal cooking temperatures. Many enzymes help digestion and are a vital necessity in extracting vitamins and minerals from food. As you can see, eating a balanced diet is absolutely no guarantee that you are getting all the vitamins, minerals and other nutrients your body and brain need.

The brain occupies only a small portion of your total body volume, yet it uses over 40 percent of the energy you produce. If you are frequently tired, you may not be feeding your brain properly. The brain also uses almost 20 percent of all the oxygen you take in your lungs. Your blood carries the oxygen to your brain. This is why the condition of your arteries can effect your memory.

■ Twenty-Year-Olds with Hardening of the Arteries

During the Vietnam War doctors who were performing autopsies on soldiers killed in action noticed that practically all the young men had plaque building up in their arteries— the beginning of arteriosclerosis (hardening of the arteries). These men were only in their twenties. Imagine how clogged your arteries are if you are over fifty.

Clogged arteries restrict the flow of the blood and therefore reduce the amount of oxygen that reaches your brain. For many years, scientists have known that reduced oxygen to the brain can cause headaches, depression, ringing in the ears and *memory loss*.

You may be thinking that because your arteries are probably partially blocked, there's no hope of correcting the lack of oxygen to your brain. This is not true. Researchers have found an uncommon nutrient that increases the blood's capacity to carry oxygen. We'll tell you more about this wonder substance, called GBE, shortly.

Considering the above facts, it is not surprising that mental illness is the fastest-growing part of the health industry. Before World War II, Alzheimer's disease was very rare according to government health statistics published in a *Los Angeles Times* article. Today, there are over 4 million cases in the United States, making it *the nations' fourth most deadly disease.* Another 8 million people suffer from senility and dementia.

Researchers believe that over 80 percent of the population over sixty has some memory problems, and scientists estimate that over 30 percent of those people will eventually develop senility, dementia or Alzheimer's. Most of the people in nursing homes are there because of mental problems. Because people with mental dysfunctions have to be watched constantly, families who would normally care for their elderly loved ones at home cannot do so, because they have to work and can't watch them all the time.

Will your memory problems inevitably get worse? Yes, if you don't alleviate the causes. Extensive research shows that deficiencies of any one of fifteen specific nutrients can cause memory problems. However, research also shows that supplementation of those nutrients cannot only stop the deterioration of your memory, but also restore your ability to recall.

The brain brings memories from their storage area to your conscious mind with substances called neurotransmitters. They are electrochemical messengers. There are a variety of these messengers that perform other essential tasks along with stimulating your memory. The major ones are acetylcholine (ACH), norepinephrine, epinephrine, dopamine and serotonin.

ACH is the most important neurotransmitter for memory and even intelligence, according to Dr. J. F. Flood. He reported in the medical journal *Neurobiology of Aging* that a shortage of ACH causes memory loss, reduces the ability to learn and restricts intelligence.

Dr. Joseph Coyle and Dr. M. R. Delong of Johns Hopkins School of Medicine reported in *Science* that they found Alzheimer's patients had 60 to 90 percent less ACH than normal for their ages. Other research indicates that a lack of ACH causes a variety of memory problems and may be the direct cause of senility.

Your body makes ACH from a nutrient called choline. In a controlled clinical test, Dr. Lozano Fernandez gave choline to 2,817 patients between the ages of sixty and eighty who had memory problems. In just two months, their memory improved 65.9 percent, headaches were reduced by 73.2 percent, insomnia by 63.5 percent, depression by 61 percent and dizziness by 73.6 percent. Even faster results can be obtained with some of the brain nutrients we will discuss shortly, but overall, the longer you take all of them, the more effective they become.

There is a nice side benefit of taking choline. It supplies the chemistry necessary for fat metabolism. Without sufficient choline in your body, fat accumulates. Women often see it as those unattractive cellulite dimples on their legs and behinds.

Unfortunately, just taking choline by itself is not the answer. First, choline needs the nutrients folate and cobalamin to be present in order for it to be converted to ACH. Second, the quantity of ACH released in the brain is often dependent on a brain protein (amino acid) called pyroglutamate (PCA). PCA is supposed to be present in all nerve cells and is a prolific neurotransmitter by itself. Normally, PCA is released in the brain when you use your memory.

Dr. S. Grioli found that when he gave patients PCA or a placebo (fake pill) in a double-blind clinical test, those taking PCA remembered a significant 17 percent more than those taking the placebo.

Even in cases where alcoholism has reduced memory substantially, Dr. E. Sinforiani found PCA helped restore part of the memory. Dr. R. Cocchi discovered that alcoholic patients automatically and unconsciously reduced their consumption of alcohol dramatically after regular use of PCA.

You may not be aware of it, but as you get older, your IQ declines (in conjunction with your memory becoming less responsive). The good news is that Dr. C. Pheiffer reported in the medical journal *Nutrition Reviews* that he found PCA to be effective in restoring the IQs of patients over the age of sixty.

PCA also has some valuable side benefits. Muscles tend

to get flabby as you get older due to a hormone called the "human growth hormone (hGH)." Clinical tests show that PCA stimulates the production of hGH, which strengthens and tones your muscles.

Dr. Lorraine Young found that PCA-supplemented patients were happier (reported less depression) and were released from the hospital sooner than nonsupplemented patients. By the way, PCA must be taken with vitamin B_6 in order to be used by the body.

Another natural substance that causes the production of several neurotransmitters is the protein tyrosine. Tyrosine is often used along with drugs in treating Parkinson's disease because it helps replace the neurotransmitters destroyed by those drugs.

As you grow older, your ability to handle stress declines. Hectic, chaotic situations fluster you more than when you were younger. One of the reasons is that stress gobbles up neurotransmitters of which you already have a shortage, according to Dr. Agharanja and his colleagues at M.I.T. Some of the neurotransmitters produced by tyrosine calm your nerves and help you handle stress better.

Your ability to handle cold weather declines as you get older, often due to poor circulation. Did you know that severe cold induces memory loss? The reason is that the exposure to low temperatures causes stress, and therefore neurotransmitters are destroyed.

Dr. David Shurtleff of the Naval Medical Research Institute was very concerned with this phenomenon because the navy's sailors are often exposed to very cold weather in northern seas. A lack of mental quickness had been observed in many young sailors.

Dr. Shurtleff conducted two studies with the same group of sailors. First, he measured their mental agility after a thirty-minute exposure to 25 degrees Fahrenheit. After two days, he gave the men tyrosine and sent them out into the cold again. Their mental agility and memory improved substantially after taking the tyrosine.

Dr. Louis Bandoret confirmed the value of tyrosine with similar tests of army personnel. Some of the men he tested showed as high as 80 percent improvement. Tyrosine must be taken with the nutrients folate, ascorbic acid, niacin and phenylalanine in order to be absorbed by the body.

There are several other benefits from taking tyrosine. It improves your mood, stops dizziness, reduces high blood pressure, alleviates depression, improves appetite and often restores virility to impotent men.

Studies done on tyrosine by Dr. Alan J. Gelenberg of Harvard Medical School as reported in the American Journal of Psychiatry also show the tranquilizing effects that tyrosine can have on patients suffering from depression. Dr. Gelenberg reported that patients showed positive responses when given oral doses of tyrosine. Over 60 percent of the patients in another study conducted by Dr. Gelenberg showed reductions in depression by at least 50 percent after receiving oral doses of tyrosine for a period of four weeks.

Dr. Eric Braverman reported two cases where tyrosine was the last resort. In the first case, a patient had been chronically depressed for twelve years. None of the mulitude of antidepressant drugs helped him. Within a month of taking tyrosine, his depression disappeared completely. Harvard researchers also found that it was very effective on their depressed patients.

The absolutely essential nutrient needed in the production of *all* neurotransmitters is vitamin B_6. It is also involved in all nerve functions. Dr. J. B. Deijen reported in the journal *Psychopharmacology* that in a double-blind, placebo-controlled test, vitamin B_6 substantially improved the memories of the patients who were over sixty years old.

Unfortunately, it is one of the hardest nutrients to get from food, because cooking and refining destroy vitamin B_6. Even whole-wheat bread, which undergoes very little refining, has lost most of the B_6 by the time it reaches your table.

Alcohol, birth-control pills, yellow food coloring (dye) and drugs such as Premarin and penicillin destroy B_6. Yellow dye is used extensively in processed food, as you will see by examining ingredient labels in your supermarket. Of all the nutrients that most people have a shortage of, B_6 stands at the top of the list—especially if they have memory or mental problems.

Many natural medicine doctors have found that patients who were taking Prozac or other antidepressants and tranquilizers actually had a B_6 deficiency. Most of the patients returned to normal after taking B_6 and throwing away the drugs.

A B_6 deficiency is the major cause of the excruciatingly painful kidney stones. Its shortage also increases the risk of heart attack and contributes to osteoporosis. A severe deficiency will show up as cracked corners of the mouth or eyes, sores that don't heal or a diminished sex drive, according to Dr. Pat Bermond at the medical school of the University of Reims in France.

Vitamin B_6 must be taken with the nutrient riboflavin in order to be used by the body. Riboflavin is also a powerful antioxidant for the nervous system, but it is not stored in the body, so it must be taken daily. A deficiency of riboflavin usually makes a person nervous, but sometimes it also causes eczema in women, and the atrophy or shrinking of the testicles in men.

Thiamine should also be included with riboflavin because it is a mental stimulant and a coenzyme in the production of ACH. Dr. John Blass at Cornell University Medical College found that Alzheimer's patients taking thiamine for ninety days showed much more mental clarity than before the treatment began.

The most remarkable substance for improving memory comes from an extract obtained from the fruit and leaves of the *Gingko biloba* or Maidenhair tree. The extract is called GBE. The Maidenhair tree is one of the longest-living trees in the world, with a thousand-year-plus life span. It was around during the time of the dinosaurs because fossils of its distinctive leaves have been found and dated as 250 million years old.

GBE is the ideal supplement for people over fifty as it solves the problem of getting enough oxygen to the brain through clogged arteries. It dilates the arteries (makes them bigger), thins the blood (which deters dangerous blood clots) and enhances the blood's ability to carry oxygen.

Dr. G. S. Rai conducted a rigid placebo-controlled, double-blind study of GBE on people between the ages of fifty and eighty-nine who had moderate to severe memory impairment. The results were spectacular. Those taking GBE recalled an amazing 46 percent more than those taking the placebo, and they answered memory questions almost 30 percent faster. The tests were conducted at the end of twenty-four weeks of daily use of GBE.

The longer you take GBE, the better the results. Dr. B. Gebner found in a double-blind, placebo-controlled trial that the quickness of recall grew faster and faster over a three-month period. However, you don't have to wait three months for results. Dr. Herve Allain found that within one hour of taking GBE, patients in his clinical trials (average age, seventy) recalled 7 percent more than those taking placebos.

GBE helps more than just your memory. Dr. H. Leroy conducted trials on moderately senile patients and found that in just one hour after taking GBE, their moods improved 140 percent, sociability went up 233 percent and alertness increased 80 percent.

Dr. G. Vorberg reported in the *Clinical Trials Journal* that elderly patients taking GBE over a twelve-month period had a significant reduction in dizzy spells and ringing in the ears. Both conditions are a result of poor circulation.

There are other bonuses with GBE. Dr. H. Schubert found that GBE caused a 50 percent drop in occurences of depression in just four weeks of taking the supplement. Dr. M. Koltai found that it reduced allergies and eczema by 62.4 percent. For centuries, Chinese doctors have used it for treating asthma and bronchitis.

There's considerable evidence that GBE normalizes circulation and breaks down clots, thereby deterring strokes. Dr. G. Thomson reported in the journal *International Angiology* that he has had tremendous success using GBE for treating intermittent claudication (pain in the calf while walking due to poor circulation). GBE increased pain-free walking distance up to 110 percent. It increased total walking distance up to 119 percent, and after two years of steady usage, walking distance had increased to almost 300 percent.

Poor circulation plays a big part in sexual activities of men and women because blood is pumped to the genitals during sexual arousal, where it increases sensitivity and stimulates lubrication. In men, blood fills the penis to create an erection. Obviously, men with circulation problems will have difficulty getting or maintaining an erection.

Dr. R. Skikora showed in clinical tests of impotent men that GBE steadily improves erectile ability. Good results began to show up after six weeks, and within six months, over half of those participating in the study had regained full potence. Dr. Skikora concluded that double dosage may increase the response time, and continued usage past six months might increase the success ratio.

GBE is a free radical fighter because it contains superoxide dismutase (SOD), the body's most powerful antioxidant. With all its attributes, it is not surprising that GBE is the best-selling over-the-counter medication in Europe where natural medicines have enjoyed popularity for many decades.

Another nutrient that helps increase the production of ACH is acetyl-L-carnitine (ALC). In separate double-blind, placebo-controlled trials, Dr. G. Rai and Dr. E. Tempesta proved that ALC significantly improves short-term memory. (Scientists don't understand why, but we don't lose much long-term memory as we age.) ALC has been used successfully in helping Alzheimer's and dementia patients improve their daily lives by retarding the progress of these diseases.

It also helps improve alertness and physical reaction time in all ages. A 1990 study of teenagers playing video games found that ALC helped quicken their reflexes and decreased the difference in reflex speed between their right and left hands.

ALC is one of the most important nutrients for the heart. Heart muscles require a lot of it for proper function and it is recommended to everyone who has a weak heart or any abnormalities. In order for ALC to be absorbed and used by your body, you must take it with ascorbic acid, nicotinic acid and vitamin B_6.

■ Brown Slime on Your Nerves!

Those brown age spots that pop up on the skin as we age are called lipofuscin. If you have any age spots, this is an indication that you have lipofuscin in your brain, where it appears as a brown slime coating the neurons. At first, it restricts the firing of the neurons, which slows down thinking and remembering. Over time, if you allow the lipofuscin to accumulate, it will dramatically slow down your mental reaction time and alertness. You'll suffer from muddled thinking, which evolves into total senility.

There are a couple of substances that reduce lipofuscin accumulations substantially. ALC is one of them, according to studies by Dr. Frank Amenta. The other nutrient that stops or slows the lipofuscin is vitamin E. Animals get lipofuscin on their brains as they age just like humans. Dr. A. Monji reported in the journal *Brain Research* that animals fed vitamin E in their diets accumulated over 50 percent less than animals not getting the vitamin.

When vitamin E is added to the diets of Alzheimer's patients it slows down the progress of the disease, which indicates that it is a good deterrent of this devastating scourge. Usually when someone has any neurological dysfunction, they have a deficiency of vitamin E, according to numerous clinical trials. Vitamin E is one of the most important nutrients required by the body, and its shortage has been implicated in heart problems and cancer.

A deficiency of vitamin E is very common among Americans. In fact, a test of *wealthy* elderly people in the midwest showed that over 45 percent had deficiencies of this nutrient. Perhaps the reason is that vitamin E is not stored in the body. If you take it in the morning, none is left in your body by evening, so you must take it twice a day.

Niacin seems to balance activities in the neurological system and is often deficient in those suffering from mental disorders. Dr. Abram Hoffer said, "I have found niacin very effective in restoring memory, increasing alertness and energy."

Extensive clinical testing that has been done on this important nutrient has revealed some amazing findings. It helps lower cholesterol, relieves migraine headaches, reduces high blood pressure, stimulates the sex drive and detoxifies the effects of drugs, alcohol and environmental pollutants.

Folate, which is required for the metabolism of tyrosine, appears to be even more involved in the brain than had been originally thought. Dr. E. H. Reynolds found that the majority of people suffering from chronic depression had deficiencies of folate.

Alcohol destroys folate in your body, and folate deficiency has also been related to various circulation problems; particularly, chronic coldness of the hands, feet and legs. Folate also has been used successfully in moderating lung damage from smoking and improving the vision of those suffering from peripheral vascular diseases.

D-phenylalanine (DLPA), which is also required for the metabolism of tyrosine, has other rather impressive qualities as a brain nutrient. Dr. H. C. Sabelli found it works well as an antidepressant, relieving over 75 percent of his suffering patients.

Dr. S. Ehrenpreis posted some dramatic results using DLPA as a painkiller in a study published in the journal *Advanced Pain Research & Therapy*. He found that patients who no longer responded to drug-type painkillers could find relief with DLPA. People with whiplash, back injuries and arthritis responded quickly, and the longer they took DLPA, the better it worked.

Another brain nutrient you need is cysteine. Its deficiency apparently triggers emotional outbursts, while supplementation calms the nerves. Generally, cysteine is a powerful antioxidant and detoxifier. It was used extensively in treating people exposed to the giant chemical spill in Bhopal, India in 1985 that killed more than two hundred people.

Each day we are exposed to more and more environmental pollutants, so taking a detoxifying nutrient daily is very prudent. Cysteine is commonly used in treating bronchitis and should be taken regularly by smokers and those exposed to smoke because it protects the lungs.

Unlike other parts of the body where old cells die and new ones are built daily, brain cells do not regenerate. *You must protect what you have.* Fewer brain cells means less memory. Memory is a key factor in thinking, because you must be able to recall experiences from the past in order to make decisions about the present and the future. Imagine how financially vulnerable you would be if you were senile. Imagine what a burden you would be on your loved ones. Imagine how awful it would be to live every day with a muddled mind, not grasping what was going on around you.

An essential acid produced in the brain called phosphatidylserine (PS) facilitates nutrient distribution to the brain cells; it activates nerve transmitter production, blocks the decline of the Nerve Growth Factor, controls cortisol production and is an important antioxidant in the brain. The production of PS declines as we get older, while free radicals increase and cortisol production goes up. Excess cortisol prevents or slows the uptake of the brain's primary energy source—glucose.

Dr. Thomas Crook conducted a double-blind, placebo-controlled study using oral PS. The 149 participants were over fifty years old and were experiencing normal age-related memory loss. Half the group took 100 milligrams of PS three times a day for twelve weeks. Those that took PS averaged a 15 percent increase in memory and learning tasks. Dr. Crook's study, which was published in the journal *Neurology*, suggests that PS compensated for twelve years of mental decline.

In studies published in 1990, another player entered the fight to treat Alzheimer's disease and other memory disorders. Dr. Eugene Roberts, a research scientist in the Department of Neurobiochemistry at the Beckman Research Institute of the City of Hope in Duarte, California, reported in his paper "Serum Steroid Levels of Those with

Alzheimer's Disease" that DHEA showed tremendous effect in enhancing memory in young and old mice.

In his paper "Cognitive Effects of DHEA Replacement Therapy," Dr. Kenneth A. Bonnet, a research scientist in the Department of Psychiatry at New York University School of Medicine in New York City, reported similar findings. He injected young test mice with DHEA and found that they showed much higher levels of memory retention and recall. Upon injecting middle-aged and old mice with DHEA, Dr. Bonnet found that their retention and recall skills, which had been remarkably lower than those of the young mice, increased to the same level as those of the young mice.

Dr. Bonnet reports of expanded studies in the paper mentioned above, detailing testing done with a forty-seven-year-old woman with lifelong multiple learning disabilities, low levels of memory retention, an inability to learn even the most simple information and recurring headaches. Among the diagnoses given to her prior to Dr. Bonnet's study were temporal mandibular joint syndrome (TMJ) and manic depression. Drugs used to treat this woman's problems before Dr. Bonnet's study had been effective for short periods of time, but her symptoms would always return eventually.

At the beginning of testing, the woman was given a standard five-part intelligence test, and her sleep patterns were evaluated. The patient's recall abilities were reported as below normal, and an EEG showed evidence of poor sleep.

Low doses of DHEA were given to the patient for one week, then she was retested. The results showed an improvement in recall ability and the patient reported feeling better rested and sleeping more soundly. The woman also reported feeling an increase in clear thinking and ability to remember.

After one month, a higher dose of DHEA was given to the woman. Testing done after this increase showed more advanced ability to recall, with long-term memory increasing also. By the end of the testing period, the patient showed a marked increase in abilities. She was able to understand material presented to her more clearly and could apply that material, and she could make judgments based on material presented to her.

Dr. Bonnet notes that the woman who was the subject of the test continued to take oral doses of DHEA and that a tolerance was not built up, as was the case with other drugs she took previously. In addition, for the first time in her forty-seven-year life, the woman was able to start up and to run a small business.

In a study completed by Dr. C. R. Merril of the Laboratory of Biochemical Genetics at the National Institute of Mental Health in Bethesda, Maryland, ten Alzheimer's patients were tested for blood-serum levels of DHEA. These levels were compared to ten control subjects of the same age group who did not have Alzheimer's disease. The results showed levels of DHEA in the Alzheimer's group to be 48 percent lower than the control group.

These findings are important because they reveal that Alzheimer's patients have much less DHEA than those without the disease. The forty-seven-year-old test patient from Dr. Bonnet's study also showed extremely low levels of DHEA when testing began. It is entirely possible that Alzheimer's patients may be able to benefit from DHEA treatment, as did the female test patient. Studies pursuing this possibility are now underway.

▪ Problems with DHEA Supplements

A few years ago, a book was released that promoted DHEA as the best thing since sliced bread. It became one of the biggest best-sellers of the year, and newspapers, magazines, radio and TV shows everywhere started hyping the benefits of taking DHEA. Naturally, drug companies jumped on the bandwagon and rushed two forms of DHEA to the stores and mail-order companies.

The "natural" form was an extract from the wild Mexican yam (no relation to the yams sold in grocery stores). It contains what the drug companies call "a precursor to DHEA," diosgenin. There's a little bit of research that indicates that a small amount of diosgenin will convert to DHEA. Most scientists say the research indicates that you would have to take an enormous amount of wild yam extract to get enough DHEA to help you.

There's another problem with diosgenin. It was the base for the first birth-control pill. It converts to progesterone (female hormone), which upsets the hormonal balance of some women. Men who take diosgenin for prolonged periods show shrinkage in their testicles and penis.

The other DHEA, which is most commonly sold in stores today, is a synthetic crystal DHEA. It is grossly ground up and packed into a pill or capsule. The drug industry calls it "plain DHEA."

What the authors of the book and the news media didn't know, or if they knew they didn't say, was that the DHEA used in *all* clinical tests was an expensive "micronized" pharmaceutical grade of DHEA.

There's a big difference between the micronized and the plain DHEA. The particles of DHEA in the miconized version are incredibly small, and the plain DHEA particles are large. In the stomach, the micronized DHEA goes directly into the bloodstream and travels throughout the body. The plain DHEA goes to the liver so it can be broken down.

A small portion of the plain DHEA gets into the blood system from the liver because the liver is unaccustomed to receiving DHEA in that form and flushes most of it out of the body.

■ DHEA Is Dangerous

Although the micronized DHEA is superior, recent studies show that *it is not the best way to increase your DHEA levels*. In fact, it can upset your whole hormonal system because it bypasses an important control in the body. (If you have been taking DHEA, your hormonal system may be out of balance. If you are healthy your body will fight to correct it, so the effects you will notice are very subtle. However, if you are not well, it could be making your condition worse or creating other problems.) In doing so, it increases the androgens, which cause facial hair in women and prostate disorders in men, according to Dr. J. F. Mortola of Harvard Medical School. He says his clinical tests also show that taking synthetic DHEA *causes your body to stop producing natural DHEA!*

■ **PN Produces DHEA in Your Body, According to Your Needs**

Dr. Eugene Roberts of the famous Beckman Research Center at the City of Hope says his studies show that it gets even worse. Supplementation of DHEA reduces the body's production of pregnenolone, the mother of all hormones.

Scientists agree that if you want to increase your DHEA naturally, you should be taking pregnenolone (PN) because it produces DHEA and all the other hormones—*according to the body's daily needs.* In other words, it keeps all your hormones in balance. The reason your DHEA levels drop as you get older is that the quantity of PN in your body diminishes at the same rate.

PN has some other jobs that are very important as you get older. It controls the adrenal glands, which effect your ability to handle stress. The stresses of driving, traveling and the demands of a job usually get more difficult to handle as you get older because your PN levels are reduced. Those taking PN daily report greater ease in adapting to stressful situations.

PN is very active in the brain. Dr. James Flood of St. Louis University medical school, who discovered DHEA, says: "PH is the most potent memory enhancer ever reported." He says the reason is that PN stimulates the amygdala section of the brain, which plays the most prominent role in memory retention.

While PN and DHEA balance and revitalize your hormonal system, and PN restores your memory, the control center of your body—the brain—still slowly deteriorates with age. One of the most critical nutrients for the brain, methionine, is deficient in most diets, according to research by Dr. Ted Bottiglieri of the Baylor University Research Center.

Methionine is converted in the body to S-adenosyl-L-methionine (SAM). SAM increases the production of the three major neurotransmitters in the brain: serotonin, norepinephrine and dopamine.

Serotonin is the daytime equivalent of melatonin, the highly publicized antiaging substance that controls the hourly cycles of body functions at night. At dusk, serotonin is converted into melatonin, according to Dr. J. Axelrod, reporting in the journal *Science*.

Serotonin is also part of our appetite-control system. When your serotonin levels drop, you get hungry—even if your body doesn't need food. Keeping your serotonin up will help you keep your weight down.

In addition, SAM is the precursor to the body's own pain relievers, enkephalin and endorphins. A lack of those painkillers is what makes us feel more aches and pains as we get older.

As a memory improver, SAM is almost as good as PN. Dr. P. Fantanari conducted a double-blind, placebo-controlled test of SAM on elderly patients at the General Hospital in Venice. After forty days of taking SAM, tests showed that the patients experienced over 300 percent improvement in memory, compared to those taking the placebo. Elderly people typically have very low levels of SAM in their blood.

Depression is about six times more common in people over sixty years old, than in those under sixty. It's easy to understand, because not feeling good physically doesn't help your mental outlook one bit. Well, SAM is *the best* natural antidepressant ever found, according to Dr. G. M. Bressa. He compared patients taking three different prescription antidepressants with patients taking SAM. The patients found SAM to be superior to the drugs in overall effect as well as the quickness in which it worked.

One of the biggest problems with prescription antidepressants is that they take up to six weeks to feel their full effects. For that reason, 53 percent of drug-related emergency-room visits are for overdoses of the feel-better prescriptions. People just keep taking more and more because they don't know the drugs take many weeks to start working.

On the other hand, clinical tests have shown that you'll start feeling the antidepressant effects of SAM in as little as four days; within fourteen days, 50 percent of the power; and the full effect within thirty days. (If you want to switch to SAM and have been taking a prescription antidepressant for a month or more, don't stop abruptly. If you do, you may have severe withdrawl symptoms. After a couple weeks of taking SAM, begin slowly to cut down the intake of drugs for the next few weeks while your body adjusts.) Most people enjoy a rapid increase in energy as well as a better mood.

SAM has also been used in hospitals to relieve the drug withdrawl symptoms of addicts and the cravings of alcoholics. It also protects and helps rebuild the liver after damage from drugs, alcohol and hepatitis.

As you get older, the fluids in your brain become denser or thicker in consistancy. The thicker fluids slow down the communication between neurotransmitters, making mental responses slower and memory poor.

Fortunately, it doesn't have to be that way, according to the research of Dr. M. Cumino, which appeared in the *Journal of Life Sciences*. He found that one of the attributes of SAM is that it thins the brain fluids to the same consistency as that of younger people.

The producer of SAM, methionine, can't begin its production unless three nutrients are present—pyridoxine, folate and cobalamin.

Italian researchers, led by Dr. Alberto Spagnoli of the Mario Negri Institute in Milan, did a year-long double-blind study of a natural compound called acetyl-L-carnitine, which has been reported to slow the deteriorating mental functioning common to Alzheimer's patients. Of the 130 patients involved in the study, the 63 who received acetyl-L-carnitine have shown improved attention span, better long-term memory and increased verbal ability with no side effects. The 67 patients involved in the same study who received placebos showed no improvement.

Acetyl-L-carnitine works as a nerve-cell stimulator, increasing the cell's ability to produce acetylcholine, proteins and new cell membranes. Tests done on animals have proven all of Dr. Spagnoli's claims, showing that acetyl-L-carnitine-stimulated nerve cells produce proteins, new cell membranes and acetylcholine.

Another substance showing promise is proanthocyanidine (PAC). It is a dietary antioxidant that crosses the blood-brain barrier to protect the brain against free radicals. Researchers feel that PAC can also aid in strengthening capillaries, thereby regulating blood pressure. Rats bred to be prone to high blood pressure and strokes lived considerably longer when given PAC. In addition, other test animals that were given chemicals to scar and damage their blood vessels showed no sign of damage if given PAC beforehand.

Dr. Peter Rohdewald of the Pharmacology Institute of the University of Munster in Germany states that PAC is not toxic, and has been used in Indian cultures for centuries with no reports of toxicity.

In a paper entitled "Fourteen Doctors Confirm L-Glutamine Improves I.Q.," Dr. Richard Passwater explains that the brain actually needs two types of "fuel." Until recently, doctors knew of only one type, glucose; but recent studies have proven that another substance exists that nourishes the brain—it's called L-glutamine. Glutamine effects brain-cell activity. When the brain is not supplied sufficiently with this substance, minor brain damage can occur.

In the book *Mega Nutrients for Your Nerves*, Dr. H. L. Newbold states that glutamine can be used to relieve depression and impotence, and works as an all-around energizer. Dr. L. L. Rogers, in *Texas Reports on Biology and Medicine*, found that glutamine improved IQ scores of mentally retarded children.

Another brain nutrient is dimethylaminoethanol (DMAE). Dr. R. Hochschild, in his article "Effect of DMAE On The Life Span Of Senile Male A/J Mice," reports that DMAE is far superior to choline in its ability to reach the location within cells where production of membranes occurs.

Although DMAE is found in such foods as anchovies and sardines, one would have to consume large quantities of these foods in order to see substantial benefit. An easier method is to take dietary supplements.

Dr. H. Murphree states in his article "The Stimulant Effect of DMAE in Human Volunteer Subjects" that DMAE produced clearer mental concentration, increased muscle tone and created positive changes in sleep patterns in the patients he studied. Dr. Ross Pelton, author of *Mind Food and Smart Pills*, found that his subjects showed better moods, improved memory and learning ability and higher intelligence after treatment with DMAE.

- ## Depression—Prozac and Its Link to Violent Behavior and Suicidal Tendencies

Until recently, for cases of severe depression the medical world has prescribed what was believed to be a miracle drug: this drug is called Prozac. Reports of violent behavior and severe suicidal impulses began to surface in connection with patients taking Prozac in 1990. Until that time, Prozac had become the nation's best-selling antidepressant, according to a report in the *New York Times*.

In the same *New York Times* article, the nonprofit Public Citizen Health Research Group was reported to have petitioned the FDA to caution the medical world strongly regarding evidence that Prozac could cause impulsively violent and suicidal thoughts and actions in some patients taking the drug. The group even asked the FDA to require warning labels on Prozac, to alert patients to possible violent side effects.

In 1990, Dr. Martin Teicher, a research psychiatrist at Harvard University, reported on six patients who showed intense, sucidal tendencies during Prozac therapy.

As of June 1992, the Citizen's Commission of Human Rights reported Prozac as having the largest number of adverse drug reactions of any drug in history (23,067, which included 1,436 suicide attempts and 1,313 deaths).

With statistics such as those listed above, it would seem amazing that the medical world would even consider the continued prescription of Prozac as treatment for depression. It becomes less amazing when one looks at the profit the drug's producer, Eli Lilly & Company, has made on the sale of Prozac. In 1990 alone, Lilly showed a profit of $385 million on the sale of Prozac.

With such huge profits involved, it is easy to see how strongly one of the nation's largest pharmaceutical giants might push the continued use of a drug like Prozac to U.S. physicians.

■ Common Nutrients That Help

Studies completed by Dr. Whitaker have determined that deficiencies in B_{12} can lead to mental illness. A study done on mentally retarded children showed that after being given large does of B-complex vitamins, IQ levels increased by 10.2 percent.

Vitamin C has been proven to aid in producing nerve transmitters and building cell structures. A study of school-children from kindergarten age to college level found that by increasing vitamin C levels in blood plasma by 50 percent, IQ levels also increased by 3.6 percent. The same study applied to retarded children showed increased IQ levels of 20 points or greater.

Tests done by Dr. Hardo Sorjatz of the Institute for Physiology in Dormstad, Germany, showed that patients taking eight grams of lecithin or choline per day scored higher on both written and oral memory tests, compared to patients taking a placebo. It should be noted that, according to Dr. Whitaker, lecithin/choline should always be taken with vitamin B_5 (pantothenic acid).

Another substance released in treatment with tyrosine is dopamine, which was discussed earlier in this chapter. Dopamine transmits nerve impulses throughout the brain and is also believed to produce a calming effect in depressed patients.

One type of depression that is particularly common in the elderly is called SAD (Seasonal Affective Disorder). Patients suffering from SAD become depressed during times of the year when daylight hours are diminished. Therapy using high-intensity light has been proven to relieve these feelings of depression. This light therapy has also been proven to increase the levels of the substance melatonin in SAD patients tested during darkened cycles.

As long ago as 1940, biotin, a component of the vitamin B complex, has been the subject of experiments with clinical depression. In a report in the *Journal of the American Medical Association*, Dr. V. P. Sydenstricker reported on an experimental study that he performed on four healthy patients. The subjects were given a diet rich in all nutrients except biotin. After living on this diet for ten weeks, all the subjects showed severe signs of depression and exhaustion, as well as nausea, anorexia and complaints of muscle pain. Immediately after supplements of biotin were given to these subjects, all symptoms vanished.

Dr. R. Levenson reported a study he did in 1983 of a patient who was experiencing depression, as well as nausea, insomnia, headaches and an overall feeling of fatigue. After five days of treatment with supplements of biotin, the patient showed a lessening of these symptoms, and continued treatment with biotin completely eliminated his feelings of depression.

Although there appears to be a trend in the United States toward the use of more natural medications by physicians, European physicians still seem to be more receptive to treatments using nature's own drugs.

One such medication, Hypericum extract, is used successfully in European countries and has finally been accepted in the United States as a front-line treatment for depression. Women from the ages of fifty-five to sixty-five who were suffering from depression were treated with the extract in a German study. The patients were tested before and after treatment to evaluate depression and anxiety levels, and were found to show highly decreased levels of depression and anxiety after the treatment was completed. Their blood levels also showed a greater quantity of dopamine after treatment. Dopamine levels are known to increase in successful antidepressant therapy.

■ Sources of Substances Mentioned in this Chapter

The following are available from health food and vitamin stores:

Acetyl-L-carnitine (ask for carnitine)
DLPA (phenylalanine)
DMAE (dimethyl-amino-ethenol)
Ginkgo biloba (GBE)
Methionine (SAM)
L-Glutamine
PAC (proanthocyanidine/it may be called phycotene)
Tyrosine
Lecithin or choline
Pregnenolone (for DHEA)
Melatonin
Phosphatidylserine (may be hard to find)
Biotin
Hypericum

Vitamins:

B_1 (thiamine)
B_2 (riboflavin)
B_3 (niacin)
B_5 (pantothenic acid)

B_6 (pyridoxine)
B_{12} (cobalamin)
C (ascorbic acid)
E (tocopheryl)

Nutrients listed under particular health food and vitamin stores may also be purchased by mail from the following:

Indiana Botanic Gardens
P.O. Box 5
Hammond, IN 46325
(219) 947-4040

6

Miscellaneous Health Problems

■ Rutin and Stroke Prevention

Scientific research has discovered that vitamins A and C, taken together with a flavonoid called rutin, cut the likelihood of strokes! Rutin comes from citrus fruit. It's an example of what are known as bioflavonoids, which are found in citrus pith. In other words, rutin is all natural and completely safe. It is surprisingly effective. Your odds of suffering a stroke when you combine rutin with vitamins A and C are cut by a whopping 75 percent! This was the conclusion of research done by nutritionists at Cornell University. A separate study done at Washington University confirmed the finding.

■ Help for Ailing Teeth and Gums

Mouthwash isn't just for kissing anymore. Recent research proves that certain kinds of mouthwash, used correctly, reduce plaque—and therefore, tartar, tooth decay, gum disease and, in all likelihood, your dental bills!

What is plaque? Lick your teeth. Feel coated or sticky? That's plaque. It's invisible and builds up primarily at night from normal bacteria, saliva and food particles. Left untreated, it will harden and become tartar. And plaque plus tartar leads to any number of more serious diseases—gingivitis, for example, (swollen, infected gums) or periodontitis, a gradual erosion of dental bone and tissue culminating in possible tooth loss.

Brushing and flossing, of course, remain important to oral hygiene, but often they are not enough. Many plaque-reducing mouthwashes are readily available in any supermarket, while others from overseas have only recently come to these shores. They may be harder to find, but are worth the search!

Here are the key active ingredients to look for: Propolis, widely tested and used in the former Soviet Union, is a sticky substance bees make from tree sap and use to line honeycombs. This "bee glue" has been shown in German studies not only to reduce plaque and gingivitis, but to heal gum injuries, tooth extractions and gangrene of the mouth. It's not sticky when found in a mouthwash. In Germany, China and Poland, propolis can be found in many mouthwashes and toothpastes. In this country, you may have to look in specialty stores and catalogs.

■ The Common Cold: Children Beware

Americans spent $1.4 billion on over-the-counter cold medicines in 1991. Over 66 percent of households reported that they stock four to eight different types in their medicine cabinets. With more than eight hundred brands to choose from, it is a very big business indeed! But a new study indicates there is more than a little truth in the old saying, "A cold will go away in a week if you treat it, but will take seven days if you don't."

Dr. Michael B. H. Smith of Izaak Walton Killam Children's Hospital in Halifax, Canada, reviewed all the scientific research on these cold medications done since 1950 and found, "There's a lot of shoddy research in this area." Of 106 studies, only 27 were scientifically valid. From those, Smith concluded that while cold medicines can relieve symptoms for adolescents and adults, they do nothing for children—especially children under six, who tend to get the most colds.

Findings for children aged six to thirteen were "weak," he said, because they neglected to take into account the placebo effect, which is considered strong, particularly in youths, according to a Johns Hopkins University study. As for children under six, "the potential side effects are such that there is no reason to have these products available for them," Smith reported.

Furthermore, the American Association of Poison Control Centers reports that over seventy-three thousand kids under the age of six overdosed on cold medicines in 1990— the number-two cause of childhood overdose, after analgesics!

But there is hope. Scientifically valid studies in Poland, Bulgaria, Romania and Russia, which did take into account the placebo effect, found that propolis—the same all-natural "bee glue" that's good for your teeth and gums—has an amazing impact on the common cold even in the youngest children.

Whether diluted in water and gargled, then swallowed; taken as a nasal spray; or mixed with honey (or anything sweet) for children, propolis has been proven to work so fast on a variety of infections it may well put the standard antihistamine and decongestant products out of business!

- **Relief from Kidney Stones**

At the Harvard Medical School, Dr. Edwin Prien and Dr. Stanley Gershoff discovered that magnesium can help dissolve these calcium-oxalate stones. Magnesium apparently bonds with oxalates as well as calcium does, but the magnesium-oxalate combination does not make stones!

Furthermore, the Harvard researchers found in 1974 that vitamin B_6 slows oxalate formation in the first place. So, taken together in even moderate doses of 300 and 10 milligrams, respectively, magnesium oxide and vitamin B_6 "are effective in prevention of recurrence of idiopathic calcium-oxalate stones," they concluded. Indeed, their studies showed incidence of these stones fell a whopping 92 percent!

Vitamin C, which had once been thought to contribute to

kidney stones, has now been found to help prevent them! It raises the acid level in your urine, which assists in dissolving stones. Actually, orange juice is even better because it contains citrate, which does the best job in dissolving stones.

■ Yeast Infections

Yeast infections affect men as well as women, the culprit being a naturally occurring bacteria called candida albicans. You'll know you've got it if your mouth or skin bleeds easily, peels or excretes a white goo—though, of course, the most common form is vaginitis.

What causes yeast infections? Antibiotics can, since they upset the balance of bacteria in your body. So can an imbalance in your nutritional intake, according to some scientists. Dr. Laurence Urdang says that doctors generally prescribe costly antifungal drugs as a solution. But evidence is mounting that there is a better way.

At a South American research center, twenty women with vaginal yeast infections douched with a natural grapefruit-seed extract twice daily for three days. According to Dr. Luis E. Todd, fifteen of them felt better after the first treatment, and by the end of the third day, the infection was gone. A study in Germany with twenty-five women confirmed the finding, Dr. G. Ionescu reports.

In this country, Dr. John Parks Trowbridge explains that a form of vitamin B called biotin can boost the body's ability to fight off and recover from a variety of diseases, not the least of which are yeast infections. "Biotin can help prevent the conversion of the yeast form of Candida to its fungal form," he writes in *The Yeast Syndrome*. He also reported that a University of Massachusetts study concluded that regular consumption of simple garlic usually prevents yeast infections.

In his paper "Therapeutic Properties of Acidophilus," Dr. C. D. Khedkar reported that Acidophilus creates various enzymes, "all of which retard the growth of Candida albicans.

- **Sources of the Substances Mentioned in this Chapter**

Vitamin and health food stores will usually carry the following items:

Acidophilus
Biotin
Propolis (as an ingredient in toothpaste or
     mouthwash for dental health, or as a nasal spray
     to treat colds in children)
Rutin

A mail-order source is:

L&H Vitamins, Inc.
38–01 Thirty-fifth Avenue
Long Island City, NY 11101
(800) 221-1152

Gero Vita International makes a natural product specifically for curing and preventing yeast infections called Candida Guard.

Gero Vita International
Dept. Z101
2255–B Queen Street East #820
Toronto, Ontario M4E 1G3
Canada
(800) 825-8482

Residents of smaller cities may not find Propolis in vitamin and drugstores. A good mail-order source is:

Beehive Botanicals
Route 8, Box 8257
Hayward, WI 54843
(715) 634-4274

7

■ ■ ■

Prostate Disorders Can Be Prevented and Even Stopped

IN 1990, FORMER president Reagan made a very public announcement that he was undergoing an operation called a prostatectomy—the removal of the prostate gland. The disclosure spawned a lot of jokes and elicited anguished expressions on men's faces across the country.

Physicians, on the other hand, applauded the announcement. It finally brought attention to one of the most common of men's health problems—prostate disorders. Unfortunately, it also created some popular misconceptions that remain today.

The prostate is a walnut-sized gland that rests under the bladder and surrounds the urethra, the canal that carries urine and semen through the penis. An accessory gland in the reproductive system, the prostate produces a large portion of a man's seminal fluids.

Because it is so intimately involved in the genito-urinary tract, an enlarged prostate is often the culprit in urinary problems and even sexual dysfunction. The prostate becomes enlarged whenever the blood circulation to it becomes poor or lymphatic fluids get blocked. The expanded prostate begins to tighten around the urethra, which can make urination difficult or even painful.

Let's face it—any problem centering around the genital area seems private at the least and embarrassing at the worst. Men with prostate irregularities often fail to come forward for treatment. Many feel guilt or shame, holding the false belief that they have done something to bring the problem on. Some simply ignore the pain.

The truth is that any man over fifty years of age stands a 60 percent chance of developing an enlarged prostate gland. Besides Ronald Reagan, presidential candidate Robert Dole and broadcaster Roone Arledge have publicly admitted needing treatment for prostate disorders. Musician Frank Zappa and actor Bill Bixby died from prostate cancer.

Although the prostate rarely causes problems for men under fifty, younger men should not ignore it. The gland may begin to enlarge at any age. Prevention should start well before any alarming symptoms appear.

Statistics show that American men are afflicted with prostate disorders more frequently than Asians and Europeans. African Americans also suffer from prostate cancer more often than Caucasians.

There are a number of signs that should warn you that you might have a problem with your prostate. The most common symptom is hard to miss. When the prostate begins to enlarge, it constricts the urethra. Urinating becomes difficult or painful.

If you need to go to the bathroom frequently throughout the night, or the urine flow is reduced to a trickle, you are experiencing other early signals that it is time for a prostate exam. In many cases the bathroom problems may seem to resolve themselves without taking any action. It's possible for this to happen, but often the symptoms become more severe.

The most common ailment of the prostate is known as benign prostatic hypertrophy, or BPH. Largely a product of the aging process, BPH refers to the noncancerous, gradual enlargement of the prostate.

A swollen prostate usually indicates that a man's body is

producing lower levels of testosterone than in previous years. Instead, the body begins producing a dangerous substance called dihydrotestosterone. The dihydrotestosterone in turn stimulates an overproduction of prostate cells. The result is a slowly expanding gland.

Research shows that half of American men age sixty or older have this condition. Some studies, such as the one conducted by Dr. M. Barry in 1990, suggest that the incidence of BPH may be even higher. A swollen prostate should cause concern, but there is little to fear. BPH is rarely life-threatening. In fact, some men can and do live comfortably with an enlarged prostate.

Even so, it should not be ignored. BPH can cause a great deal of discomfort, and an inflamed prostate may be a sign of something much worse. Another common malady of the prostate is known as prostatitis. Unlike the natural enlargement that happens with BPH, prostatitis is caused by a bacterial infection and men of all ages can contract it.

Prostatitis is an acute inflammation of the prostate. The symptoms are much more severe than those of BPH. The flow of urine can be partially or totally blocked, which often causes urine retention in the bladder. The infected urine can weaken the bladder, or cause urinary infections. In chronic cases, the bacteria can pass into the bladder and spread upward to other vital organs.

Signs that an infection has become advanced include difficulties or irritation during urination, blood in the urine, or pains in the lower back or between the scrotum and rectum. Severe cases need immediate treatment.

Prostate cancer is the third most common cancer found in males. One in eleven American men will develop cancer in their prostate, and it kills more than 30,000 people annually. Studies indicate that prostate cancer is on the rise in the United States. For instance, in 1970 research showed that 60 men out of 100,000 were infected with prostate cancer. In 1990, the number increased to 120 out of 100,000. That's a rise of 100 percent!

Like the other prostate disorders, symptoms occur because of an enlarged prostate. The difference here is that deadly cancerous cells cause the swelling. Warning signs of prostate cancer are the same as they are for BPH and pro-statitis—the number-one reason why you should never ignore painful urine flow.

A digital rectal exam can determine whether or not a prostate is cancerous. A healthy prostate has a firm, rubbery feel to it. Cancer causes the organ to stiffen to a woodlike density. Physicians recommend that every man over the age of forty should have a prostate exam at least once every three years.

Considering the prevalence of BPH, it seems every man will seek treatment for a prostate disorder sooner or later. The *New York Times* reported in 1990 that American men spent over $3 billion annually on prostate surgery.

Urologists tend to follow two time-honored paths when combating a prostate problem. The first is to employ a sys-tem of "watchful waiting." The second is the more aggres-sive approach of surgery.

The prostate generally enlarges very slowly. If the level of discomfort is not very great, some men choose to wait and see if the symptoms improve without treatment. Urine flow often returns to normal levels because men unwittingly adapt to the problem by strengthening their bladder muscles.

Patients should never decide to take this approach on their own. Always consult with a doctor to ensure that symp-toms have improved or stabilized. Having a doctor monitor a problem can really pay off. Seventy-five percent of the men who wait a year to put off surgery find that the proce-dure becomes unnecessary.

Presently, surgery is the preferred method for treating prostate disorders. In 1990 alone, doctors performed more than four hundred thousand prostatectomies. The standard procedure in 95 percent of the operations performed in the United States is called a transurethral resection of the prostate, or TURP.

The TURP is a relatively simple procedure that requires no incisions. It's a bit like scooping out the innards of a sliced melon. A urologist winds a tiny, tubelike instrument called a resectoscope through the penis and up into the urethra. An electrified wire inside the scope scrapes away the excess tissue.

Because the procedure is so unintrusive, a man typically is back on his feet the day after surgery. A catheter is needed to urinate for a few days, but usually is discarded before a patient is discharged from the hospital.

The TURP procedure has been touted as virtually risk-free. That certainly accounts for its popularity with urologists, but some doctors are beginning to seek alternative methods for treating patients with BHP.

When the diagnosis is cancer, surgery is probably unavoidable, but with BHP, a TURP might not be as effective or as risk-free as once believed. Most reports state that the chance of death following a TURP is a low 1 percent. Recent federal studies of Medicare patients indicate a slightly higher mortality rate that varies between 3 and 9 percent. The discrepancy depended upon the hospital.

Dr. John E. Wennberg, an epidemiologist at Dartmouth Medical School, conducted an independent study in 1990 that produced some surprising results. Urologists generally believe that early surgical treatment to combat BHP helps patients live longer. Yet the Wennberg research indicated that, rather than help, the preemptive surgery actually lowers life expectancy!

More alarming still, the Wennberg report, published in the Spring 1990 edition of the *New England Journal of Medicine*, showed that TURP patients were more likely to suffer heart attacks than those who chose a different procedure.

In addition to these new concerns, the operation does cause some side effects. According to Dr. Herbert Lepor, an associate professor at the Medical College of Wisconsin in Milwaukee, about 6 percent of patients, or approximately twenty-five thousand in 1990, who had a TURP, suffer from impotency. Though it's difficult to judge whether that is the result of surgery or a related psychological problem.

A more frequent postoperative problem is retrograde ejaculation, commonly referred to as a dry orgasm. After the procedure the bladder often fails to close around the urethra properly during ejaculation. The semen shoots back into the bladder rather than out the penis—infertility is the obvious result.

An embarrassing side effect, but one that occurs with less frequency, is incontinence—the inability to control urination. Five percent of men who have the operation report incontinence, although the problem usually resolves itself over time. Surgery itself is not a cure for a prostate that slowly enlarges with age. Even when the procedure is successful, the condition can reoccur. Ten percent of men who have a TURP need a second operation within five years.

There are a handful of alternatives to the TURP that offer relief from symptoms of an enlarged prostate. Some have such a short track record that it is impossible to tell what their long-term effectiveness may be at this juncture.

A procedure quickly gaining in popularity is one where surgeons insert a tiny balloon into the urethra to the prostate. They inflate the balloon at high pressure, which works to reopen the clogged passageway. At present the method only works well for patients with advanced BPH symptoms. The drawback is that it seems to offer only temporary relief.

A microwave treatment inserts a wire into the urethra that heats and destroys excess prostate tissue. A similar procedure, used by Terrance R. Malloy, chief urologist at Pennsylvania Hospital in Philadelphia, uses ultrasound to bombard the enlarged prostate. The intense sound waves break away prostate cells, which are then sucked away with an aspirator.

Considering the expense of surgery, not to mention stress factors, patients and doctors have sought a way to treat an enlarged prostate without resorting to an operation.

In 1987, Abbott Laboratories, located near Chicago, introduced a drug called Hytrin, a pill used primarily for people with high blood pressure. Called an alpha-blocker by scientists, Hytrin relaxes muscle tissue like the kind found in arteries and the prostate. Early research shows that Hytrin provides immediate relief of many BPH symptoms in about two-thirds of the patients who use it.

Although Hytrin was not specifically developed for prostate disorders, physicians can prescribe it for BPH.

Patients who use it report good results, though it does cause mild side effects such as dizziness, fatigue and occasional fainting spells.

The alleged breakthrough in a prostate medication came in 1992 with the introduction of Proscar. Developed by the pharmaceutical giant Merck & Company, Proscar has received a lot of attention in recent years. Officials at Merck estimate that over five hundred thousand men already take the drug every day. They'll take it for the rest of their lives, if it proves as effective as touted.

Proscar blocks the agents that cause the hormone testosterone to convert into dihydrotestosterone, the catalyst that promotes prostate cell growth. It can't help people with prostate cancer, but its makers claim it can reduce the swelling caused by BPH.

Questions remain about Proscar's effectiveness and its costs. A study published in the October 1992 edition of the *New England Journal of Medicine* compared three hundred men with enlarged prostates who took Proscar against a group who took a placebo pill.

The tests showed that Proscar did help relieve some of the symptoms of BPH. The catch was that the drug does not have an impact until a patient takes it for six months to a year. Further, the research indicated that the improved urine flow increased only by about 17 percent, compared with the 50 percent rise afforded patients who choose surgery. Considering the costs of the drug—about two dollars per pill—Proscar treatment would amount to an outlay of $730 per year—an expensive solution indeed.

Proscar does not, however, bypass the side effects that earlier drugs created. Sexual dysfunction can still be a problem. As many as five percent of the sample subjects reported that Proscar lowered the sex drive and the amount of ejaculate, and even caused impotence.

Merck warns that Proscar damages semen and has caused birth defects in laboratory animals. Couples are advised to use contraception when the male takes the drug. It is impossible to determine yet if long-term use causes any other side effects.

Clinical tests were conducted recently comparing Hytrin and Proscar. The *New England Journal of Medicine* published the results in 1996 that showed Hytrin did give significant relief, but Proscar was no better than a placebo or sugar pill.

It's surprising that so much time and research was spent in producing prescription drugs for prostate disorders. Though physicians in the mainstream still push drugs for these conditions many others believe that natural solutions are the key to solving this age-old problem.

Prostate disorders are clearly on the upswing in American men. The aging of the population is a contributing factor, but an often overlooked suspect, nutritionists believe, is the type of foods available. Most store-bought items undergo an extensive amount of processing. All this processing destroys a very important ingredient in the male diet—zinc.

Scientists have learned that the prostate uses ten times more of this mineral than any other organ in the body. Zinc picolinate does naturally what drugs like Proscar try to do with chemicals: block the body's production of dihydrotestosterone. Dr. Earl Mindell, author of the best-selling book *The Vitamin Bible*, writes, "Most zinc in food is lost by processing, or never exists in a substantial amount due to nutrient-poor soil."

Further support of this claim comes from Dr. Denham Harman, professor emeritus at the Nebraska School of Medicine and the developer of the free radical theory of aging, who says, "Some 90 percent of the population consumes a diet deficient in zinc." It's no wonder that prostate disorders are on the rise.

Two research teams published recent studies that confirm zinc picolinate's contributions to a healthy prostate. Dr. M. Fahim and Dr. J. Harman reported in a government medical journal that zinc was effectively used to reduce prostate enlargement. It also controlled many of the painful symptoms.

A separate investigation by Dr. G. D. Chisholm, published in the *Journal of Steroid Biochemistry*, also confirmed the view that zinc picolinate prevents swelling of the prostate. Iron has long been held as a necessary mineral for women's health. These studies indicate that zinc may soon become known as the "man's vitamin."

Men with prostate problems, and those who want to prevent them from occurring, should consider taking zinc supplements. Zinc can provide additional benefits; according to observations by Dr. Mindell, "I have even seen success in cases of impotence with a supplement program of B_6 and zinc."

It is important to note that Dr. Mindell suggests a combination of zinc and vitamin B_6. A study by Dr. G. W. Evans published in the *Journal of Nutrition* showed that B_6 (pyridoxine) enhances the body's ability to absorb zinc. The additional supplement ensures that the prostate gets the healthy amount of zinc it needs.

Another natural ingredient that has a long association with prostate health is the saw palmetto berry. Formally known as serenoa repens, this short species of palm tree can be found throughout the lower half of the United States.

The Native Americans used it in a number of ways. The seeds were eaten as food, the leaves ground into powder and applied as a poultice for wounds and the berries were thought to be a mild aphrodisiac, as well as a cure for urinary problems.

Even though it has been listed in pharmacology books for over eighty years, scientists are just now beginning to reexamine serenoa's healthful properties. In 1984, Dr. G. Champault completed a double-blind study that tested serenoa's ability to combat the hormonal imbalance that causes prostate growth.

Champault's report, written in the British *Journal of Pharmacology*, showed that serenoa had a dramatic impact on urine flow for men with BPH symptoms. More interesting still was that serenoa proved much more effective than Proscar. Even so, the FDA has ruled that makers of serenoa extracts may not even hint that it can help men with prostate disorders. Indian medicine men obviously know something that the FDA doesn't want to believe.

During an allergy experiment in 1989, two doctors accidentally discovered that amino acids are important to prostate health. The physicians administered a mixture of three amino acids—glycine, 1-alanine and glutamic acid—to a group of patients suffering from allergic symptoms. As tests continued, one of the subjects volunteered that his urinary problems had suddenly disappeared.

The disclosure prompted Dr. K. W. Donsbach to initiate a new study. This time the amino acid mixture was given to patients with urinary disorders. Forty men were used in the three-month experiment. Twenty received the amino acids, and the others were given a placebo. The results were dramatic.

More than 90 percent of the subjects experienced a reduction in the swelling of the prostate. Almost a third had prostates that returned to normal size. An overwhelming majority urinated more quickly and less frequently, and most reported a much improved urine flow.

Subsequent controlled studies supported Donsbach's results, but there was one caveat. As soon as the subjects stopped taking the supplements, the symptoms slowly returned. The amino acid treatment is a good preventative, but not a cure for BPH.

An extract from the bark of an evergreen tree that grows in Madagascar (*Pygeum africanum*) has recently been proven to be the most effective weapon against BPH with no significant side effects.

In France, Germany and Italy, 672 men suffering from prostate disorders were given either *Pygeum* or a placebo for six months in double-blind studies at thirteen hospitals, three university research hospitals and four other research facilities. Supervising the tests were thirty-eight of Europe's most prominent medical scientists, who concluded that *Pygeum* corrected the prostate disorders in 66 percent of the cases studied. Several prestigious medical journals published the results of this amazing new medicine which is now available in the United States.

Then scientists at the University of Munich and Warsaw School of Medicine found that if they added a particular polysaccharide and an isolectin from the root of the *Urtica dioica* plant, the results were almost twice as good. *Urtica* is the common nettles weed, which grows wild in many places in the world.

There were good reasons this combination worked so well. The *Urtica* ingredients tested in vitro showed that they gave the immune system a tremendous boost by substantially increasing antitumor lymphocytes. In fact, Dr. Hans Wagner reported in the medical journal *Phytomedicine* that the *Urtica* extract was "markedly superior" to the anti-inflammatory drug Indomethacin.

Dr. A. Frisen of the urology department of Munich City Hospital conducted a double-blind, placebo-controlled clinical trial of the *Urtica* extract. He found that *Urtica* reduced urination problems by 83 percent and increased urine flow by 87 percent. Overall, 91 percent of the patients taking *Urtica* experienced improvement in their prostate health.

What puzzled scientists for a while was why men in Italy and Greece had about 45 percent fewer prostate problems than other Europeans or Americans. This is where American scientists got to show their stuff.

The most abundant carotenoid in the prostate are "lycopenes." American scientists discovered lycopenes in the skin of tomatoes. Italians and Greeks have a much heavier diet of tomato products than other people in the world.

Dr. Edward Giovannucci at Harvard Medical School led a research team that followed the eating habits of 47,894 doctors for six years. Those that had ten meals or more per week which included tomato products had about 30 percent less occurances of prostate cancer. There's not many lycopenes in tomatoes, and their preventive effects were apparent even in those that ate only three or four tomato products per week. They had about 15 percent less occurrances of cancer.

In the Orient, the powers of ginseng have been lauded for centuries. Indeed, ginseng is cited as a cure for almost any ailment imaginable. Recently, scientists have reported that as far as the prostate is concerned the claims might not be so outrageous.

Dr. W. S. Fahim studied the effect ginseng had on the prostate. His research showed that panax ginseng increased testosterone levels in test animals, while decreasing the size of the prostate. This confirmed what many older Asian men have believed for centuries—that ginseng improves virility, stamina and improves sex life overall.

Modern medical research too often resorts to artificial or chemical means to find cures for common ailments. Many times solutions or preventative measures can be found in natural products or vitamin supplements. They are safer, less expensive and generally come free of any side effects.

If your prostate is giving you problems, it's a good idea to investigate natural solutions before scheduling any surgery or taking prescription medication. Natural products can be the most effective and inexpensive way to improve your health and promote a better quality of life.

■ Sources of the Products Mentioned in this Chapter

The following supplements are available in vitamin or health food stores:

B$_6$ (pyrdoxine)
Ginseng
Glutamic acid
Glycine
L-alanine
Pygeumaftricanum
Saw Palmetto (Serenoa repens)
Urticadioca (nettles)
Zinc picolinate

One company, Gero Vita International, has combined the proper quantities of each of these ingredients into one pill, called "Prostata."

Gero Vita International, Dept. Z101
2255–B Queen Street East #820
Toronto, Ontario M4E 1G3, Canada
(800) 825-8482

8

■ ■ ■

PMS, Menopause and Osteoporosis—Relief Is Available and Safe

OFTEN WHEN WOMEN are suffering through premenstrual syndrome (PMS), they get little help from doctors, who tell them it's just another mysterious "female problem." Rather than do the research or take the time to educate themselves about PMS, many doctors prefer to keep their patients—and themselves—in the dark about the causes and available treatments.

Scientists have found that PMS may be caused by the drastic drop in progesterone levels in a woman's body in the week preceding her period. The preeminent scientist on PMS, English physician Katharina Dalton, who coined the term "premenstrual syndrome," first theorized about the role of progesterone. Because of her research, thousands of women with PMS have found relief with progesterone treatments.

Progesterone works to buffer the negative effects that elevated estrogen levels can have. During the phase of a woman's cycle when progesterone drops most rapidly, unbuffered levels of estrogen can lead to PMS symptoms, such as low blood sugar, salt and water retention, increased body fat and reduced oxygen levels in the cells.

Synthetic progesterone is expensive, can only be obtained with a physician's prescription and causes many undesirable side effects. Synthetic progesterone inhibits a woman's production of natural progesterone, which can worsen hormonal imbalance.

Also, some synthetic progesterone is two thousand times stronger than the natural hormone and can lead to salt and fluid retention and blood sugar imbalances; worse, it can increase the risk of cancer.

Few doctors are aware of natural progesterone because it can't be patented by pharmaceutical companies, so no drug company is going to launch a multimillion dollar ad campaign to get the word out. But there are natural sources of progesterone that are safe, effective and inexpensive.

One natural medicine, Ovatrophin, can help raise progesterone levels in a woman who still has her ovaries. It is a glandular medicine made from bovine ovaries. The usual dosage is three pills per day for three weeks and then two pills per day for the next week. The dosage can often be cut down to one pill per day for maintenance after a month of treatment.

A half-century ago, American scientist Russell Marker discovered a way to extract natural progesterone from wild Mexican yam plants. Traditionally, the wild yam had been used by local people to treat menstrual cramps and prevent miscarriage.

Now, the yam extract is available in a blend of aloe vera, vitamin E and vegetable oil. The product is a medicinal cream called Pro-Gest Moisturizing Cream. Multiple studies have found that topical use of the cream significantly raises progesterone levels. As a result, Pro-Gest can be a vital treatment for PMS—and for menopause and osteoporosis, too.

Pro-Gest has the extra benefit of being plant-based. Dr. Cynthia Watson, a clinical faculty member at the University of Southern California, has found in her medical practice that botanical hormone supplements are preferable to any other source, because they do not have the side effects of synthetic and animal-based hormones, and they are more easily metabolized.

It is generally recommended that Pro-Gest be applied twice daily. In the week before menstruation begins, the cream can be applied up to five times per day if needed. Once menstruation begins, however, the cream should not be used again until bleeding stops.

About one-fourth to one-half teaspoon of Pro-Gest should be applied to the abdomen, chest, face or back of the neck. If the appropriate amount of cream is used, it will be absorbed through the skin in three to five minutes. If it disappears in less than two minutes, then more should be used. Once the cream is absorbed, it will change from white to transparent.

By the third month, PMS symptoms should be alleviated, and then Pro-Gest should be used only in the week prior to menstruation. Again, the dosage should be one-fourth to one-half teaspoon applied two times per day. More cream can be applied if symptoms are still severe. While some women choose to use the cream for a few days each month on a long-term basis, many no longer need it after three or four months.

It is the job of the liver to eliminate excess estrogen, and it needs sufficient amounts of vitamin B_6 (pyridoxine) and magnesium to do this. B_6 is considered by experts to be one of the most important defenses against PMS. Usually women are advised to take a B-complex vitamin daily with one hundred milligrams of B_6 and four hundred to eight hundred milligrams of magnesium.

The *Journal of Reproductive Medicine* reported that many women with PMS are lacking in the minerals and nutrients they need to produce progesterone naturally. For instance, the *Journal of the American College of Nutrition* reported that daily doses of 150 IU of vitamin E can raise progesterone levels. However, keep in mind that high daily dosages of vitamin E can actually *lower* progesterone levels, so keep your dosage below 200 IU per day.

Drawing from the results of animal studies, the journal

Feedstuffs reported that beta-carotene can increase the synthesis of progesterone. The recommended dosage of beta-carotene is five hundred milligrams per day.

A team of scientists reported in Hawaii Medical Journal that bromelain, a pineapple extract, aids the production of progesterone, which is needed to balance out excess estrogen. Another study, published in the *American Journal of Obstetrics and Gynecology*, found that bromelain relieves menstrual cramps.

The journal *Recent Advances in Clinical Nutrition* reported that evening primrose oil can also be used to treat PMS because it works much like bromelain in aiding the production of progesterone. The recommended dosage of evening primrose oil is usually five hundred milligrams three times a day.

Usually when a woman begins menopause, her doctor will prescribe supplemental estrogen because this is the time in her life when estrogen levels naturally begin to decline. But it is often more effective to use supplemental progesterone to treat the symptoms of menopause.

Not only is Pro-Gest Cream good for treating PMS, it can also be a real lifesaver for women suffering through the symptoms of menopause. When hot flashes occur, one-half to three-fourths teaspoon of Pro-Gest Cream should be applied topically four times during the hour following the hot flash. At this dosage, symptoms should stop within one week to a couple of months, with individual variations. Once symptoms are under control, a maintenance program can begin with the topical application of one-fourth to one-half teaspoon each day.

Many women experience a drop in their vaginal lubrication after menopause. It has been reported that when applied to the vaginal area, Pro-Gest Cream can increase a woman's natural lubrication. As an added plus, for some women Pro-Gest Cream has smoothed out wrinkles and faded age spots.

As long ago as 1945, Dr. C. J. Christy published in the *American Journal of Gynecology* the results of his study on menopausal women. Dr. Christy found that when treated with vitamin E, the women experienced significant relief from menopausal symptoms, with no side effects.

A few years later, Dr. H. Ferguson reported in the *Virginia Medical Monthly* the research he did on sixty-six women with severe symptoms associated with menopause. Dr. Ferguson found that when treated with 15 to 30 IU of vitamin E every day, the women experienced complete relief from their symptoms.

So, if the benefits of vitamin E were proven almost fifty years ago, why is the therapy still underused? Because vitamins aren't patentable, and no patent means little profit for pharmaceutical companies, says Dr. R. Passwater, a leading expert on menopause.

■ Osteoporosis Afflicts Twenty Million Older Americans

Osteoporosis, or brittle bone disease, is a horrible and crippling disease plaguing the nation's elders. A few years ago at the International Symposium on Osteoporosis held in Denmark, a specialist warned, "More women die from osteoporosis-related fractures than from cancer of the breast, cervix and uterus combined, and in the United States hip fracture health care costs up to $10 billion annually, causing 200,000 deaths."

This debilitating disease causes severe weakening of the bones, often leading to a loss in bone mass of as much as 30 to 40 percent. Millions of fractures occur every year because of this disease. A study carried out in Knox County, Tennessee, found that the number of fractures resulting in hospitalization doubled every five years in people over fifty.

Thousands of people break their wrists and suffer collapsed spinal vertebra, a painful and disfiguring problem. But the most devastating injury is the hip fracture: one out of three women and one out of six men after the age of retirement will suffer hip fractures.

Women most likely to develop osteoporosis are those who don't get much exercise, have small frames, have kidney disease, smoke and drink alcohol, use steroids or thyroid medication, had their ovaries taken out before they were forty years old, have family members with osteoporosis or are of Northern European, Latin or Asian background.

For people who suffer hip fractures, often the most devastating part is the loss of independence. Half will never again be able to walk without assistance. Many have no choice but to stay in a convalescent hospital, where they may end up feeling more frail and burdensome.

■ Profiteering with Estrogen Therapy

The medical establishment has for years run a one-track campaign insisting that all postmenopausal women should receive estrogen therapy for the rest of their lives. Because of this, pharmaceutical companies manufacturing estrogen are raking in the profits hand over fist.

Research has shown that long-term synthetic estrogen use does prevent further bone deterioration. But Dr. Cynthia Watson of the University of Southern California reports that the hormone is really only effective in fighting bone loss during the first five years after menopause. And some researchers are finding that standard estrogen replacement therapy may be helpful in only 25 percent of the cases. Most importantly, estrogen *cannot* replace bone that had been lost already before treatment; it merely slows further deterioration.

Artificially raising the levels of estrogen in postmenopausal women runs against the grain of nature. The body's natural balance is designed for a decrease in the hormone. Disrupting the natural balance can lead to very serious consequences.

Researchers have found that artificially high levels of estrogen can lead to high blood pressure, abnormal blood clotting, diabetes, cancer and liver and gallbladder disease. Women who take estrogen are as much as fourteen times more likely than other women to develop uterine cancer.

In fact, even the manufacturers of Premarin, one of the most prescribed estrogen replacement therapies, admit that the drug increases a woman's risk for uterine and breast cancer and can cause a whole host of deleterious side effects, including hair loss, tumors, migraines, depression and worsening of heart disease.

Progesterone derived from plants has been proven to play a vital and unique role in treating osteoporosis. Amazingly, it can reverse the damaging bone loss caused by the disease. In fact, no treatment that *excludes* natural progesterone has been able to improve bone density and strength in people with osteoporosis.

Medical researcher Dr. John Lee studied the effects of Pro-Gest Cream when used along with a common treatment plan for osteoporosis. He found that over the course of six months of treatment, bone density increased by up to 10 percent. When treatment was continued, bone density improved at a rate of 3 to 5 percent per year until plateauing at the level generally found in healthy thirty-five-year-old women, as reported in the prestigious British medical journal *Lancet*.

Most importantly, Dr. Lee's regimen, which included one hundred postmenopausal women aged thirty-eight to eighty-three, improved bone density across the board—regardless of age or time elapsed since menopause. This is a critical advantage over an estrogen-only program, because estrogen has been found to help only in the first five years after menopause.

Remarkably, women who began Dr. Lee's study with the most bone deterioration experienced the most improvement over the course of the program. In addition, none of the women in the study suffered bone fractures. Many of the women in Dr. Lee's program found that their sex drive returned to normal and that they had more energy, more mobility and less aches—with no side effects!

We all know that children should drink calcium-rich milk for strong bones, so the same must go for adults, right? Wrong. Americans drink more milk than anyone else in the world, but we also have the highest occurrence of bone ailments. Obviously, milk alone isn't the answer. Dr. N. M. Lewis of the University of Wisconsin Department of Nutritional Sciences studied people on dairy-rich diets and found that they excreted the majority of the calcium they consumed.

Worse yet, Dr. R. R. Recker reported in the *American Journal of Clinical Nutrition* that the large amounts of protein and phosphorous in milk cause the body to *lose* more calcium than it gains.

Calcium supplements alone can't do the job of protecting you from osteoporosis because the mineral can be absorbed into the body only when the stomach produces a healthy level of acid.

Dr. M. Grossman reported in the journal *Gastroenterology* that about 40 percent of postmenopausal women have extremely low levels of stomach acid. And Dr. R. R. Recker reported in the *American Journal of Clinical Nutrition* that people with low acid levels can absorb only 4 percent of an oral dosage of calcium carbonate. Healthy people absorb about 22 percent.

When calcium is taken with other nutrients and minerals, absorption improves. Dr. Recker found that people deficient in stomach acid could absorb calcium citrate at more than ten times the rate of calcium carbonate.

Researchers have found that special combinations of other important minerals, such as zinc, copper, boron, magnesium, manganese, silicon and even strontium, can help build bone and increase density. Dr. Cynthia Watson recommends the supplement *Osteo Health*, which provides many of these necessary nutrients.

■ Boron Is Key in Fighting Osteoporosis

Vegetables, kelp, nuts and fruits as easy to find as grapes and apples all contain the vital mineral boron. Nutritional expert Dr. Earl Mindell reports that boron may slow down bone loss in postmenopausal women. Boron's beneficial role is twofold: it helps the body retain dietary calcium, and it can greatly increase the levels of natural estrogen.

Dr. F. H. Nielsen found in his study on boron that deficiencies in the mineral leads to abnormal bone formation. He estimates that people need one to two milligrams of boron daily.

The *Journal of the American Geriatrics Society* has published two independent studies concluding that people over sixty-five are commonly deficient in vitamin B_6, vitamin B_{12}, and folic acid. These important studies, conducted by Dr. H. Barker and Dr. C. Infante-Rivard, were able to establish a link between low levels of these nutrients and osteoporosis.

Women who have taken birth-control pills are particularly at risk because the pill causes vitamin B_6 deficiency. To avoid the health problems of long-term B_6 deficiency, including bone disease, women taking birth-control pills should supplement their diets with at least fifty milligrams of B_6 per day.

Both vitamins C and K are important for building a strong matrix within bones, and deficiencies can lead to bone disease. A study of patients with osteoporosis found they had vitamin K levels of only 35 percent of healthy people of the same age. Other studies have found that vitamin K supplements increase bone growth after a fracture and also reduce the amount of calcium excreted in the urine by up to 50 percent.

Vitamin D is needed to absorb calcium. The level of vitamin D in the elderly tends to be half that of younger people. Dr. R. M. Francis reported in the *New England Journal of Medicine* that vitamin D deficiency can lead to serious bone loss. Although some vitamin D treatments can be expensive and difficult to manage, studies have found that the minerals magnesium and boron can naturally boost levels of the vitamin in the body.

Medical problems associated with PMS, menopause and osteoporosis seem very scary and overwhelming—but they don't have to be. You don't need to get an M.D. or pay a lot of money to make or keep yourself healthy. All you need is a little knowledge—which you now have from reading this chapter—and the courage to help yourself. So don't let the pharmaceutical companies pull the wool over your eyes. Stay informed of safe and inexpensive alternative treatments, and you'll be doing yourself and your body the favor of a lifetime.

■ Sources of the Medicines Mentioned in this Chapter

The following can be found in most health food and vitamin stores:

Vitamin B_6, B_{12}
Beta Carotene
Boron
Bromelain
Calcium Citrate
Vitamin D
Vitamin E
Evening Primrose
Vitamin K
Osteo Health

Pro-Gest Cream is made by Professional and Technical Services, Inc., located at 3331 N.E. Sandy Blvd., Portland, OR 97232. For information on ordering, call their main office at (800) 648-8211 or (503) 231-7244.

Ovatrophin is produced by Standard Process Laboratories and can be ordered by contacting the company at 1200 W. Royal Lee Dr., Palmyra, WI 53156. You can also order Ovatrophin through the Vitamin Shoppe at (800) 223-1216 or by contacting a doctor who specializes in nutrition.

Another natural alternative to conventional estrogen replacement therapy is PMSupport, which contains natural estrogens. It is available from Gero Vita International, Dept. Z101, 2255-B Queen Street East #820, Toronto, Ontario M4E 1G3, Canada. Or call (800) 825-8482.

9

■ ■ ■

Enjoy a Healthy Sex Life
Even in Old Age

ALTHOUGH VIAGRA AND the other new sexual drugs seem to promise the ultimate answer to impotence and other sexual problems, new drugs usually start showing long-term side effects only years after they've been approved for use by the public. Essentially, these drugs work by opening a valve to allow blood to flow to the penis. They stimulate some women who take them in the same way; they allow more blood to flow in the genital area, increasing sexual sensitivity. The concern we have is that the drugs do not correct the cause of the problem. Many scientists suspect that the cause of sexual problems is a hormonal imbalance brought on by nutritional deficiencies. Therefore, this chapter covers the clinical studies that have shown success in overcoming sexual problems with nutritional adjuvants rather than drugs. This chapter is on the sexual problems of both men and women. It would be useful if men and women read the entire chapter so they will have an understanding of their partner's problems and what can be done to treat them.

For centuries people have equated sexual virility with good health, strength and overall vigor. Elderly men or women who remain sexually active seem more youthful. To maintain that edge, people throughout the world have sought sexual stimulants—aphrodisiacs.

Oats have a long history as a folk remedy for an ailing libido. The ancient Greeks were perhaps the first to associate the grain with sex. A sheaf of oats almost always accompanied any depiction of Eros, the Greek god of passion.

The Romans, who borrowed much of their culture from the Greeks, also picked up on the connection. Steaming bowls of oats were the preferred nourishment that attendants would serve to revelers following an afternoon of orgiastic partying.

Perhaps that's why the phrase "feeling your oats" is considered a connotation for sexual vigor. Most people today feel that anyone who believes that oats can help with a sagging libido is falling for an old wive's tale. However, recent research indicates that maybe the ancients understood more than anyone thought.

■ The Carp Miracle

Chinese farmer Lee Zhang was a practical man. In addition to growing grains and vegetables typical to most farms, Zhang raised carp in a pond on his property to trade at his local market. The colorful fish also served as emergency rations for his own family when money was tight.

Feeling his son needed to help out more with the day-to-day chores of the farm, Zhang asked the boy to start feeding the carp before he went off to school. The boy did as he was told and began giving them food from a bag stored in the barn.

After a few weeks the boy ran out of food and dutifully told Zhang that they needed to buy some more. Zhang was surprised. He knew the feed supply should have lasted much longer. After investigating, Zhang saw that the bag holding the carp feed was still full. A bag that once held green oats, however, was now empty. His son had fed the carp the wrong food.

Zhang, fearing the worst, immediately checked up on the fish. He was shocked at what he saw. The carp obviously enjoyed their new diet. Hundreds of baby carp swam around in the now crowded pool. Furthermore, the older carp seemed much livelier and quite healthy—very unusual for a fish that is normally a lazy breeder. Zhang concluded that the green oats somehow caused the fish to mate much more aggressively.

During trips to the market, Zhang mentioned the story of the miracle carp to his fellow farmers. Word spread of the amazing discovery. The tale eventually caught the ears of researchers who decided to test the oats for themselves.

Chinese scientists first examined Zhang's carp to see if the story had any validity. They found that various hormone levels in the fish were more than one-third above the norm.

Next they obtained a quantity of the oat mixture to see if they could duplicate the effects in humans. The green oats, along with an amount of a stinging nettle, were ground up into powder and stirred together with water to form a broth.

The Chinese researchers conducted an unofficial experiment by consuming the strange cocktail themselves. The results were surprising. All the scientists reported having more energy. They also noticed that they had much firmer and larger erections than ever.

The oats were not the typical farm brand, but a similar strain known as *Avena sativa*: not an unusual variety, but only a fresh batch proved capable of working its magic.

The stimulating qualities of *Avena sativa* were noted as early as two centuries ago by German physicians, who wrote about its positive effects in a pharmacopoeia of the time. A common medicine in folk remedies, oats allegedly cure allergies, eczema, and circulatory and digestive problems.

Added to the oats were a few grains of a stinging nettle known formally as *Urtica dioica*. Another therapeutic plant, *Urtica dioica* has a history of use as an aid for a host of problems, ranging from urinary tract disorders to a cure for anemia.

Even though researchers learned what was in the grain, they were unable to reproduce the original results. Oats alone did nothing; the same was true with a pure nettle extract. For some unexplained reason, the aphrodisiaclike properties only seemed to work when just the right amount of the two grains was added to water.

Academics became skeptical of the extract's powers. New studies focused upon whether or not a measured batch of the mixture truly worked as an aphrodisiac. The Chinese themselves initiated a more rigorous double-blind experiment a year after the initial discovery.

In it, nearly two hundred men took a stabilized formula of the mixture for several weeks. An astounding 90 percent of the sample subjects reported that it increased their desire to have sex, and even claimed it improved their performance.

A Hungarian scientist, Dr. Robert Frankl of Budapest University, conducted an independent study in 1984. Twelve male subjects consumed the mixture for several weeks. Dr. Frankl confirmed that the formula helped the men increase their aerobic power and muscle strength. It also increased the testosterone levels of the subjects.

Scientists at the University of Texas studied the extract's effect on horses. Tests verified that it was an effective energy stimulant, and also improved the animal's endurance.

A similar test that used humans as subjects was developed by researchers at the College of Medicine of Northwestern Ohio University. Here, the data was more conclusive. Experiments showed that the nettle and oat mixture helped sexually dysfunctional men develop and sustain an erection. The blood hormone levels of these men markedly increased by 30 percent.

All of these experiments eventually caught the eye of scientists at the Institute for Advanced Study of Human Sexuality, a nonprofit research organization based in San Francisco.

Researchers at the institute wanted to determine whether or not the nettle-oat extract actually produced any sexual benefits. The results of a six-week double-blind study using forty subjects were impressively in favor of the nettle-oat extract.

Using urine samples as an indicator, researchers confirmed that the testosterone levels of men and women participating in the experiment increased an average of 105 percent. Men suffering from impotency reported they could now perform. Women who claimed they had little or no desire for sex felt pangs of sexual excitement for the first time in years.

Testimony of the participants lent further support for *Avena sativa*'s usefulness for men and women. A twenty-eight-year-old woman said she "felt better, more intense orgasms," and had "more sexual dreams." A twenty-five-year-old female subject felt the mixture really helped stimulate her sense of touch. "You are supersensitive to touch, sexual and nonsexual, especially in your mouth," she reported.

The report also raved about the formula's impact on men. "The overall effect for the men who reported improvement can be summarized as a generalized sense of well-being with an increased ability to function sexually." Most men claimed that the stimulation they felt was "reminiscent of their youth."

The most dramatic reports came during a live taping of the syndicated *Geraldo* TV program. The host, Geraldo Rivera, interviewed Loretta Haroian, Dean of Professional Studies at the institute, along with several people who took part in the experiment.

Ray McIlvenna, a sixty-eight-year-old male participant in the study, provided the show's greatest moment when he announced that after taking the formula his erections became "larger than ever in my life." Geraldo's reaction: "Well, God bless."

Researchers at the Institute for Advanced Study of Human Sexuality recognize that there is still much to learn about *Avena sativa*. "We will continue," say the institute's administrators, "to investigate and supervise the research of physicians who are willing to hold the scientific hypothesis that this particular extract of oats or some derivative thereof can restore sexual vigor and enhance the sexual experience of men and women."

▪ Another Successful Approach for Men

If you are a man who has problems getting and maintaining firm erections or have decreased sexual desire, you are not alone. There are millions of men just like you—about 52 percent of those over forty.

Most men just accept the situation, assuming that it is a result of getting older. This is unfortunate, because men are capable of firm erections well into their eighties. Fortunately for everyone, male scientists get older and often have the same sexual problems as other folks. That means many scientists, for clearly personal reasons, conduct research on sexual dysfunctions as they get older. A scientist at Stanford University remarked recently, "Sexual inadequacy is the most researched and up-to-date area in the medical science field—for obvious reasons."

In the 1800s, the famous psychologist Sigmund Freud convinced the world that 90 percent of sexual problems are psychological. However, in the last decade, modern scientists have proved in many clinical tests that over 90 percent of the problems are of organic origin and only 10 percent are psychological. In the last few years, the discoveries in this field are of enormous consequence.

Technology has made it possible for scientists to determine specifically what causes the body to function or malfunction sexually in most cases. The majority of impotence or erectile inadequacy cases are caused by three conditions.

First, all men need a sufficient amount of testosterone, the primary male hormone, in their system. If testosterone levels are low, there's little desire for sex and no ability to get an erection. Second, high cholesterol is associated with impotence. For every ten-point rise in cholesterol above normal, there's a 32 percent increase in the risk of impotence.

Third, there are nerves in the brain called alpha-2-adrenergic receptors. If these receptors are activated, they will prevent the blood valves to the penis from opening. As some people get older, these receptors stay active, probably due to the normal deterioration of the brain with aging. Scientists have found very effective ways to correct those three major causes, and more importantly, neither chemical prescriptions, shots or invasive surgery is necessary.

■ Oysters on Your Wedding Night

One of the answers is strictly nutritional. Male sex organs use more zinc than any other part of the body. It's no wonder, then, that so many men have sexual problems, according to professor emeritus Denham Harmon, M.D., Ph.D., of the University of Nebraska School of Medicine. He said, "Some 90 percent of the population consume diets deficient in zinc."

The reason for this is nutrient-depleted soil. The plants we eat extract zinc from the soil, yet commercial fertilizers don't replace the zinc. Over decades of farming, no zinc is left in the soil, so the food we eat is devoid of this important nutrient.

Dr. Earl Mindell, a famous pharmacologist, says, "If there's any zinc in food, much of it is lost in food processing systems."

Zinc deficiency in children causes delayed sexual development, according to studies conducted by Dr. S. Z. Ghavami at the Pediatric Department of New York's Nassau County Medical Center.

Dr. U. Mehta reported in the *Journal of Experimental Biology* that his clinical tests showed that the testes and penises of animals atrophied and shrank when fed diets devoid of zinc. They also exhibited no desire to mate.

On the other hand, the testosterone levels of men given zinc supplements rose dramatically, according to clinical studies conducted by Dr. A. T. Crockett at the University of Rochester School of Medicine. Dr. H. G. Kynaston showed in a clinical study published in the medical journal *Urologia* that infertile men given zinc supplements for four to eight weeks produced 45 percent more sperm than before.

Zinc also stops the pituitary gland from producing prolactin, according to research done by Dr. Alan Judd at the University of Virginia Medical School. Prolactin stops testosterone production and causes dihydrotestosterone to be produced. Dihydrotestosterone is the main culprit responsible for prostate enlargement—one of the male sex organ's deadliest enemies.

For many centuries, bridegrooms have been encouraged to eat oysters on their wedding night. When this began, there was no scientific basis for this suggestion, but the wisdom of the ages was right. Modern analysis of the oyster shows that it is loaded with zinc.

■ High Cholesterol Injures More Than Your Heart

High cholesterol levels are common in impotent men. Scientists are still studying the interrelationship with sexual performance. In the meantime, Dr. Charles Day, a biologist for Audex Laboratories, has made a significant discovery. He found that plant sterols, particularly beta-sitosterol, block the intake of cholesterol by 62 to 72 percent. Beta-sitosterol is found in a nutritional substance called cholestatin.

This plant sterol is also a precursor or raw material for the production of testosterone in the body, according to Dr. Cynthia Watson, an expert on sexual dysfunction and the author of the best-selling book *Love Potions*.

Another plant sterol that helps the body make testosterone is *Smilax officinalis*. It comes from the root of the plant that also gives us the flavoring called sarsaparilla. *Smilax* lowers cholesterol and is very popular with body builders because it increases energy and endurance.

In bars around stadiums where rodeos are held, macho cowboys show off their masculinity by eating pickled bull's balls, which are known as "Denver oysters." They joke about how virile they are as a result.

In some cultures centuries ago, men often ate the testes of powerful animals, such as lions, tigers and buffalo. Leaving no stone unturned, scientists recently analyzed the content of bull and rat testes. They found a substantial amount of testosterone in each. The big question was whether man would get any benefit if he ingested them.

A group of scientists, led by Dr. A. P. Rommerts, measured the testosterone of male rats and then fed them with the fluid and tissue from rat testes. Much to their surprise, the rats' testosterone levels rose. Further tests of calf and bull testes revealed similar results.

Dr. M. P. Hedger reported in the medical journal *Biology of Reproduction* that testicular fluid and tissue (orchic tissue) contain testosterone-stimulating factors for men. So those cowboys at rodeo bars are loaded with testosterone.

Twenty years ago, most scientists laughed when anyone suggested that ancient "medicine men" and "witch doctors" had effective curatives for many ailments. Their medicines were basically plant concoctions. Back then, most scientists thought all the answers to human ailments would be found in synthetic chemicals they could cook up in their labs.

In the last ten years, the scientific community has done a complete about-face. A tremendous amount of research has been done on the old medicine mens' formulas, and literally hundreds of valuable and beneficial substances have been found.

There is so much enthusiasm for this concept that medical scientists have become the leaders in the activist drive to save the rain forests. Their major contention is that valuable plants that don't grow elsewhere will be lost. Those plants may contain the cure for cancer, AIDS and dozens of other diseases.

Two amazing substances that alleviate sexual disorders have been found in South American and African witch doctors' brews. For several centuries in South America, when a man felt he had lost his sexual drive or had trouble getting a firm erection, the witch doctor would give him an extract from the plant *Pthychopetalum ocaloides*.

The natives called it Muira Puama. The French government assigned Dr. Jacques Waynburg, one of the world's foremost authorities on sexual functioning, the chore of testing it. At the Institute of Sexology in Paris, Dr. Waynburg assembled 262 male patients who complained of lack of sexual desire or inability to get or maintain an erection. Half of the group were given a placebo, and half were given Muira Puama for only two weeks. The results were quite astounding: 62 percent of those taking Muira Puama claimed it had a dynamic effect on their sexual desire and performance, with no side effects.

The results of this carefully controlled, double-blind study were published in the prestigious American *Journal of Urology*. Now scientists around the world are involved, and numerous long-term studies are under way.

The second plant extract, used by ancient doctors up to a thousand years ago, comes from a tree in Camaroon, Africa, called *Pausinstalia yohimbe*. A substantial number of clinical tests on this substance have shown it to be the most powerful sexual stimulant ever discovered. The FDA recently approved its use in a prescription drug. It is sold under the brand-names, Prohim and Yohimex.

Dr. Robert Margolis published an extensive study of over ten thousand impotent patients taking *yohimbe* in the medical journal, *Current Therapeutic Research*. He found that up to 80 percent of the patients reported good to excellent results. Almost 55 percent of the patients were between fifty and eighty years of age.

The tests of those patients were conducted over a period of ten weeks. Although some patients' sexual ability improved significantly within a couple of weeks, others took longer to see the effects. However, the statistics show that the effect grew steadily stronger over the ten weeks.

Dr. Francesco Montorsi, professor of the Urology Department at the University of Milan School of Medicine in Italy, conducted a smaller, double-blind, placebo-controlled study of impotent patients for eight weeks. Their ages ranged from thirty-five to seventy-eight. Almost 71 percent of the patients claimed positive results. Dr. Montorsi said, "Yohimbe is a very effective and safe way to treat impotent men."

Dr. A. J. Riley analyzed all results from the extensive testing of *yohimbe* and concluded, "It is now possible to restore usable erections for up to 95 percent of men with erectile inadequacy. . . . "

Doctors say that most patients using *yohimbe* claimed that overall sexual pleasure increased with more intense orgasms. Some men said they felt warm, pleasant pelvic tingles within an hour after taking it.

One of the clinical studies that Dr. Riley found particularly indicative of the power of *yohimbe* was with castrated rats. Castration stops the desire for sex unless hormone replacement is done. In this study, when the castrated rats were given *yohimbe*, they tried to mate with female rats.

A team of scientists at Stanford University led by Dr. Julian Davidson were amazed by their tests on laboratory rats. Normal rats given *yohimbe* mated as much as forty-five times in fifteen minutes. Impotent rats regained interest in sex and started mating. Scientists have no doubt that *yohimbe* promotes sexual activity in humans as well as in animals.

Technology today allows scientists to follow any drug or nutrient through the body and observe the reactions. After following *yohimbe* through the body, scientists concluded that its most profound effect is in stopping the alpha-2-adrenergic receptors (discussed earlier) from interfering with the erection process.

The clinical tests of *yohimbe* didn't work on 20 to 28 percent of the men taking it—probably because that's all they took. As mentioned earlier, there are three major causes of erectile inadequacy and impotence. *Yohimbe* is effective for only one of those causes. Zinc deficiency, low testosterone levels and high cholesterol must also be corrected for a man to regain optimum sexual performance.

Although some men taking yohimbine, *Smilax,* zinc and orchic tissue feel a significant difference within a couple of weeks, clinically *it takes eight to ten weeks to experience the full effect*. Of course, you'll want to maintain your sexual health, so you should continue taking it as a daily regimen.

In South America, the bark from the *Aspidosperma quebracho*, a hardwood tree in the dogbane family, has a similar reputation. The drug quebracho has an equivalent chemistry to yohimbine, so it should be no surprise that its sexual enhancing properties are nearly identical.

Physicians have learned that the blood flow that causes

the penis to swell is controlled by the release of the enzyme norepinephrine. Yohimbine and quebracho have proven effective as sexual stimulants because they impact the sympathetic nervous system—which regulates norepinephrine flow. The upshot of all these chemical reactions is more frequent erections.

Another extract that has shown some efficacy as an aphrodisiac is the humorously named horny goat weed. Daniel Reid, author of Chinese Herbal Medicine, writes that horny goat weed increases "sperm count and semen density" in men. Tests also show that it enhances blood circulation, particularly in thin capillaries like those found in the penis.

It seems strange to think of animals having sexual performance problems, but veterinarians, ranchers and farmers say that it has always been a common problem—especially as the animals get older. Obviously, the animals are not much different than human men.

One out of four men over the age of fifty is impotent; by the age of sixty-two, the number has grown to almost 50 percent. When men reach retirement age, most of them have erection malfunctions in varying degrees.

As humans, we learn to live with those conditions, but for ranchers and farmers, their animals' inability to have sex lowers their income—a serious situation.

Those that raise cattle, sheep and hogs depend on the mating of the animals to renew their herds as market-ready animals are sold. Until recently, if a male animal was unable to mate, there was nothing that could be done about it.

■ Spanish Fly Is Not a Sexual Stimulant

Earlier in this century, reluctant female animals were given "Spanish fly" to encourage them to mate. Spanish fly is not a sexual stimulant. It causes a terrible itching and burning in the vagina of the animal, prompting a desire for something to be inserted in the vagina to rub the itch.

Although the "fly" often caused the animals to mate, the damage they did to themselves, fences and barns, in their uncontrollable frenzy, clearly made the fly an undesirable stimulant.

No stimulant existed for male animals, and this was a bigger problems than reluctant females. No matter how enticing females in "heat" were, and how much problematic males tried, they could not achieve penetration.

The problem was narrowed down to low testosterone (male hormone) levels in the males. Once they were fully grown, each year the testosterone levels dropped until they could no longer perform.

The same thing happens with men. From the age of thirty-five, a man's testosterone level drops from .5 to as much as 2 percent each year, according to specialist Dr. Anna Grey. Dr. R. Greenblatt said that between the ages of seventy and eighty many men's testosterone levels are similar to those of men who have been castrated.

Several years ago, Bulgarian veterinarians were studying old folk literature in search of a sexual stimulant for aging animals. They found several references to a plant called Devil's Thorn—*Tribulus terrestris,* a shrub that grows at high altitudes up to ten thousand feet.

The veterinarian scientists obtained some of the plants and made an extract to the specifications in the folk literature. They gave the extract from the Devil's Thorn bush to old boars (male hogs) that were either totally impotent or had very low sexual ability.

The boars were put in pens with sows (female hogs) who were in heat. After five days of giving the extract to the boars, the scientists were astounded at what they saw. *All* of the boars were performing like young hogs. Even most of the totally impotent old hogs were taking their share of the young females—71 percent fully regained their sexual ability.

Other farm animals were tested with the Devil's Thorn extract with equal success, so older scientists began thinking, "will it work on men?"

News of this potent potion spread throughout the medical research groups in Bulgaria. Soon tests on men began at two government facilities, the Higher Military Medical Institute and the Medical Academy's Institute of Endocrinology, Gerontology and Geriatrics. The men chosen for the placebo-controlled tests all had sexual problems, such as poor erections, inability to maintain an erection, impotence and more severe sexual problems.

The men were monitored for sixty days, and the results were nothing short of spectacular. There was an average increase in testosterone levels of 114 percent, according to professor E. Bozadjieva, who led one of the government research teams. And *unlike the testosterone injections*, sexual ability and performance climbed by an equivalent percentage.

The subjects' volume of sperm increased a phenomenal 3 million per milliliter on average. The movement of the sperm increased 45 percent above the average, and their speed rose 116 percent. Even more amazing was that the activity of the sperm lasted over thirty minutes longer than normal.

Professor Ivan Viktorov, who led another group, reported the amount of semen ejaculated increased an average of 125 percent, and the test subjects claimed they felt twenty years younger.

If you have any friends or relatives who are trying to have a baby and having trouble, tell them about this. It is not only a sexual stimulant, it is a fertility potion—like no other.

The research groups concluded that the Devil's Thorn extract was the most amazing sexual stimulant ever found, and there were several very beneficial side effects. The test subjects experienced lower cholesterol, improved moods, increased self-confidence, measured 45 percent less fatigue (on average), higher mental alertness and increased muscular strength.

You are probably wondering why, if the Devil's Thorn extract is such a fantastic substance, you haven't you heard about it in the United States until now? Well, there's a very interesting reason that will probably surprise you.

Until recently, most of the small Eastern European countries were behind the iron curtain. Any accomplishment they made technologically was kept within the countries' borders. Their only contact with the free world was through international athletic events. Consequently, the only way to show their national pride was superiority in sports. That gave them bragging rights much like you would have if you lived in Denver as a fan of the Super Bowl champions and met someone from another major city.

So winning a gold, silver or bronze metal in an international sporting event makes a whole country the envy of their neighbors—to a much higher degree than we experience in our sports competition with other cities, states and countries. If fact, it is so important in the Eastern European countries that *the military controls and nurtures their country's athletes with an unlimited government budget!*

Professor Viktorov is the chief doctor for the Higher Military Academy of Bulgaria, which means that he is very much involved with the country's athletes. Shortly after the testing of the Devil's Thorn extract was completed, the government clamped a top secret order on the results.

The Bulgarians excel in weight lifting events in the Olympics and other international contests. Ever since steroids were outlawed in athletic competition, the Bulgarians have been searching for a natural substitute. The Devil's Thorn extract was just the substance they were looking for because it *increased testosterone, which means it also increased muscle strength!*

Apparently the thinking went, *"the hell with farmers, ranchers and men who have sexual problems."* They wanted to win gold medals—and no one was going to know their secret!

Meanwhile, scientists in the Orient, who were quietly investigating a plant extract used for treating people for asthma or chronic bronchitis, found a very unusual side effect. People taking the extract told the researchers that it made them feel very sexy! The extract came from a common house plant, *Epimedium grandiflorum,* generally known as Bishop's Hat because of the shape of its flowers.

A careful investigation of the people taking the extract showed that it did, indeed, increase the sex drive of both men and women, according to Dr. Y. Zhu. Dr. S. M. Yeung reported that *Epimedium* seemed to stimulate sensory nerves, thereby increasing sexual desire.

Dr. H. M. Chang found that it also stimulated the production of testosterone in men, and through some unknown mechanism, it helped alleviate menopausal problems for women. Dr. Chang also found *Epimedium* very useful for those suffering from high blood pressure. It caused blood pressure to drop by almost 30 percent within two hours of taking it.

Scientists in Bulgaria's neighboring country, Hungary, were working on another sexual problem. Men who take antidepressants, which affect the production of serotonin in the brain, often lose interest in sex or cannot raise a sufficient erection to perform—regardless of their age. Occasionally, even without taking antidepressants, some men develop the same problem due to a malfunction in brain chemistry. This usually happens to men over the age of fifty.

Dr. T. T. Yen at the Semmelweis University Medical School in Budapest, Hungary, found an ingredient in the root of the houseplant *Policias fruticosum* that not only corrects the problem, but does something quite extraordinary. For decades, scientists tried to find something that would stimulate the part of the brain that controls sexual behavior. Dr. Yen finally found it.

Dr. Yen gave the root extract to male animals that were at the age where most of them have very little interest in sex because they lack the ability to get an erection or ejaculate.

Within three months of taking the *Policias* extract, the number of animals that could get erections and ejaculate jumped a whopping 657 percent! These old animals acted like they were young again—a fantastic discovery.

In the meantime, men who were privy to the "top secret" Devil's Thorn research were using the extract to regain their youthful sex drives. Wives talk, and the men probably had trouble containing their enthusiasm from their new-found rejuvenator. However it happened, the secret eventually leaked beyond the borders of the country.

Bulgarian weight lifters and athletes were scoring impressively in international events, and eventually people started to wonder why. With the iron curtain gone it was hard to keep the secret for very long. Soon bodybuilders, scientists and men looking for sexual rejuvenation began visiting Bulgaria by the hundreds. The military leaders, realizing they no longer had a secret, decided to capitalize on the Devil's Thorn formula by selling it on a royalty basis to pharmaceutical companies.

■ Sometimes Women Need a Sexual Stimulant, Too!

As you may know, after menopause your body can play a lot of tricks on you. These include a loss of sexual interest and desire, loss of sensation and lack of lubrication. Obviously, the inability or desire to respond honestly to sexual overtures from one's mate can erode one's relationship as well as eliminate one of life's greatest pleasures.

Throughout history most of the search for sexual stimulants for women has been for the benefit of men. Men have looked for the magic substance that would make women fall to their knees begging for sex. Older men have long sought the potion that would give them the virility of a twenty-year-old.

Up until the last few decades, women have been largely forgotten, but thanks to the advancement of science, hormone therapy has made it possible for many women to maintain normal sexual activity after menopause. Unfortunately for some women, therapy doesn't stimulate their sexual desire and sensitivity, but instead brings on undesirable and aggravating side effects along with the threat of cancer.

As far back in history as the Aztec period, women in traditional societies in tropical areas of Central and South America have relied on a plant to correct their hormonal problems. It's quite astounding when you realize that out of thousands of plants they had to choose from, that they were able to single out those with curative powers.

The Aztec women brewed a tea from the leaves of the *Turnera* plant (generally called Damiana), which they drank to alleviate their menopausal problems as well as stimulate their sexual desires. If their daughters had irregular menstrual cycles, the tea also corrected that problem. In rural areas, the practice still goes on today.

Homeopathic scientists discovered this bit of medical

folklore early in this century and found that extracts from the *Turnera* plant actually stimulated the body to produce hormones naturally that regulate and activate the sexual system with no side effects.

As usual, modern mainstream scientists were the last to discover this phenomenom. They are still puzzled by how women of traditional societies knew to choose this plant. Today, thankfully, there are a lot of scientists who know that a person's hormonal balance is very delicate. Aside from menopause, drugs, illnesses or any kind of trauma can upset that balance.

Many female doctors feel that harsh drugs work against the balance of our bodily systems rather than with it, as natural medicines do. Thanks to technology and advanced testing methods, today we can really see that this is true.

Dr. Hiroshi Hikino at Tohoku University Medical Center in Japan recently found that an extract from the flower of the *Angelica sinesis* plant stimulates sexual functions and prevents or fights vaginal infections naturally without any side effects.

Dr. Steven Dentali discovered an ingredient in wild yams called diosgenin, which produces estrogenic effects in postmenopausal women. In other words, diosgenin causes the body to produce female hormones without side effects. Why take hormones when your body can produce its own from certain foods?

Most people think of the hormone testosterone as being strictly a male hormone. Men certainly have a substantial amount, but women also have this hormone, which is produced by the ovaries. In fact, it is responsible for a good portion of a woman's sex drive. However, after menopause the production of this hormone drops considerably.

Dr. Julian Whitaker, a prominent natural medicine scientist and editor of the most popular health newsletter in this country, recently stated, "Testosterone increases the sex drive of both women and men. Women with higher testosterone levels have more sex and orgasms and tighter bonds with their mates. They have a radience of sensuality."

Of course, if women are injected with testosterone, it

could cause facial and body hair to sprout. The safest way to increase it is to stimulate your own body to produce it. Normally, your body won't produce an excess, so there's no danger of causing facial-hair growth.

Dr. Barbara Sherwin, a scientist at the prominent research laboratories of McGill University in Canada, has conducted extensive tests of the effects of testosterone on postmenopausal women. She has concluded that it is absolutely necessary for optimal sexual functioning.

An extract from the *Panax ginseng* plant has been proven to stimulate the production of this hormone in women. *Panax* also helps reduce stress and stimulates better mental functioning.

Another natural plant substance that stimulates women's bodies to produce testosterone is extracted from the licorice plant *Glycyrrhizae radix.* Dr. Robert Bradford, a scientist and the director of the famous Bradford Research Institute, says, "Glycyrrhizae also helps prevent tumors and candida as well as lowering cholesterol."

Note to candy lovers: don't rush out and buy licorice candy. It only has the licorice flavor and none of the testosterone-producing ingredients.

What is available is a product called Damiana that contains extracts from *Angelica sinesis, Panax ginseng, Glycyrrhizae radix* and *Turnera* plants that also includes diosgenin. It is formulated in the proper proportions for the most effective results.

■ Sources of Substances Mentioned in this Chapter

The following are readily available in vitamin and health food stores. Ask sales people to show you samples of:

Angelica
Boron
Cholestatin
Damiana
Ginseng
Glycine
Horny Goat Weed

Licorice Extract (not flavoring)
Muira Pauma
Nettles
Pyridoxine (vitamin B_6)
Quebacho
Similix
Yohimbe
Zinc Picolinate

The second product is called Exsativa, and is carried by some health food stores. It only contains nettles and oats.

Horny goat weed, Devil's Thorn (*Tribulus terrestris*), Bishop's Hat (*Epimedium grandiflorum*) and *Policias fruticosum* may be found in herb shops, but a few larger health food stores may carry them.

You may have problems finding orchic tissue and oat extract. Vitamin stores that cater to weight lifters may stock these or can order them for you.

Two vitamin companies have developed *avena sativa* and nettle extracts in pill form. Gero Vita International produces Sexativa, which is available by mail or phone order. In addition to the nettle and oat mixture, Sexativa also contains zinc, glycine and boron. Write to Gero Vita International, Dept. Z101, 2255–B Queen Street East #820, Toronto, Ontario M4E 1G3, Canada, or call 800–825–8482.

There's a product called Testerex that contains *yohimbe*, Muira Puama, cholestatin, *Smilax*, orchic tissue, zinc picolinate and pyridoxine. Write or call S & G Laboratories, 892 E. William St., Dept. Z101, Carson City, NV 89701, (800) 406-1307.

Damiana is a brand name that contains Angelica, ginseng, licorice extract, damiana and diosgenin. Write or call Lifeforce Laboratories, 561 Keystone Ave., Dept. Z101, Reno, NV 89603, (800) 637-8447.

10

■ ■ ■

To Eliminate Fatigue and Increase Energy, Your Body Needs Racing Fuel

As YOU AGE your body becomes less efficient at producing some essential nutrients. Some metabolic processes also slow down. Each year your body tends to work a little bit harder to maintain itself. This natural aging process is a big factor contributing to fatigue.

Famous athletes today have the best scientific help available to assist them in achieving optimal performance. Literally hundreds of tests of various foods and nutrients have been done on athletes to determine what nutritional supplements make for peak performance of mind and body. Now that information is also available to you.

It is generally agreed that the B vitamins are helpful for stress. Two B vitamins are specifically for enhancing energy. The first is pantothenic acid, also known as B_5. In a recent double-blind study reported by Dr. D. Litoff in *Medicine and Science in Sports and Exercise*, well-trained distance runners were given pantothenic acid daily for two weeks. These athletes outperformed the athletes who received placebos. The runners who took the pantothenic acid used 8 percent less oxygen and had nearly 17 percent less lactic acid buildup than the placebo group—quite a significant difference.

The other important B vitamin is para-aminobenzoic acid (PABA), which is essential to the body for the breakdown and utilization of proteins and in the formation of blood cells. Dr. Robert Atkins, author of *Dr. Atkin's Superenergy Diet*, recommends para-aminobenzoic acid for alleviating fatigue and achieving optimal energy.

The two minerals that make a difference in energy levels are magnesium and potassium. Magnesium and potassium are involved in just about every major biologic process, including the production of nucleic acids and protein, the metabolism of glucose and the release of cellular energy. They are also necessary for muscle contraction, nerve conduction, the beating of the heart and regulation of vascular tone.

Deficiency of one or both of these important minerals can lead to high susceptibility to fatigue. In a study of individuals diagnosed with chronic fatigue syndrome (CFS)—sometimes called the "Yuppie Flu" or Epstein-Barr—it was found that all participants diagnosed with CFS had abnormally low levels of magnesium in their blood. In the double-blind study, those who received magnesium sulfate injections responded with increased energy, decreased pain and improved emotional states compared to those who received the placebo.

Other studies in Sweden on well-conditioned athletes found that when the athletes took potassium-magnesium aspartate prior to an exercise stress test they showed an astounding 50 percent increase in their endurance.

With thousands of new cases of CFS appearing each month, medical researchers have been investigating the cause of this mysterious disease which can leave its victims debilitated by fatigue for months or years. The prevailing theory at this time is that CFS is related to an imbalance in the immune system and that less severe cases of fatigue can also be related to immune weakness.

Studies have shown that CFS weakens the immune

response of a type of lymphocyte (white blood cell) called a natural killer cell, but have also found that alkylglycerols found in shark-liver oil boost the production of these white cells.

Another substance, N,N-Dimethlyglcine (DMG), based on the amino acid glycine, is also a powerful energy-builder and immune enhancer. Several Japanese medical studies have shown that a protein-rich substance found in some algae, phycotene (phycocyanin), assists in the replacement of leukocytes—essential to proper immune functioning.

Another powerful immune stimulator is Echinacea. Echinacea was one of the most popular medicinal plants in the United States in the 1800s, and it has recently attracted renewed interest. Commonly known as coneflower, Echinacea has natural antiviral properties and is also helpful in combating bacterial and fungal infections.

From the natural cornucopia of the Brazilian rain forest comes Suma, an herb that makes us energetic and helps the body adjust to stress. Suma has been reported by Dr. Paul Lee, director of the American College of the Healing Arts, to combat fatigue, prevent colds and flu, speed healing, regulate blood sugar and stimulate the sex drive. Dr. Michael Tierra, author of *The Way of Herbs*, reports that his most consistent use of Suma has been in the treatment of chronic fatigue and low-energy conditions.

Suma contains substantial vitamin A, C and germanium—a known immune enhancer. It is also rich in two plant hormones, sitosterol and stigmasterol, which prevent cholesterol absorption and improve blood circulation. Studies have shown Suma to increase both energy and strength while at the same time triggering the body to find its own unique state of balance.

Yet another powerful energy-enhancing plant makes its home in the Brazilian rain forest. This one is *Paullina cupana*—known as guarana by the natives. Used by the Brazilians for hundreds of years, the herb, served in tea form, was introduced to European explorers who brought it back to their homelands. Today it is consumed in liquid form to combat fatigue, increase alertness and decrease hunger.

Although *Paullina cupana* does contain caffeine and tannin, it has several other active ingredients. According to Dr. L. Grieve: "It is a gentle excitant, useful for the relief of fatigue or exertion." Most users report experiencing increased energy and decreased fatigue without the typical "letdown" of other stimulants.

Adenosine triphosphate (ATP) stores energy in the body's cells, and its production is stimulated by allantoin. When ATP levels are low you feel sluggish and tired. Many people do not have sufficient allantoin in their diets for efficient ATP production, partially due to the eating of refined grains, which lose allantoin during processing.

Symphytum, commonly known as comfrey, is a rich source of allantoin as well as vitamins A and C, potassium, magnesium, phosphorous, iron, sulfur, copper, zinc, eighteen amino acids and protein.

■ RNA Makes People Look Fifteen Years Younger

Ribonucleic acid (RNA) builds protein in the body. As you age there is an increasing probability of shortages and breakdowns in nucleic acid in your body, leading to errors in RNA and protein synthesis. Dr. Benjamin Frank explained in his book *Nucleic Acid Nutritional Therapy* that dietary nucleic acids are essential for optimal health. He noted that individuals who take RNA supplements on a regular basis appear five to fifteen years younger than their actual age.

Dr. Milton Fried reports many beneficial results for individuals taking RNA supplements: less fatigue upon physical exertion; improved tolerance of extremes in temperature; better near vision; enhanced immunity; and tighter, more radiant skin.

Another supplement, coenzyme Q10 (CoQ10), plays an important catalytic role in the process of cellular energy production. Dr. Peter Mitchel and Dr. Karl Folkers, who discovered its vital role, were awarded the Nobel Prize and the Priestly Medal of Honor, respectively.

Recent studies, including those conducted by researchers at the Institute for BioMedical Research at the University of Texas and at the Methodist Hospital in Indianapolis, have shown that CoQ10 has improved heart-muscle metabolism and is effective in the treatment of congestive heart failure and coronary insufficiency.

It has been found that most people over the age of fifty, and individuals with heart disease, cancer, gum disease or who are obese have low levels of CoQ10. The addition of CoQ10 to their diets has resulted in increased vitality, faster healing, improved immunity, strengthening of the heart and normalization of blood pressure.

■ Sources of Substances Mentioned in this Chapter

The following supplements mentioned above are available from health food or vitamin stores:

B_5
DMG
Echinacea
Panothenic acid
Para-aminobenzoic acid (PABA)
Paullina cupana (guarana)
Potassium-magnesium aspartate
RNA supplements
Shark-liver oil
Suma
Symphytum (comfrey)

11

■ ■ ■

Skin Care Takes a
Giant Leap Forward

WE'LL ALL HAVE problems with our skin at some point or
another. We may not remember the diaper rash of our cradle
years, but few of us can forget acne, which many of us suffered to at least some degree in our teen years. And those of
us who are not already experiencing the mid-adult years can
look forward to age spots, wrinkles and permanent bags or
circles under our eyes as our skin begins to show the weari-
ness of age.

The skin of an average-sized adult would cover about
twenty square feet if laid out flat, writes Dr. D. Chapman in
The Biochemical Journal. Our skin is, as a matter of fact, the
largest organ of our bodies. It is a complex organ with three
primary functions: regulating body temperature, protecting
us and acting as a tactile organ (i.e., giving us our sense of
touch). Each of these layers of skin is susceptible to disease
and photo-aging (sun damage), wrinkling, yellowing and
mottling or splotching.

Beauty may be only as deep as this thin organ, but many
of us are concerned about its health and appearance. Fortunately, relief is available from several little-known products

for such problems as acne, scars, painful or itchy skin diseases, varicose veins and especially our inevitable wrinkles. Some of these wrinkle-fighting health products offer additional antiaging benefits, which include help for the fight against gray or thinning hair, brittle nails and age spots. Others can help reduce cellulite or scars, as well!

Wrinkles and other signs of aging skin can be caused or enhanced by several culprits. Stress, a lack of sleep or exercise, illness, smoking, poor nutrition and pollution are some of these, but one of the worst premature skin-aging villains is the sun, according to Dr. Allen Lassus, a researcher in the Department of Dermatology at University Central Hospital in Helsinki, Finland.

Dr. Attila Dahlgren was a child prodigy who received his medical degree at the young age of twenty-five. Working with his associate Manuel Haipern, a heart and aging specialist from the University of Lisbon, Doctor Dahlgren studied the damaged, wrinkled skin of patients aged twenty through eighty. He discovered that ultraviolet (UV) radiation from the sun often causes heliodermatitis, a low-grade inflammation in the lower two layers of skin. If we continually expose ourselves to UV rays, Doctor Dahigren explained, the heliodermatitis becomes chronic.

Chronic heliodermatitis congests the skin's capillaries. Since capillaries feed nutrients from the blood to the skin's membranes, congested capillaries equal starved skin. Protein fibers that hold the skin together, keeping it smooth and healthy, break down when the skin becomes malnourished. This fiber breakdown, in turn, causes the skin to lose its ability to retain moisture. The visible result is that the drier the skin gets, the deeper its creases become. We all reach that day when our laugh lines show even when we're not laughing. Many of us consider face-lifts at this time. But there are several simpler ways to ease creases and other signs of aging than facing the pain and expense of plastic surgery.

Your dentist has one key to unlock youth's door: procaine, also known as Novocain. The positive results of procaine on such aging signs as wrinkling, hair loss, graying and hardened tissues have been well documented. Between 1930 and 1951, in fact, more than 165 studies were published revealing procaine's benefits in the fight to combat aging, according to an article in *Anti-Aging News*.

The components of procaine are available in a chemical-free antiaging skin cream called Gero Vita GH3 Mature Skin Revitalizer. In the periodical *Cosmetics & Toiletries*, Dr. J. A. Hayward states that the famed Geriatric Institute of Romania used a similar cream as its primary form of treatment for wrinkles. Since treatments could cost $10,000 a week or more, the institute catered only to those who could afford it, including celebrities such as Elizabeth Taylor, Kirk Douglas, Aristotle Onassis, Marlene Dietrich and Cary Grant.

Procaine is created in the laboratory by bonding two vitamin nutrients with gigantic names: para-aminobenzoic acid (PABA) and diethylaminoethanol (DEAE). According to Dr. D. Chapman in *The Biochemical Journal*, when procaine is taken into the human body, it is broken down into PABA and DEAE as well as an additional nutrient by-product, dimethylaminoethanol (DMAE).

DEAE and DMAE enhance tissue circulation and stimulate the production of phosphatidylcholine, one of the building blocks of cellular membranes. Dr. Chapman states that "cellular membrane degradation" is one of the primary causes of aging. PABA is a B vitamin that helps form metabolizing proteins and healthy blood cells. It also works as an aid to keep hair, glands and intestines in optimum condition.

Mature Skin Revitalizer cream mixes PABA, DEAE and DMAE with liposomes—tiny spheres made from various lipids, explains Dr. Ronald DiSalvo, research director for Paul Mitchell Cosmetics and one of the developers of the cream. (Lipids are organic substances that store reserve energy in the body.) "When applied topically, these liposomes are able to penetrate and reach aging skin tissue," DiSalvo says.

In order to minimize contamination, Gero Vita GH3 Mature Skin Revitalizer is not sold in jars; rather, it is distributed in bottles with special noncontaminating applicators. The reason for this is simple: creams can lose their potency when they come in contact with dirt, oils and emollients from fingers. Mature Skin Revitalizer's noncontaminating applicator ensures that remaining cream is never touched when a dose is applied to the skin. This maintains the cream's potency.

- An Antiaging Cream That Fades Scars

Another nonprescription cream can help heal sun-damaged skin, fade age spots and other blemishes and diminish small wrinkles; and in addition to such antiaging qualities, it helps fade scars as well! Skin Secrets Glycolic Renewal is the name of the cream. Its active ingredient is a natural derivative of sugarcane: glycolic acid.

Dr. James Leyden, a professor of dermatology at the University of Pennsylvania, tested forty people with creams containing glycolic acid. "We saw improvements in all of the test subjects," he attested. "The thin wrinkles disappeared and their skin was smoother and fresher looking."

Glycolic acid has properties that help to slough away dead cells from the skin's surface. This gives new cells a chance to emerge and show themselves off in the form of smoother, younger-looking skin. The application of creams containing glycolic acid will generally bring about noticeable skin improvements within three to seven days. Daily use of such products over a period of six to twelve months can mean dramatic improvements—diminishing deep skin creases and virtually eliminating fine lines.

Susan Akin—Miss America of 1986—testified glowingly about the effects of Skin Secrets Glycolic Renewal. Akin suffered multiple cuts on her face in a car accident in 1987. Additionally, Akin's nose was "slashed and smashed sideways," she told reporters. "The tip of my nose was actually touching my left cheek," she continued. "I was rushed to a hospital [for] extensive facial surgery."

After Akin's injuries had healed, scars remained on her nose and under her eyes. Akin had resigned herself to living with the scars permanently until she read an article about the glycolic product. For the first seven days after receiving her supply of the cream, Akin says, she used it twice daily, as recommended by the company. She began using it three times a day after seven days, however, because the improvement to her face was so dramatic. She said her scars faded completely within thirty days.

- ## Fountain of Youth Found in Fish

Wrinkles, as we stated earlier, are caused or enhanced by sun damage. Similarly, as hair and nails use many of the same nutrients as skin, many women with sun-damaged skin also have fragile nails and hair.

Imedeen is an oral restorative for UV-damaged skin that has also proven effective in combating brittle hair and nails! It is produced by combining nutrients essential for healthy skin with extracts from various marine plants and animals. These deep-sea nutrients include marine-plant proteins and extracts from certain types of fish cartilage and the shells of shrimp and crab.

One protein extracted from marine organisms is NADG (N-acetyl-D-glucosamine). Studies have shown NADG to have a repairing effect on skin. NADG is commonly used by dermatologists for treating dermatitis and other skin rashes, and one form of it has been successfully used to create artificial skin for burn victims.

Research conducted by Dr. R. L. Ruberg has shown that a cofactor in the production of many enzymes necessary for healing damaged skin is zinc gluconate, a special form of zinc. Skin healing can be retarded by even a minor zinc deficiency, Doctor Ruberg's studies have shown. The chapter on prostate disorders explained why the diets of approximately 90 percent of Americans are deficient in zinc. With this in mind, it's no wonder that skin damage can be reversed when zinc supplements are taken!

Calcium is another mineral needed by our skin (as well as our bones, nails, hair and other connective tissues) to maintain its healthiness. Our bodies convert organic silica to a form of calcium readily used by our skin and connective tissues. Silica dioxide is used in Imedeen because it is one of the richest sources of organic silica.

One vital protein for healthy skin is collagen. L-ascorbic

acid is a rare variation of the nutrient ascorbic acid, which, when taken orally, stimulates the production of collagen. One of America's leading dermatologists, Dr. Sheldon Pinnell of the Dermatology Department of Medicine at Duke University Medical Center, published research on l-ascorbic acid's collagen stimulating effects in the *Yale Journal of Biology and Medicine*. NADG, zinc gluconate, silica dioxide and l-ascorbic acid are the essential ingredients in Imedeen.

The aforementioned Dr. Allen Lassus published his research on Imedeen in the *Journal of International Medical Research*. In this journal, Dr. Lassus reports: "Photodamaged skin shows a wide spectrum of structural changes. A conspicuous feature is a huge accumulation of tangled, thickened and strikingly abnormal elastic fibres. This condition, termed 'elastosis' . . . is accompanied by a great loss of collagen. . . . "

Dr. Lassus conducted double-blind, placebo-controlled studies of Imedeen. The study group was divided into subgroups. One of these subgroups consisted of women with moderate to severe solar elastosis who were treated with half a gram of Imedeen daily for ninety days. A similar group of women was treated with placebos. There was a "statistically significant" difference in the nonplacebo group, Dr. Lassus concludes, "an improvement in wrinkles, mottles and dryness was observed.

"All patients with brittle hair and nails showed normalization. Both skin thickness and the elasticity index increased. Imedeen repaired clinical signs of solar elastosis, the effect of treatment usually evident after sixty days. No adverse effects were reported by the patients or observed by the investigators." Additionally, several women in Dr. Lassus's study reported a reduction in cellulite, which is essentially a skin problem.

■ Dermatein: An Improved Version of Imedeen

The essential formula for Imedeen is now incorporated in a pill manufactured in the United States. This pill goes by the trade name Dermatein and is billed by its manufacturer,

Gero Vita Laboratories, as a "significantly improved version of the original beauty from within a pill."

Gero Vita has added to its formula vitamin A, a nutrient important to the healthy metabolism of our outer layer of skin. Vitamin A also functions as an important antioxidant. Another antioxidant addition to this newer formula is Dl-alpha tocopheryl acetate, which stops free radicals. Research has shown that free radicals are the major cause of aging because they kill cells of the organs. As a major organ, our skin is most vulnerable to free radical attacks, which can cause age spots and deepen wrinkles.

The "oral cosmetic" phycogene, also known as proantho-cyandine or PAC, was originally used to treat skin and vein diseases. It was later found to prevent early facial wrinkles! When Dr. Jacques Masquelier of Bordeaux University in France began his PAC studies, he researched the drug's effects on eczema, ulcerated varicose veins and related disorders. Later research prompted Dr. Masquelier to report in two medical journals that PAC, when taken soon enough, can prevent early facial wrinkles.

This is how PAC helps prevent wrinkles: Collagen is the underlying protein of our skin which maintains its texture and elasticity. PAC reacts with damaged collagen to bind its fibers and protect it from such harmful elements as free radicals and collagen-degrading enzymes. In so doing, PAC realigns the collagen fibers into a form that gives skin a smoother, more youthful appearance. In addition to collagen's benefits on wrinkles and skin and vein conditions, the research of Dr. Stewart Brown, a gastroenterologist at the University of Nottingham in England, has shown that PAC helps to prevent stomach ulcers.

Many of us find it difficult emotionally to deal with the cosmetic aspect of skin blemishes. As former Miss America Susan Akin put it, "My self-esteem and self-confidence really suffered [due to facial scars]. People stared at me, and I couldn't handle people feeling sorry for me."

Skin diseases, however, are often more difficult for people to endure than scars or the process of aging. In addition to any emotional trauma, victims of skin disorders must deal with annoyances ranging from itching to mild discomfort to severe pain.

■ New Hope for Shingles Sufferers

Shingles (herpes-zoster) is one such painful skin disease. It effects nerves. Symptoms usually include pain and small skin blisters that form directly over the nerves involved. The nerves most commonly affected are those of the face, ribs, chest and spine. Conventional treatments for shingles include painkillers, tranquilizers, steroids, ultrasound and hot-and-cold packs. Less conventional treatments are acupuncture, chiropractic adjustments, biofeedback and bee propolis. A chiropractor can sometimes stop the disorder if it is diagnosed early enough. But unfortunately, while most remedies bring some relief to shingles symptoms, they don't treat its cause.

A study published recently in the *Journal of the American Academy of Dermatology*, however, documents the seemingly miraculous relief experienced by shingles sufferers who used the salve Zostrix. The active ingredient in Zostrix is the cayenne pepper extract capsaicin. Capsaicin has long been known to improve circulation and relieve intestinal gas when taken internally.

Twelve shingles patients at Case Western University participated in a capsaicin study conducted by Dr. David Bickers. The patients were instructed to apply a salve containing .025 percent capsaicin to their diseased skin five times daily the first week, followed by three times daily for an additional three weeks. At the end of four weeks 25 percent of the patients reported that their pain was completely gone! Another 50 percent gained substantial relief.

Echinacea has been used by people throughout the world and the ages as a virtual cure-all for skin ailments. Several studies have been recorded that document echinacea's benefits when either mixed in an ointment and used topically or when ingested orally. A German study of 4,598 patients documented an echinacea ointment's relief of an incredible array of skin conditions. The study reported an overall success rate of about 85 percent when the ointment was applied to skin areas affected with varicose leg ulcers, eczema (also known as dermatitis), wounds, abscesses, herpes simplex and foliculitis (inflammation of hair follicles).

"Generally the symptoms of pain, irritation, itching, etc., were gone within four days," Dr. David Williams, editor of the *Alternatives* newsletter, reported. "In almost 90 percent of the cases involving wounds, burns, and herpes simplex the associated lesions disappeared within seven days. Significant improvement was seen in 83 percent of the eczema patients and 71 percent of those with leg ulcers."

A study cited in the journal *Planta Medica* documents echinacea's usefulness for stimulation of the immune system's production of interferon. Interferon consists of one or more proteins formed when cells are exposed to viruses. It combats viral infection in the body. The study also concluded that echinacea stimulates production in our bodies of T-lymphocytes (or T-cells) and other white blood cells. (Lymphocytes provide cellular immunity by acting against antigens such as bacterial toxins.)

Echinacea is an effective medicine for treating a wide array of skin conditions associated with toxicity, such as acne, skin eruptions and boils. This is because our lymphatic system will often become overworked when our bodies harbor infection and disease. Echinacea stimulates macrophage activity, which keeps our lymphatic system running at a healthy pace. Macrophages are large cells in our lymph nodes that act like battle submarines: they seek the enemy and filter and destroy bacteria and other foreign particles circulating in our lymph fluid.

What do acne, warts, burns, bedsores (decubitus ulcers) and herpes all have in common? They can all be treated—and benefited—by propolis. Propolis is a brownish, resinous, waxy substance that is collected by bees from the buds of trees and used as beehive cement. It contains high concentrations of flavonoids, which are aromatic compounds that include many common pigments. Some of the flavonoids found in propolis are extremely potent antioxidants.

Propolis has incredible skin-healing properties. Extensive studies on hundreds of patients in Russia have testified as to this beehive cement's antibiotic, bactericidal, anesthetic and regenerative qualities. One Russian study demonstrated that a 30 percent propolis ointment applied to severe skin conditions twice a day brought on better, faster healing than sulfur-based creams or the commonly prescribed antibiotic tetracycline!

In Russian hospitals during the 1960s, the most commonly used topical healing salve was an ointment made of 15 percent propolis in a vegetable fat base. The Russians also use it as a remedy for chronic inflammatory diseases and various kinds of ulcers. These include skin ulcerations of the lower legs, varicose ulcers, ulcerating bedsores and ulcerations brought on by arteriosclerosis.

Bulgarian doctors have reported that propolis, when used to treat burns, demonstrated better, faster skin regeneration than most traditional treatments! Propolis ointment dressings have an added plus: they don't stick to burn wounds, making dressing changes simple, quick and, best of all, painless! Bulgarian scientists are also reporting that a derivative of propolis has been very effective in enhancing the immune systems of laboratory animals.

At Poland's Silesian School of Medicine, studies have shown that yet another propolis derivative protects animals from gamma radiation. Researchers at London's National Heart & Lung Institute have found that propolis combats the potentially fatal TB virus, *tubercle bacilli*! When used topically, propolis can fight acne, warts and at least two herpes viruses: herpes zoster (shingles) and herpes simplex (which causes fever blisters and cold sores).

Propolis can potentially cause allergic reactions. Users should test just a small amount at first. Be aware that topical application of the beehive cement will cause temporary inflammation to the treated area. As with all medications you should first consult a doctor—preferably one who is nutritionally oriented—before taking propolis.

■ Sources of Other Substances Listed in this Chapter

The following may be found in many health food and vitamin stores:

Echinacea ointment (pure Echinacea liquid extract)
Propolis
Vitamin A ointment (retinol cream)

Propolis can be obtained from beekeepers or purchased through a mail-order firm, C. C. Pollen Co., 3627 E. Indian School Rd., Ste. 209, Phoenix, AZ 85018-5126. Their toll-free phone number is (800) 875-0096.

Gero Vita GH3 Mature Skin Revitalizer and Dermatein are available by mail from Gero Vita International, Dept. Z101, 2255-B Queen Street East #820, Toronto, Ontario M4E 1G3, Canada, or call (800) 825-8482.

Skin Secrets Glycolic Renewal's name has been changed to "New Cell Therapy" and is available from L & H Vitamins. Call (800) 221-1152. L & H Vitamins also stocks vitamin A ointment.

Imedeen tablets are produced by Ime-Enterprises of Switzerland. They are available in the United States from Health Fest, 74 20th St., Brooklyn, NY 11001.

Zostrix is produced by the GenDerm Corporation of Northbrook, Illinois, and is also available without prescription at many drugstores.

12

■ ■ ■

New Scientific Ways to Lose Weight and Keep It Off

AT ONE TIME or another just about everybody has wanted to lose some weight. Sometimes the reason for losing weight is personal, like looking good for the upcoming summer bathing-suit season or next month's wedding reception, or just being able to bend over and tie one's own shoes. Sometimes the reason for weight loss is medical: heart problems, high blood pressure, diabetes. But how we love to eat: pizza, hot fudge sundaes, fried chicken, cheesecake, eggs Benedict, duck à l'orange and lasagne.

Of course, we have all heard that the only way we can lose weight and keep it off is to start a strict exercise regimen and to cut calories. And we all know that exercise requires a major time and energy commitment, not to mention the fact that low-calorie diet foods are no fun at all. If only there were some pill or magic formula we could take to get the weight off!

Remember how our mothers would always tell us that breakfast is the most important meal of the day? Well, many people ignore what mom said and try to cut back on the amount of calories they consume each day by skipping breakfast. Guess what? Studies show that mom was right about breakfast!

According to a study of dieters by Vanderbilt University scientist Dr. David G. Schlundt, published in the *American Journal of Clinical Nutrition*, breakfast eaters lost more weight than breakfast skippers. The study noted that contrary to the breakfast skippers' aim of cutting calories, the actual result was that passing up the morning meal induced hunger and encouraged high-calorie snacking later.

Dr. Schlundt determined that "meal skipping may influence adherence to calorie controlled diet by encouraging overeating later in the day or by increasing between meal snacking on foods with poor nutrient density." In other words, if you skip meals you will end up being so hungry that you'll eat a whole lot of fattening junk food.

The human body has a fat-producing trigger mechanism that seems to be left over from the Ice Age. As reported in the publication *Intelli-Scope* in an article titled "Natural Fat-loss," humans developed the ability to store energy in the form of fat in order to survive thirty thousand years ago. This ability came in handy since there were long periods of famine due to scarcity of food during long winters. This stored body fat gave us the warmth and energy we needed to survive. The fat-producing survival mechanism is still part of our genetic makeup, and it is triggered when we skip meals.

"The bottom line," says noted author and life-extension scientist Durk Pearson, "is that, if you want to get rid of body fat, caloric restriction—not eating when you're hungry—is the ultimate unnatural act. Your genes are telling you you're going to die if you do this, and in fact, when people lose weight too fast with any technique, the master control center in their brain will actually alter their metabolism to make it very difficult to lose further fat, because that fat is their Ice Age life insurance policy."

Dr. Schlundt points out that eating breakfast, in addition to minimizing impulsive snacking, seems to provide many benefits that include reducing a person's daily intake of fat, maintaining a more constant blood-sugar level and improving strength and endurance.

Eating breakfast, Dr. Schlundt concludes in his weight-loss study, "may be an important part of a weight reduction program." Further, he recommends that "individuals attempting a weight loss program include a breakfast that is low in fat and high in carbohydrates as part of their weight loss regimen," since eating the morning meal discourages snacking in general and encourages healthier snacks when snacking does occur.

And, as reported in *Intelli-Scope,* about 95 percent of those people who lose weight using the calorie deprivation method gain all of those lost pounds back within a year. Now we know that if we torture ourselves by avoiding meals and cutting calories, our chances at permanent weight loss are poor. It is beginning to seem hopeless, so what can we do to lose weight permanently?

One of the more conventional solutions to the weight-loss dilemma is thyroid supplements, which speed up the activity of the thyroid gland and burn off weight. Unfortunately, thyroid medication must be administered under a doctor's care and is generally given only to obese people with underactive thyroids.

Nonprescription dietary weight-loss supplements fall into two basic categories: appetite suppressants and fat burners. DL-phenylalanine (DLPA) is a natural appetite suppressant and an essential amino acid. DLPA causes the brain to release cholecystokinin (CCK), a hormone that inhibits appetite. CCK has a gradual affect that makes eating seem less important, rather than causing outright rejection of food. The hormone tends to make a person feel full on much smaller amounts of food than they would normally need.

Recently, researchers have come across a brain chemical called galanin. Galanin, it seems, increases the desire to eat fat. "Galanin," says Dr. Sarah Leibowitz of Rockefeller University in New York City, "is the only brain chemical found that directly correlates with fat intake." Its discovery, she states, has important implications for medical problems that revolve around obesity and eating disorders. The finding of and testing for galanin, according to Dr. Leibowitz, may help doctors determine which children will be most susceptible to high-fat diets. Dr. Leibowitz also found a substance that blocks the effects of galanin. Testing has been done and that magic pill to suppress our fat craving may be just a few years away.

Studies have found that medium-chain triglycerides (MCTs) reduce fat deposits by converting them into energy. MCTs change the pattern of fat metabolism so that more fat is burned for energy and much less fat is stored.

"MCTs," says nutritionist Dr. Allan Geliebter, "may have potential for dietary prevention of human obesity." A study of animals given MCT showed that these animals gained less weight and had a lower fat content than the group that was not fed MCT.

The study was conducted at Harvard Medical School's Nutrition/Metabolism Laboratory and headed by Dr. Pei-Ra Ling. "MCT reduces the fat deposition without reducing the whole body protein content," concluded Dr. Ling.

L-carnitine, an amino acid that is essential for fat metabolism, can be used in conjunction with MCT. Studies show that L-carnitine significantly lowers blood-fat levels and is very powerful when taken in combination with MCT.

Chromium picolinate is a mineral that is more than just an effective weight management tool. Studies show that it reduces body fat while building lean muscle. In a Louisiana State University study, women taking chromium picolinate gained 80 percent more lean muscle and had significantly greater increases in measurement of chests, arms and thighs than women taking a placebo. In addition, chromium picolinate provides the added advantages of lowering cholesterol and blood-sugar levels.

DHEA is a naturally occurring steroid hormone produced by your body; however, it can be taken as a diet supplement. It enhances the body's thermogenic process, thereby transforming food into energy and preventing fat from accumulating. A study at Temple University's School of Medicine found that DHEA caused weight loss without a change in appetite. Weight loss occurred because calories were converted to heat rather than to fat.

Dr. Terence T. Yen, a biochemist at Eli Lilly, conducted a

study that showed significant weight loss in obese mice who were fed DHEA. Although our bodies produce DHEA naturally, at about age twenty-five production begins to decline, necessitating DHEA supplementation, which is best done by taking pregnenolone, the producer of DHEA in our bodies. Studies of mice indicate that in addition to the weight-loss benefit there are other reasons to take DHEA. The hormone increased life expectancy and reduced the risk of developing several forms of cancer. Dr. Schwartz reported that DHEA reduced body fat by one-third, prevented atherosclerosis and mitigated diabetes.

Lipase is an enzyme that aids the body in breaking down fats and removing fat from storage. Without a sufficient amount of this enzyme, fat stagnates and accumulates not only in the obvious places, but also in the arteries. The fats in the arteries contribute to cholesterol and arteriosclerosis.

Dr. David Galton at the School of Medicine of Tufts University tested people weighing an average of 230 pounds. He found that every one of them was lacking enzymes in their fatty tissue.

Doctors Berker and Meyers tested a group of older people averaging seventy-seven years of age for blood enzyme levels. The results showed that they had half the amount of enzymes of a normal twenty-five-year-old. Those with arteriosclerosis, high blood pressure and high cholersterol were deficient in the enzyme lipase.

Veterinarians conducted an interesting experiment with hogs. One group of hogs was fed only raw potatoes, and another group only cooked potatoes. The group eating raw potatoes lost weight quickly, but those eating cooked potatoes gained weight. This clearly shows the effect of enzymes on weight, because although potatoes are high in enzyme content, cooking destroys them.

In the past few years, technology has made it possible for scientists finally to understand the mechanism that causes us to gain or lose weight. Basically, our appetites are controlled by the brain.

When you eat carbohydrates, they cause the production of insulin, which allows tryptophan to enter the brain.

Tryptophan stimulates the production of a neurotransmitter called serotonin. Serotonin makes us feel good. This change in mood is so subtle, we are not consciously aware of it. But, apparently the people who are chronically overweight have become subconsciously addicted to the serotonin-stimulated feelings.

Most snack foods are carbohydrates, such as potato chips, pastries and sweets. *The subconscious desire to feel good* causes people to eat more carbohydrates. That same desire causes people to eat more food than necessary, which becomes a habit. The calories in excess of our energy needs are stored as fat. Protein, on the other hand, does not stimulate production of serotonin, and people rarely overindulge in protein-type foods.

■ Serotonin Is an Obesity Control

The notorious Fen Phen and Redux diet drugs, which were taken off the market, worked effectively because they caused an increase in the production of serotonin. Unfortunately, these drugs also had very adverse effects on the heart, lungs and liver. Yet there are safe, natural food supplements that increase serotonin equally as well as or better than those drugs—without dangerous side effects.

With plenty of serotonin in the brain, people don't have much desire for carbohydrates and don't eat as much, so they lose weight. Dr. Richard J. Wurtman, a scientist at M.I.T., reported in the medical journal *Obesity Research* that animals given serotonin-releasing stimulants would not overindulge in carbohydrates when given the choice of carbohydrates and proteins. This proves that *serotonin is the obesity control in our bodies*.

An extract from the plant *Hypericum perforatum* has been used for many years in Europe as an antidepressant. In fact, according to *Prevention* magazine, doctors in Germany prescribe *Hypericum* more often than all the antidepressant drugs combined, such as Prozac and Valium, because there are no significant side effects, and *Hypericum* works better.

Instead of flooding the body with dangerous drugs to increase serotonin, *Hypericum* increases serotonin naturally by inhibiting an enzyme in the brain called monoamine oxidase (MAO). MAO destroys serotonin and norepinephrine (another important brain neurotransmitter related to fat removal). Dr. S. Perovic reported in the medical journal *Drug Research* that *Hypericum* also keeps serotonin active between meals to prevent snacking.

Most people view dieting and losing weight as a very difficult chore that will continue to make them miserable until they stop. *Hypericum* has just the opposite effect due to its antidepressant qualities. You'll feel happy, comfortable and won't have to fight the cravings and hunger pangs.

■ Some Beneficial Side Effects

Dr. E. U. Vorbach conducted a double-blind study where half the people were given a popular antidepressant drug and half were given *Hypericum*. *Hypericum* reduced depression by 56 percent, whereas the drug only reduced it by 45 percent.

There are more advantages in taking *Hypericum* because it strengthens your immune system against several ailments. Dr. H. Thiede reported that *Hypericum* effectively inhibited Herpes type 1 and 2 viruses, type A and B influenza viruses and was useful in ameliorating stomach virus, Epstein-Barr, mononucleosis and Chronic Fatigue Syndrome.

One very big reason cigarette smoking is so addictive is that nicotine stimulates serotonin production. People who try to quit are moody, crave sweets and snack foods and usually gain weight because they are accustomed to feeling better because of the excess serotonin. *Hypericum* can help compensate for the nicotine if you are a smoker wanting to quit and don't want to gain weight.

■ Lack of Exercise Not the Cause

People who live in climate zones where winters are cold often gain weight during the winter. Until recently, it was generally thought that lack of activity and exercise were the reasons for the weight gain.

Now, scientists know that many people in cold climates suffer from mild cases of Seasonal Affective Disorder

(SAD) in the winter. SAD causes a depression of mood, so those effected tend to eat more carbohydrates in a subconscious effort to improve their moods. But unfortunately, they also gain weight.

Dr. B. Martinez reported in the *Journal of Geriatric Neurology* that he was able to reduce the depression of SAD patients by 72 percent with *Hypericum*. Then, of course, they felt better and didn't have a desire for snack foods.

As technology makes it easier for scientists to understand bodily functions, they find the body more complex than anyone believed. For example, for serotonin to be produced by the body, there must be sufficient tryptophan available (which the body manufactures), but tryptophan requires the essential vitamin pyridoxine to be present to round out the metabolism.

Pyridoxine is one of the hardest vitamins to get from food. Therefore, it is not surprising that depressed people and those with nerve problems are deficient in this nutrient. Also, drinkers and women on the pill are usually deficient in pyridoxine because alcohol and the pill flush it out of the body.

Our bodies have two kinds of fat cells: white fat cells (where energy is stored) and brown fat cells that burn the white cells, releasing their energy. The fat-burning process is called thermogenesis, and anything that can increase this natural process makes it possible for us to lose weight without dieting.

The basis for all thermogenic enhancers is the Ephedra herb, an herb that has been used for centuries in the Orient, often in the form of Ma Haung tea, for relief of asthma, nasal congestion and gastric cramps. Clinical studies with obese individuals showed that the Ephedra's effects are enhanced by extended use. Without either dieting or exercising subjects lost an average of one pound a week for twelve weeks.

The National Health Federation recommends Vita Trim, a natural thermogenic dietary supplement that contains Ephedra sinica and Camellia sinsensis. The two herbs suppress appetite as well as increase the rate at which the body burns fat.

Vitamin Research Products (VRP) provides several weight management formulas that contain Ephedra. Thermo "T" is an instant herbal tea, while Thermogenic Enhancer combines Ephedra, niacin and caffeine in a capsule. Another VRP product is ThermaLoss, which blends Ephedra, L-carnitine and taurine, an antioxidant.

Dymetadrine 25 is an over-the-counter drug that is used to treat bronchial spasms, but it is actually pure natural ephedrine, the drug derived from Ephedra.

The fat on your body is created when your liver has an excess of glucose (glycogen). Any starches and sugars (glucose) existing in your body at that time are converted to fat and stored, which you recognize as weight gain.

Recently, scientists found an ingredient called (-) hydroxycitric acid, or simply, (-)HCA, in the rind of the Malabar tamarind fruit that does an amazing trick on the liver-glucose mechanism. (Tamarind, which is technically called *Garcinia cambogia,* has been used as a condiment on food in Thailand for centuries.)

(-)HCA is a godsend for people who want to lose weight. It stops the glucose from being converted to fat, which causes the liver to signal the brain to turn off the appetite. According to Dr. M. F. McCarty in an article in the medical journal *Medical Hypotheses,* several studies have shown that (-)HCA causes food consumption to drop by 10 to 24 percent. The reduction in food intake causes the stored fat to be drawn out of fatty tissue and used to create energy—all without you feeling even the slightest bit of hunger.

Dr. R. M. Rao reported in the medical journal *Nutrition Research* that his tests of (-)HCA on animals showed a 27 percent drop in fat accumulation in a short time. Dr. McCarty says that (-)HCA causes cholesterol to drop along with triglycerides, and there's no loss in lean muscle or any side effects.

People often build tolerances to diet drugs quickly (sometimes in a few days), after which the drug doesn't work. (-)HCA, on the other hand, continues working steadily to lower your weight.

The combination of *Hypericum* and (-)HCA are so powerful at appetite control and fat removal that you are probably wondering if you will have an appetite at all. Actually, it varies considerably from person to person, but most people feel full rather quickly when they eat. Even though you won't have a strong desire for much food, it is important to balance your diet with a full range of nutrients at each meal—and to eat three small meals each day.

During the process of thermogenesis, your body needs another nutrient, inositol hexanicotinate. This is a form of a B vitamin that assists in breaking down the fat into soluble lipids. There's a side advantage to this thermogenesis generator. Dr. Neil Stone, a professor at Northwestern University School of Medicine, found that hexanicotinate reduced LDL (bad cholesterol) by 17 percent while increasing HDL (good cholesterol) by almost 30 percent.

Gaining weight has a cascade effect on your health. As you gain weight, you tend to become less active. Less exercise accelerates weight gain. Overweight people tend to have more ailments. People who live most of their adult lives 10 percent overweight or more shorten their lives by 10 percent.

Numerous scientific studies have shown that being overweight by as little as 5 percent substantially increases your risk of heart and vascular disorders, hypertension and diabetes. *Time* magazine reported approximately three hundred thousand deaths each year where being overweight was a major contributing factor.

■ Sources of Substances Mentioned in this Chapter

The following can be obtained from some health food and vitamin stores.

l-carnitine
Chromium picolinate
CoQ10
D1-phenylalanine (DLPA)

(-)HCA
Hypericum
Inositol hexanicotinate
MCT
Pregnenolone
Pryridoxine

Thyroid supplements are available with a doctor's prescription.

A mail-order source of the foregoing and Thermo T, Thermogenic Enhancer and ThermaLoss is:

Vitamin Research Products (VRP)
3579 Hwy. 50 East
Carson City, NV 89701
(800) 877–2447

Some vitamin shops may carry the enzyme lipase, but usually it will be in a multienzyme formula like Phytozyme. The other enzyme ingredients will help digestion, which is important in weight loss.

Eurothin, a product manufactured by Gero Vita International, contains *Hypericum,* (-)HCA, pyridoxine and inositol hexanicotinate. A multienzyme called Medi-Zyme N and Vita Trim can be purchased by mail or phone-order from:

Gero Vita International
2255 Queen's Street East, #820, Dept. Z101
Toronto, Ontario M4E 1G3, Canada
(800) 825-8482, Ext. Z101

13

New Remedies for Arthritis and Rheumatism

MORE THAN 32 million individuals, approximately 14 percent of the nation's population, suffer from one form or another of arthritis—an inflammatory joint affliction. Sixteen million have been diagnosed with osteoarthritis, a disease of joint cartilage with associated secondary changes in the underlying bone. Some 6.5 million others are diagnosed with rheumatoid arthritis, also known as rheumatism.

Osteoarthritis commonly affects the hip, knee and thumb joints. It is most prevalent in people who are middle-aged or older and results from degeneration of the protective cartilage surrounding the joint through years of use or injury. Eventually the rough, unprotected surfaces of bone painfully rub against each other.

According to the American Rheumatism Foundation, rheumatoid arthritis is most common in the hips, elbow, shoulders, fingers and wrists, and found less often in the knees, sacrum, heels and toes. This type of arthritis destroys the cartilage and tissues in and around the joints. Scar tissue replaces the destroyed tissue, with the space between the joints fusing together in the later stages of the disease. Both types of arthritis can cause extreme pain, due to inflammation of the affected joints.

Rheumatoid arthritis has been related to a dysfunctional immune system. The body's antibodies are in some way deficient and unable to distinguish between invading organisms and healthy cells, and thus attack both. A variety of immunological organisms are typically present in the joint fluid and serum.

The disease is systemic and initially appears with general immune-related symptoms such as fatigue, weakness, poor appetite, low-grade fever and anemia. Unlike osteoarthritis, which generally is found among older people or former athletes, rheumatoid arthritis tends to strike individuals in their thirties and forties and is far more common among women than men. Because it is a systemic condition, rheumatoid arthritis can progress from one joint to many others.

The Arthritis Foundation estimates that Americans spend more than $5 billion per year to ease the pain of their arthritis. The physician's conventional approach to arthritis is the prescription of costly nonsteroidal anti-inflammatory drugs (NSAIDs).

In a recent study by Dr. Kenneth D. Brandt at the Indiana University School of Medicine that was reported in the *New England Journal of Medicine*, it was shown that osteoarthritic patients who took over-the-counter medications did just as well as those who took the expensive, prescribed NSAIDs.

NSAIDs, when used on a continous basis, can be extremely dangerous. Each year twenty-five thousand people suffer from gastrointestinal tract bleeding as a direct result of ingesting prescribed NSAIDs.

The very drugs that are being prescribed for arthritis can in actuality accelerate cartilage destruction. In a recent Norwegian study of osteoarthritic patients taking Indocin, a strong NSAID, it was found that those taking the drug had far more rapid destruction of the hip than the group that was not taking Indocin or any other NSAID.

In a recently published report in the *Journal of the Amer-*

ican Medical Association, physicians based in New York and Boston reported on the severe liver damage caused by Voltaren, one of the NSAIDs most frequently prescribed for arthritis in the United States. Patients developed hepatitis within four to six weeks of taking the medication, and one died from liver damage several weeks after starting on the drug.

Even over-the-counter anti-inflammatories and analgesics (pain relievers) such as Anacin, Bufferin, Bayer (containing aspirin), Advil, Motrin, Nuprin (containing ibuprofen), Tylenol, Datril and Pandol (containing acetaminophen) can have disastrous side effects.

The chemical mechanisms of ibuprofen and acetaminophen are actually the same as those of prescription NSAIDs—they block the action of prostaglandins, chemical messengers involved in the inflammatory process.

Prostaglandins, however, have other, more useful functions in the body—one being to maintain the protective mucosal lining of the stomach. Twenty percent of the twenty million Americans who take large doses of these nonprescription NSAIDs for arthritis develop serious gastric ulcers. Each year ten thousand of these individuals die from hemorrhages. Kidney failure is another alarming potential side effect of NSAIDs, particularly in individuals whose blood flow is diminished by age or other medications.

None of the prescription and over-the-counter medications attempt to alleviate the cause of the problem. Many scientists believe the cause can stem from two sources: an injury or bump to the joint and/or low immune response which allows inflammation to grow unabated.

■ Don't Believe "Your Joints Are Worn Out"

Beware of the doctor who says, "There's nothing more I can do for you except operate."

For many years, mainstream doctors have been telling osteoarthritis patients that their joints *"can't be repaired."* Keep in mind that most doctors are in medicine for the money and joint-replacement surgery is very, very expensive and profitable. So either the doctor is giving you a line to get you to go for joint-replacement surgery, or he or she didn't listen very well in medical school.

All doctors are taught in school that cells in many parts of your body wear out and are replaced daily——right up to the moment you die. Even if you are one hundred years old with one foot in the grave, you are replacing a billion skin cells every day.

All the constituents of your joints—the cells of your cartilage and bones—are being replaced daily. The quicker you stop the inflammation and the drugs, and the more you give the joints the food they need (MSM and collagen II), the faster you'll repair those joints.

Also, joint-replacement surgery is not a piece of cake. It is estimated that over 50 percent of those who have this kind of surgery still have pain and restricted mobility. Many have worse problems than they did before the surgery. Even if you are one of the lucky ones, the new joint will start giving you problems in about four years and have to be replaced in about eight years. The most important thing to consider is that the cause of your joint problems has not been corrected, so other joints in your body will continue to deteriorate.

One of the most prolific substances in your body is collagen. It is the stuff that holds your body together. Your skin is made from collagen. It knits together calcium to form bones. Your blood vessels are lined with it. Tendons, ligaments, cartilage and even the corneas of your eyes are made from collagen.

There are fourteen types of collagen that function in different ways in the body. Type II collagen could be characterized as the glue that holds cartilage together. Cartilage lines your joints.

Rheumatoid arthritis is also known as rheumatism, but throughout this chapter, it will be referred to as R. arthritis. If you have R. arthritis your immune system, in this case the white blood cells that kill bacteria and viruses, start attacking the collagen in your joints. Thus, the essential cartilage that makes your joints move smoothly is being destroyed. Inflammation, pain, swelling and difficult movement are the results. The current arthritis drugs and over-the-counter medications may lessen the pain, but many of them accelerate the destruction of cartilage.

In 1958, Dr. John Prudden was an associate professor of surgery at Columbia University's medical school. In a very roundabout way, Dr. Prudden found a way to stop the immune system from attacking the collagen. He was experimenting with various ointments, trying to find one that would speed the healing of surgical wounds. He found that collagen II, taken from young chicken sternums, would heal wounds almost twice as fast as any other substance.

When Dr. Prudden told his colleagues about his success, one suggested that he try collagen II on a hospital patient suffering from severe skin ulcers caused by psoriasis. Nothing the doctors had tried worked.

The next day, Dr. Prudden met the patient and applied collagen II to his skin ulcers. Within three days, the ulcers started to heal and close up. The doctors at the hospital were astounded, and the word spread. Within the next few months, Dr. Prudden treated sixty patients with wounds that wouldn't heal. Collagen II worked quickly in fifty-nine of the cases.

All of the wounds or ulcers were inflamed. It occurred to the doctor that arthritic joints are inflamed. He thought, Maybe collagen II could help arthritis victims.

Dr. Prudden decided to inject collagen II into the joints of some R. arthritis patients. He was amazed at the results. All of them got worse! At first it didn't make any sense until the doctor started thinking about the problem in depth. If the body is attacking collagen in the cartilage, the immune system must think collagen is a foreign substance. It has its wires crossed.

Then, Dr. Prudden had a brilliant idea. A food or foreign protein entering the body through the stomach is not rejected because the immune system suppresses any response to it. In other words, the first time you eat steak, the immune system recognizes it as food; otherwise, the next time you had steak, you would become violently allergic to it.

Because collagen II is obtained from a chicken, our body considers it food and does not reject it. Dr. Prudden figured that if he gave R. arthritis patients a pill or two of collagen II, the immune system would assume it was food and *signal the white cells to stop attacking collagen II in the joints.*

He arranged for a few R. arthritis patients to take collagen II orally three times a day for a month. Before the month was over, their symptoms began to subside. He was right. *What an amazing breakthrough!*

Dr. Arthur Johnson, a professor at the University of Minnesota's medical school, heard about Dr. Prudden's discovery and set up animal tests to verify Prudden's theory. His tests confirmed it was true.

Dr. S. J. Thompson, a specialist in immunology at Kings College medical school in London conducted clinical tests that showed collagen II could actually block the causes of R. arthritis. This is fabulous news for younger people who suffer the ravages of this awful ailment. Researchers at Harvard medical school led by Dr. Jenny Zhang also tested the amazing concept and came to the same conclusion.

Dr. T. E. Trentham of Harvard put together a group of patients with severe R. arthritis to test collagen II against a placebo in a double-blind setting. Within three months, the majority of the patients taking collagen II showed excellent improvement, with an astounding 14 percent in complete remission (no pain, or other symptoms). Dr. Trentham said that it dramatically reduces inflammation and greatly suppresses the severity of the ailment.

Scientists are still not exactly sure why R. arthritis begins, but Dr. A. Oikarinen says that as we age, the body's production of collagen II drops continually, and certain drugs reduce production even more. Some researchers suspect that aspirin or other drugs may trigger the start of R. arthritis.

Chicken collagen II contains not only collagen but glucosamine sulfate (GS) and chondroitin sulfate (CS). Scientists have separated GS and CS from collagen II and given it to patients with various kinds of arthritis to determine what each one does.

Dr. E. Paroli conducted clinical tests on arthritis patients at the University of Rome Medical Center. He found that CS caused degraded bones in the joints to begin a repair process through its ability to increase absorption of calcium.

Dr. Prudden discovered that CS coats and protects the cartilage by blocking an enzyme called elastase, which destroys collagen. Dr. A. E. Kingston gave animals CS and then tried to cause arthritis with a rare arthritis-causing bacteria. The animals were protected by CS.

The test results for GS were almost identical to those for CS. Dr. J. M. Pujalte reported in the journal *Current Medical Research and Opinion* that GS totally eliminated swelling, and the pain decreased by an average of 80 percent in a three-month treatment period. Other clinical tests showed similar results with walking speed increasing 72 percent. Many patients were symptom-free in six months.

Long before chicken collagen II was identified, the basic therapy for arthritis in Europe was GS and CS, according to comments by Dr. G. Rovetta of the Institute of Rheumatology in the journal *Experimental Clinical Research*.

All types of arthritis are complex, and curing them should be approached from all possible angles. Dr. Harry Diehl found a new cure angle and a possible preventive. While a researcher at the government's National Institute for Health (NIH) in Maryland he was given a research assignment to test arthritis drugs on animals. Earlier, scientists had found a very rare bacteria that caused arthritis in some animals. So he injected the bacteria into some Swiss albino mice to prepare for the drug tests.

Then something remarkable happened. The mice didn't get arthritis! So he injected them again with a much higher dose of the bacteria. Still nothing happened. His supervisors told him to use another species of mice that they knew was susceptible to the bacteria.

Dr. Diehl followed their instructions, but it bothered him that the Swiss mice didn't get the disease. Months later, he convinced his bosses to let him explore why those mice didn't get R. arthritis. After hundreds of tests, Dr. Diehl finally discovered that the Swiss mice made a substance in their bodies called cetyl myristoleate (CMO), which stopped the onset of R. arthritis.

CMO seemed to keep the immune system in control by not letting it attack the collagen in the joints. Also, CMO was a super lubricant which softened the cartilage, making it more pliable and helping joints glide smoothly.

CMO occurs naturally and is a combination of ceytl alcohol, which is found in coconut and palm trees, and myristoleic acid, which is found in tiny amounts in a few vegetables and nuts.

Dr. Diehl was astounded at the results because CMO had an awesome potential for stopping R. arthritis, as well as deterring its onset. He presented his findings to his superiors at NIH with a request for testing on humans or at least baboons, whose bodies are almost identical to humans in function.

However, his request was turned down. Yet the results were sent to various drug companies. Dr. Diehl hoped that at least a drug company would do the tests and offer CMO to the millions of arthritis sufferers who needed it. His hopes were dashed when he learned the drug companies weren't interested because CMO was a natural substance, and they couldn't patent it.

Dr. Diehl retired many years later, and in 1991, he developed osteoarthritis (I'll call it O. arthritis). He had never forgotten the debacle of CMO at NIH. Shortly after his doctor told him he had O. arthritis, he made up a batch of CMO and started taking it.

Within a couple months, he was totally free of any symptoms and started treating friends, who also recovered quickly. Dr. Diehl was determined for scientists worldwide to learn about his amazing discovery, so he submitted his research findings to the *Journal of Pharmaceutical Sciences*, which published them.

As soon as Dr. H. Siemandi, a specialist in arthritis research, read about CMO, he began setting up a double-blind, placebo-controlled clinical test of CMO on humans. The results were amazing. The patients taking CMO showed almost 90 percent improvement in three months. Also, the time between outbreaks of pain increased substantially.

Although CMO and collagen II are really fantastic,

there's another discovery that may be important to use with them in repairing damage to your body.

If you would like to learn how bad our drug company-controlled medical system is, sit down and talk to a veterinarian who treats farm animals (not a city doctor who treats dogs and cats). You'll be surprised to find that most farm vets rarely ever visit a human medical doctor for their own problems. They treat themselves with animal medicine.

There's no health insurance for farm animals, and ranchers and farmers can't afford expensive drugs and surgeries. After all, how much can they afford to spend on a chicken that's worth $2, a sheep that's worth $100, a hog worth $200 or a bull valued at $1,000?

Consequently, vets rarely use drugs or surgery or treat symptoms. Unlike human doctors, they look for the cause and try to eliminate it by natural means. Aside from antibiotics, their medical bag contains mostly natural medicines.

Dr. John Metcalf is a farm vet who became quite well known among racehorse owners because he could correct afflictions of expensive Arabian horses that other vets couldn't. Arabian horses are high-strung but delicate and develop many more ailments than the average horse. Over the years, Dr. Metcalf has treated horses for everything from arthritis to ulcers to infertility.

His favorite medication for many problems is methyl-sulfonyl-methane (MSM). Plants obtain MSM, a form of sulfur, from the soil and pass it on to humans in the foods we eat. Every cell in your body has sulfur in it, and sulfur has literally hundreds of functions in your body. It is like T-bars that hold all your connective tissue together—skin, cartilage, tendons, ligaments and muscle.

Collagen can't be made in the body unless sulfur is present, so this means your joint cartilage can't be repaired without sulfur or MSM. Unfortunately, synthetic fertilizers used today don't contain sulfur, so it isn't replaced in the soil.

What little MSM that is available in vegetables, meat and milk is lost in cooking because heat destroys MSM. Additionally, milk available in most grocery stores is heatpasturized. That means that unless you eat uncooked vegetables, raw meat or fish and drink unpasteurized milk, you probably have a deficiency of sulfur or MSM.

Mineral deficiencies cause problems more quickly than vitamin deficiences, and the problems are more severe. For example, if you fail to get a millionth of an ounce of iodine in your diet daily, your thyroid will enlarge. That's why salt sold today is "ionized." Iodine is added to it because we can't get it from plants or meat. Dr. Metcalf often saw mineral deficiencies as the cause of many problems in animals.

Throughout his life, the vet had been very healthy, rarely suffering from even a cold, but in his late fifties, he began having occasional back pains. At first, he thought it was from bending over too much, but by his sixtieth year, he realized he had spondylitis—a type of R. arthritis concentrated in the spinal area.

Dr. Metcalf was aware of studies by Dr. R. Rizzo, which showed that arthritic cartilage has two-thirds less sulfur than normal. He thought to himself, *I've treated arthritic horses successfully with MSM—why not myself?* After a few months of taking MSM regularly, Dr. Metcalf's back problems had disappeared.

A friend visited with an old Labrador dog that was so stiff and crippled with arthritis it could not get up without help. The vet gave his friend MSM to give the dog in its food because it is odorless and tasteless. Within five weeks, the dog was getting up by himself and walking again.

Dr. R. J. Herschler, a research scientist, learned about the amazing effects of MSM from Dr. Metcalf and began extensive clinical tests on humans. He found it not only relieved all types of arthritis, muscle aches, day- and night-type cramps, but it also suppressed a multitude of other afflictions, from allergies to migraine headaches. MSM is not related to sulfa drugs, so if you are allergic to those drugs, you can use MSM.

■ The Side Benefits of MSM

When Dr. Herschler's research was being conducted on arthritic patients, they reported all sorts of side benefits of

MSM. Some said their skin became softer, smoother and more pliable; nails less brittle; and hair more radiant and healthy.

It seemed that whatever their minor afflictions were, MSM brought relief. The typical ones were constipation, yeast infections, breathing difficulties, migraine headaches, high blood pressure, poor circulation and depression. Many found that MSM relieved ulcer problems better than Tagamet and Zantac. Scientists believe the reason is fairly obvious because every cell in the body needs sulfur to function properly. A deficiency would cause many organ malfunctions.

People with allergies were particularly impressed with MSM. Most allergies are caused by an oversensitive immune system. Clinical tests show that MSM normalizes oversensitivity, allowing the allergy-causing particles to be flushed from the body. People with allergies to certain foods, such as milk, cereal, shrimp and wheat lost their allergic response to those foods.

A double-blind study was conducted on patients given MSM and a placebo after surgery. Those taking MSM healed much faster. That goes to prove the old cliche that a balanced diet is the key to good health. Unfortunately, today it is practically impossible to get enough nutrients out of a balanced diet because of nutrient-depleted soils and nutrient-poor processed foods. Obviously, supplementation with MSM and other nutrients is necessary.

Anyone who has any type of arthritis either is or has been taking over-the-counter or prescription drugs for his or her problem. Well, those drugs may have relieved their pain somewhat, but they created other problems. Not only do those drugs accelerate the destruction of the cartilage, they stop the production of one of the most important healing mechanisms in your body—prostaglandins.

There are two kinds of prostaglandins—good and bad, much like cholesterol. The bad prostaglandins cause inflammation of the joints. Normally, in any other part of the body, inflammation is an important trigger in the healing process. In a damaged joint, however, the inflammation-type prostaglandins interfere with the good guys, the "healing" prostaglandins. Most arthritis drugs stop both prostaglandins, and joint damage worsens.

Scientists have discovered a remarkable substance in the pineapple plant called bromelain. There's not much bromelain in the pineapple fruit; it's concentrated in the stem or stalk. Bromelain serves a fabulous biochemical function that every arthritis sufferer needs. It stops the bad prostaglandins and doesn't affect the good ones. Dr. H. Winter reported clinical tests that show bromelain lowers inflammation by 60 percent in a very short time.

In the journal *Clinical Medicine*, Dr. M. G. Cirelli reported that he had used bromelain extensively for five years, in over seven hundred cases, on all types of arthritis, muscle and back pain, as well as on patients before and after various kinds of surgery. He said arthritic patients quickly regained movement and had much less pain, swelling and inflammation. His surgery patients got out of the hospital 30 to 50 percent quicker than normal.

Dr. A. Cohen told the *Pennsylvania Journal of Medicine* that his tests of bromelain on arthritic patients produced very impressive results with a high majority reporting greatly increased mobility and dramatically reduced swelling of the joints.

To find the extent of bromelain's healing power, Dr. J. L. Blonstein conducted a double-blind, placebo-controlled test of bromelain on 146 Olympic boxers. No matter how good their physical condition, boxers suffer bruises when fighting.

Dr. Blonstein found the seventy-three boxers who were taking bromelain healed over three times faster than those getting the placebos. The bromelain users said their soreness went away almost overnight.

Most arthritis and pain-relieving drugs cause stomach problems, particularly ulcers. Bromelain is well known as a digestive aid, and it also accelerates the healing of ulcers. Dr. G. E. Felton reported in the *Hawaiian Medical Journal* that his clinical tests show many unusual benefits from regular consumption of bromelain. It reduced blood clotting and blood pressure and blocked the development of varicose veins. It increased lung capacity and subdued coughs and bronchitis. Almost 85 percent of those suffering from sinus problems found relief. Dr. Felton says it also helps in weight reduction by accelerating the release of fat from the body.

Many of you have heard that free radicals are one of the major causes of aging because they destroy cells and our bodies' defenses against them diminish as we age. There are various kinds of free radicals in the body. The most common ones are oxygen and peroxide free radicals. In the joints, a different free radical is at work: nitric oxide.

According to Dr. Marion Chan of Rutgers University, nitric oxide radicals create a tremendous amount of damage in the joints—especially where there is inflammation. In fact, Dr. D. R. Blake reported in the British medical journal *Lancet* that his studies indicate that free radicals in the joints may be the trigger that causes R. arthritis.

Fortunately, scientists have found a natural substance that particularly likes to go after nitric oxide radicals. It is called curcumin and is found in the root of the turmeric spice plant. Turmeric is commonly used as a spice in curry-type dishes. Dr. V. K. Shalini says that curcumin is twice as powerful as beta-carotene and vitamin E in stopping nitric oxide free radicals.

To give you an idea how much nitric oxide radicals contribute to arthritic problems, Dr. S. D. Deodhar gave arthritis patients curcumin for thirty days. The curcumin alone reduced swelling by over 25 percent, decreased morning stiffness by 10 percent and increased walking time by 15 percent.

Curcumin has numerous side benefits. It is particularly protective of the liver and is used in Europe and India for treating hepatitis. It also breaks down fats in the liver, helping with weight reduction. Some doctors use it to stop inflammation from asthma and bronchitis. Others find it deters blood clots and suppresses digestive gases from forming following the consumption of gas-causing foods. One of the great benefits of curcumin is that it contains methionine—a very important nutrient.

Dr. Nancy Francis of the federally funded National Institute of Health and Dr. Carl Nathan of Cornell University Medical College reported in the *Journal of Experimental Medicine* that the amino acid arginine also destroys the nitric oxide free radicals.

Arginine is recognized among scientists as a stimulant or precursor of the human growth hormone (HGH). Until we reach the age of about twenty-five years, HGH is primarily responsible for our growth. After that it continues to stimulate the thymus gland which builds our bodies' defenses against disease, according to clinical studies by Dr. J. Barbul published in the *Journal of P. & E. Nutrition*. Dr. Barbul stated, "We believe that supplemental arginine may provide a safe, nontoxic nutritional means of boosting immune response in these patients."

■ Other Promising Arthritis Relievers

Dr. Seymour Ehrenpreis, a pharmacologist at the University of Chicago School of Medicine, found that if given in sufficient quantity (375 milligrams) a common amino acid acts as a fantastic painkiller.

In a double-blind test, this amino acid, dl-phenylalanine (DLPA) was given to arthritic and rheumatic patients as well as those with back pain and migraines. All had previously been treated by conventional methods for two years or more with no appreciable relief. After taking DLPA for only five days, nearly 80 percent were relieved!

Doctors at the famous Royal Infirmary in England (where the queen goes for treatment) duplicated Dr. Ehrenpreis's study with patients who were resistant to drug treatment. The results were similarly spectacular.

Dr. Reuben Balgat, an anesthesiologist at the University of Chicago School of Medicine, was curious as to why DLPA worked. He eventually found that DLPA was causing the brain to increase its production of endorphins, the body's own natural painkillers—absolutely the safest painkillers! Dr. Ehrenpreis found that people with chronic pain have much lower levels of endorphins than healthy folks.

DLPA also has a powerful anti-inflammatory effect on

arthritic patients. Dr. Ehrenpreis tells of a woman who had been suffering from rheumatoid arthritis for eighteen years. The joints in her hands were swollen so badly that her knuckles were not visible. Conventional treatments had not helped her. Within ten days after she began taking DLPA, the swelling greatly subsided, her hands became flexible again and she could hold cooking utensils for the first time in years!

DLPA has been found effective in treating gout and bursitis as well as being an excellent natural antidepressive. The *Journal of Neural Transmission* reported that tests showed 95 percent of depressed patients taking DLPA responded positively (80 percent reached a normal state and 15 percent were significantly improved).

No side effects have been observed with DLPA, and it is not addictive. Also, you don't build up a tolerence as you would with many prescription drugs. In fact, the opposite is true because it still has an effect long after you stop taking it.

Dr. Ehrenpreis treated a man who had a whiplash injury two years before he began treatment. Nothing had been able to stop his pain. He took DLPA for three days. The pain steadily diminished until it totally stopped. The doctor called him six months later and found there had been no reoccurance of the pain.

Another amazing substance, capsicum, has been the subject of over 650 scientific studies of its properties as a painkiller. It has been shown effective in the treatment of all types of pain from headaches to arthritis. This plant extract, when rubbed on the skin area where the pain is felt, penetrates and goes to work on the nerves that transmit pain. A chemical in the nervous system called Substance P is responsible for transmitting the pain that you feel. Capsicum inhibits its production.

A study at Case Western Reserve University Medical Center showed that 80 percent of those treated with capsicum felt relief within two weeks. Apparently it takes a week or two for nerves to deplete their reserves of Substance P. After that period, regular use of capsicum will inhibit production of substance P enough to provide pain relief.

Dr. G. A. Cordell reported in the medical journal *Annals of Pharmacotherapy* that in a double-blind test of 277 patients with severe arthritic-related symptoms, over 70 percent of those treated with capsicum experienced significant pain relief.

Swedish scientists reported in the *Scandanavian Journal of Rheumatology* that capsicum also causes the body to produce its own anti-inflammatory agent. This natural event causes a reduction of inflammation at the source of the pain for those suffering from osteo and rheumatoid arthritis.

In the search for more effective and safe anti-inflammatory agents, the benefits of an extract of the New Zealand shellfish, *Perna canaliculus*, have been proven in two carefully controlled double-blind trials at the Victoria Infirmary and Glascow Hospital in Scotland.

Dr. Sheila Gibson, one of the doctors who conducted the separate clinical tests, stated, "In our experience of treating over 500 patients, *Perna canaliculus* extract has proven to be a very effective preparation for the treatment of osteo and rheumatoid arthritis."

In the medical journal *The Practitioner* Dr. Gibson reported, "We have obtained X-ray evidence of reversal of rheumatoid joint pathology, an effect which has not been previously reported with other substances. It reduces the amount of pain and stiffness, improves the patients' ability to cope with life and apparently enhances general health. The fact that many disabled and crippled patients can return to an active working life speaks for itself!"

Dr. R. A. Couch confirmed Dr. Gibson's findings in clinical trial results published in the *New Zealand Medical Journal*. Dr. Couch concluded that the *Perna canaliculus* extract did have genuine anti-inflammatory effects.

If you have arthritis, you are probably nutritionally depleted as well. Dr. George Moore, head of six arthritis clinics in Southern California and a recognized arthritis expert, notes that the majority of the arthritic patients seen at his clinics are malnourished, exhibiting deficiencies in zinc, B vitamins and vitamin C.

The levels of vitamin C were found to be significantly

decreased in the leucocytes and plasma of rheumatoid arthritis patients in a study reported by Dr. Mullen in *Proceedings of Nutritional Science*. This finding, the study proposed, was probably due to increased degradation and excretion of vitamin C in response to inflammation.

Dr. Linus Pauling, in his book *How to Live Longer and Feel Better*, explains that in diseases like rheumatoid arthritis, substances are released into the blood that interfere with phagocyte mobility. Vitamin C supplements have been found by many investigators to improve the activity of these immune cells.

One of the most dramatic and well-known examples of the power of vitamin C therapy was the case of Norman Cousins, the former editor of the *Saturday Review* and later a prominent medical lecturer, researcher and author of *Anatomy of an Illness, The Healing Heart* and *Head First*.

Cousins successfully overcame a particularly crippling form of arthritis—ankylosing spondylitis—through a combination of high dosage vitamin C infusions and laughter. He checked himself out of the hospital and into a hotel room, where he received high dosage vitamin C intravenously and watched comedy videos. He recounts this experience in the book *Anatomy of an Illness*.

The mineral zinc is essential for the normal functioning of joints. It is no surprise, then, that lower levels of serum zinc are found in rheumatoid arthritics than in nonafflicted individuals. A study by Dr. W. Niedermeier in the *Journal of Chronic Diseases* and a later study by Dr. S. P. Pandey in the *Indian Journal of Medical Research* validate this finding.

A double-blind study conducted by Dr. P. A. Simkin and published in *Lancet* reported significant initial reductions in morning stiffness and joint swelling in those subjects taking zinc supplements. The benefits to the treatment group (given zinc sulfate) continued, which was not the case with the control group.

Another double-blind study by Dr. O. J. Clemmensen of patients with psoriatic arthritis (inflammatory arthritis coupled with the skin disease psoriasis), published in the *British*

Journal of Dermatology, reported similar relief of rheumatoid symptoms with zinc supplementation.

Anemia may be one of the symptoms of rheumatoid arthritis. Dr. W. Niedermeir reported in the *Journal of Chronic Disease* that patients with rheumatoid arthritis had significantly reduced levels of iron in their blood serum compared to those without the disease. A recent study in the *Scandinavian Journal of Rheumatology* by Dr. M. Hansen notes the positive results achieved in patients with rheumatoid arthritis who received iron supplements.

■ Dangers of Cortisone and Prednisone

Perhaps you've wondered why your doctor says he or she can only give these drugs to you for a short time. Cortisone and Prednisone are usually only given to patients who won't respond to any other treatment for pain, and there's a very good reason.

Both of these drugs cause the production of cortisol, which scientists often refer to as the "death hormone." The main reason is that cortisol severely depresses your immune system. With a depressed immune system, you are vulnerable to all kinds of bacteria, viruses and other disease-causing agents. Also, cortisol thins your bones, causing osteoporosis, high blood pressure, diabetes and mental problems—just to name a few of the dangerous side effects.

■ How Soon to Expect Results

While the treatments discussed above are effective, be aware that it takes time to reduce the inflammation and rebuild damaged tissue. You are not going to be totally pain-free until the tissue is rebuilt. Obviously, everyone's situation is different. That is, individuals suffer from different degrees of damage, and show a wide range of general health, diet, exercise and age. The older you are, the slower the rebuilding process.

Some people begin noticing the effects within a week or two, but most people start seeing definitive results in about six weeks, and then the progress is steady. You must remember that the damage to your joints didn't happen overnight, and the repair won't happen overnight either.

All the clinical tests show that for best results, you should continue treatment for a minimum of three months. If you are not in total remission (symptom-free) in three months, continue taking it until you are. Then you should lower the dosage to deter the ailment from coming back because it was probably caused due to lack of nutrients in your diet.

You may continue taking pain medications during the first month of treatment; however, after that point, try to wean yourself by cutting back for the next two weeks. Then take it only when absolutely necessary because the drug will hinder your progress due to the damage it causes to cartilage and the prostaglandin system. Some people don't need any pain medication after two or three weeks. Most people find that the pain frequency and intensity declines steadily for about six weeks.

■ Sources of Supplements Mentioned in this Chapter

The following supplements mentioned in this chapter are available from health food or vitamin stores:

    bromelain
    vitamin C
    capsaicin (cayenne)
    cetyl myristoleate (CMO)
    curcumin
    Dl-phenylalanine (DLPA)
    iron
    l-arginine
    Lipase (enzyme to help digestion of CMO and
        curcumin)
    methyl-sulfonyl-methane (MSM)
    pantothenic acid

Chicken collagen II is more difficult but not impossible to find in health food stores. Some stores will have bovine collagen II, which is about 80 percent as effective as the chicken collagen. A good mail-order source is:

The Vitamin Shoppe
4700 Westside Avenue
North Bergen, NJ 07047
(800) 223-1216

Gero Vita International makes a product called Arthro 7 that contains the proper amounts of each of the following: chicken collagen type II, which contains naturally occurring glucosamine sulfate (GS) and chondroitin sulfate (CS); methyl-sulfonyl-methane (MSM); cetyl myristoleate (CMO); bromelain; curcumin; vitamin C; and lipase.

Gero Vita International, Dept. Z101
2255–B Queen Street East #820
Toronto, Ontario M4E 1G3, Canada
(800) 825-8482

14

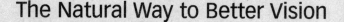

The Natural Way to Better Vision

OUR EYES ARE our windows to the world. Yet nearly 143 million Americans suffer from vision problems that affect their view of the world. Unfortunately, many of these individuals are unaware of the array of natural substances that can help them maintain healthy eyes and good vision.

Numerous medical research studies confirm what many have believed for a long time—that nutrients are effective in treating a wide variety of eye difficulties ranging from fatigue to night blindness to cataracts. The scientific community is just now recognizing that many natural substances have legitimate medicinal applications for treating eye problems.

For hundreds of years, the bilberry plant (*Vaccinium myrtillus*), which grows wild in Northern Europe and Asia, has been used to make fresh jam. But it wasn't until World War II that the jam was discovered to have medicinal purposes. British Royal Air Force pilots found that when they ate bilberry jam before flying a mission, their night vision and visual acuity improved.

Since World War II, doctors and scientists all over the world have demonstrated the effectiveness of the bilberry fruit for treating a variety of visual problems. More than fifty scientific studies have been published confirming the value of the bilberry.

Anyone who suffers from eye strain or scratchy, blurry, fatigued eyes can benefit from the healing effects of the bilberry plant. In Europe, bilberry anthocyanosides are the main ingredient in many over-the-counter treatments for eye problems.

The extract can help soothe tired eyes, which are problematic for many of those who read a lot, work at computers for long periods of time, drive long distances at night or have difficulty adjusting to dim or bright light.

The modern theory of vision is that how well you see and the ability of your eyes to adapt in dim light is directly related to the amount of rhodopsin (visual purple) in the retinal rods of your eyes. Dr. J. P. Baillart reported in the medical research journal *Le Medicine de Reserve* that one's store of rhodopsin is depleted when one strains his or her eyes or when the eyes have to adjust to the dark.

As you age, your supply of rhodopsin steadily decreases, resulting in poor vision. Anthocyanoside, the active ingredient in the bilberry fruit, has been found to *stimulate* the production of rhodopsin in the eye. In experiments with monkeys, Dr. R. Alfieri determined that the bilberry extract accelerated the replenishment of rhodopsin and increased the speed at which the eye adapts to dark.

Dr. M. Ala El Din Barradah at the Ophthalmology Department of the University of Cairo substantiated the earlier findings of Baillart and Alfieri. Dr. Ala El Din Barradah's own research showed that bilberry extract could stop the development of nearsightedness and even reduce severe nearsightedness. According to a published report in the Bulletin of the Ophthalmological Society of Egypt, in only ten days, anthocyanoside improved visual acuity and night blindness in 100 percent of the severely nearsighted patients studied.

Other scientific studies have yielded similar results. A team of French scientists headed by Dr. G. E. Jayle found that bilberry extract improved visual acuity and improved vision during prolonged exposure to light. The study also concluded that human subjects also experienced some improvement of vision in low light.

In addition, bilberry provides relief for tired eyes, according to Dr. E. Gil Del Rio in a study published in a French ophthalmological journal *Gazzette Med De France*.

In a series of scientific studies published in *Biology and Biochemical Pharmacology*, Dr. C. Cluzel reported that the bilberry extract improved retinal functioning. As stated in the book *Guaranteed Potency Herbs: Next Generation Herbal Medicine*, "Bilberry anthocyanosides have a favorable affect on the operation of crucial enzymes in the retinal cellular metabolism and function. . . . "

This amazing extract also tested positively for preventing the eye diseases associated with hypertension and diabetic-induced glaucoma, according to a study by Dr. B. Bever documented in the *Journal of Crude Drug Research*.

The results of clinical research reported by Dr. G. Zavarisse indicate that the bilberry ingredient also reduces sensitivity to light or day blindness. In addition, Dr. Zavarisse noted that no side effects to the bilberry treatment were experienced.

When taken orally, bilberry extract is completely non-toxic. Several other scientific trials uncovered corroborating evidence that the anthocyanocides provide relief for eye conditions without side effects, and that the effect of the herb gradually wears off over time. For medicinal substances, these are generally believed to be favorable attributes.

The *New England Journal of Medicine* reported startling evidence of a correlation between heavy aspirin consumption and macular degeneration (breaks in the blood vessels of the retina that can eventually lead to blindness).

Research indicates that bilberry and other nutrients, such as vitamin C, selenium and zinc can reduce clotting as well as aspirin can, without the risk of hemorrhaging that can lead to a loss of vision. Bilberry is one of the few treatments found effective in fighting this degenerative disease.

Adding to the value of the bilberry, Dr. G. Demure published the results of a study in the European medical journal *Medicine Clermont*, which demonstrated that the bilberry is more productive than other flavonoids (collectively known as vitamin P) in fighting the breakdown of the capillary walls.

The bilberry extract has also proven more effective than vitamin P in stimulating the production of rhodopsin (necessary for good vision), according to a study published by Dr. H. Pourrat in the journal *Chemical Therapy*.

Proper dosage is dependent on the individual and the severity of the eye problem. For treating most eye conditions, two to four twenty-five milligram capsules per day are recommended. For temporary or mild eyestrain, one day of treatment should provide appropriate relief. Higher doses have not been found to produce any negative side effects.

However, bilberry alone is not the answer. Studies indicate that there are other nutrients that are also essential for preventing visual disorders and maintaining healthy eyes.

It is estimated that 50 million people worldwide suffer from cataracts. A cataract is buildup of protein on the lens of the eye resulting in blurred vision and sometimes blindness. According to a study by the World Health Association, cataracts cause half the blindness in the world.

Most young people do not develop cataracts because normal eye functioning clears the excess protein from the lens. However, exposure to the sun and dangerous ultraviolet rays can cause protein to build up on the eye and form cataracts over time.

New scientific evidence indicates that antioxidant nutrients, such as carotene, vitamin C and vitamin E, can protect eyes against the damage caused by ultraviolet light. According to Dr. H. Gerster in a report published in the Swiss medical journal *Ernahrungswissenschaft*, "Different animal species have demonstrated a significant protective effect of vitamins C and E against light-induced cataracts. Sugar and steroid cataracts were prevented as well. Epidemiological evidence in humans suggests that persons with comparatively higher intakes or blood concentrations of antioxidant vitamins are at a reduced risk of cataract development."

Nobel Prize winner Dr. Linus Pauling states in his book *How to Live Longer & Feel Better*, that "the importance of ascorbate (vitamin C) for good eye health is suggested by the fact that concentrations of this nutrient in the aqueous humor of the eyes is very high." He adds, "There is much evidence linking low intake of ascorbate to cataract formation. . . . "

Research dating back to 1935 by Dr. Monjukowa found that patients with cataracts had a low level of vitamin C in their blood plasma. He concluded that deficiencies in vitamin C were not the result of the disease, but rather the cause of the cataract formation.

While the symptoms have usually been treated with eyedrops or the like, researchers are finally recognizing the benefits of correcting the root of the problem; that is, giving your body the nutritional supplement it lacks.

In a study conducted by Dr. D. S. Devamanoharan of the Department of Ophthalmology at the University of Maryland, intake of vitamin C (ascorbate) has clearly proven effective in treating cataracts.

Dr. Passwater of the University of Western Ontario, found that daily supplements of 400 IU of vitamin E and 300 IU of vitamin C is a practical treatment for cataracts. The study concluded that a treatment combining both vitamin E and C supplements has an even greater effect on cataract prevention.

A report by Dr. S. B. Varma in the *American Journal of Clinical Nutrition* demonstrated similar findings. Dr. Varma stated: "The cataractogenic effect . . . can be thwarted by nutritional and metabolic antioxidants such as ascorbate, vitamin E and pyruvate. These agents, therefore, may be useful for prophylaxis or therapy against cataracts."

Vitamin E (tocopherol) has also tested effective in preventing cataract formation, according to a report in the *Journal of Nutrition* by Dr. G. Bunce. In a study of pregnant rats, Dr. Bunce found that a diet deficient in vitamin E resulted in cataracts in one-fifth of the newborns. Other scientific findings reported by Dr. W. Ross in the *Journal of Experimental*

Eye Research indicate that vitamin E also delays or reduces the risk of cataracts.

The results of a serum analysis confirmed that a very high percentage of patients with cataracts had low levels of vitamin E and C. In a recent Canadian study, reported in the *American Journal of Nutrition*, Dr. J. Robertson concluded that "consumption of supplementary vitamins C and E may reduce the risk of senile cataracts by about 50 to 70 percent."

These findings have significant implications, considering there are more than one million cataract operations being performed annually in the United States. According to a recent report by the Associated Press, government guidelines are encouraging eye doctors to consider alternatives to surgery. The U.S. government spends $3.4 billion on cataract surgery for Medicare patients each year.

"Have you ever seen a rabbit with glasses?" Believe it or not, the question has more scientific significance than you may have imagined. In a study of rabbits, scientists have uncovered a link between the nutrient beta-carotene from carrots (which is converted to vitamin A in the liver) and good eyesight. Dr. D. M. Geller, of the Department of Ophthalmology at Mount Sinai School of Medicine, found that carotene and vitamin E prevented cataracts in rabbits.

Clinical trials have also uncovered the value of vitamin A in the treatment of an assortment of other eye disorders. Harvard researchers have reported that vitamin A may be the first successful treatment of retinitis pigmentosa (RP). RP is an inherited disease characterized by degeneration of the retinal function. According to the results of a study by Dr. E. L. Berson of the Berman-Gund Laboratory for the Study of Retinal Degenerations at Harvard Medical School, vitamin A therapy will help alleviate the disorder and allow people with RP keep their vision longer.

While this is not a cure, it provides good news for the one-in-four-thousand people who suffer from the disease. However, be advised that researchers warn against self-treatment without the supervision of an eye doctor.

According to the *Textbook of Anatomy and Physiology*, a

deficiency in vitamin A is also linked to night blindness, softening of the cornea and conjunctivitis (pinkeye). Dr. G. Milkie reported at the annual meeting of the American Academy of Optometry that beta-carotene can help prevent blindness as well as corneal lesions. Milkie also commented that lack of zinc oxide deters the eyes ability to adjust in darkness. Dr. K. Seetharam Bhat, an Indian researcher, found that zinc and copper may be associated with the formation of cataracts.

The latest findings about "new" treatments often come from remedies that have been used for centuries. Goldenseal root (Hydrastis canadenis), used by Native American Indians, can significantly reduce inflammation of the eye and treat eye infections. Dr. Gibbs and Dr. Nandkarni confirmed in separate studies that the herbs have potent antibiotic and antiseptic qualities.

An extract from the eyebright plant (*Euphrasia officinalis*), a European plant that grows wild, has been used for two thousand years for treatment of eye infections. In the book *The Scientific Validation of Herbal Medicine*, Dr. Mowrey states: "Most cases involve sore and/or inflamed eyes in which there is considerable stinging and irritation associated with watery-to-thick discharges, or conjunctivitis (pinkeye). The herb may help relieve other symptoms that often accompany inflamed eyes, such as a runny nose, earache and sneezing. Science has been remiss in not investigating this herb."

Researchers have now backed up the treatment with scientific evidence that eyebright alleviates sensitivity to the light and soothes acute and chronic inflammation of the eyes. Eyebright may be used as a topical eyewash or compress. For best results with topical applications, the whole herb should be dried before being used. For relief of conjunctivitis and blepharitis, it should be taken orally.

■ Sources of Substances Mentioned in this Chapter

The following are available in many vitamin and health food stores.

Ascorbate (vitamin C)
Beta-carotene (vitamin A)
Billberry anthocyanosides
Eyebright
Goldenseal root
Tocopherol (vitamin E)

Gero Vita International, a nutrition company, has developed Ocu-Max, an oral daily supplement, which contains many of the substances mentioned in this chapter in addition to other ingredients. The supplement contains tocopherol (vitamin E), carotene (vitamin A), ascorbate (vitamin C), zinc oxide, vanadium, cuberic oxide, selenium, molybenum, eyebright and bilberry extract.

Gero Vita International, Dept. Z101
2255-B Queen Street East #820
Toronto, Ontario M4E 1G3, Canada
(800) 825-8482

BioEnergy Nutrients sells a product guaranteed to contain 25 percent anthocyanosides (bilberry extract).

BioEnergy Nutrients
6395 Gunpark Drive, Ste. A
Boulder, CO 80301-3390
(800) 627-7775

15

■ ■ ■

Heart Disease Is Four Times More Dangerous Today Than in 1900

DISEASES THAT CAUSED death in 1900, such as tuberculosis, enteritis, diarrhea and diptheria, have been practically eliminated thanks to advances in medicine. On the other hand, heart diseases cause over four times more deaths today. Many scientists believe nutrient-depleted soils and heavily processed foods are the major reason.

The heart is the most active muscle in the body, so its nutritional demands are very high. Chronic deficiencies in certain nutrients may cause the heart to get weaker and weaker until one finally succumbs to a heart attack.

Doctors often misdiagnose women with heart disease because they think of it as a "man's disease." To make things worse, women are more likely to delay calling nine-one-one when they have signs of a heart attack because many don't think they are susceptible to heart disease, according Dr. Joann Lindenmayer, assistant professor, Brown University School of Medicine.

Probably more money has been spent on the research of heart problems than on any other affliction, since it is the biggest killer of humans in North America. Of the 1.5 million people who suffer heart attacks each year, *only 23 percent survive!* Now, the combined efforts of hundreds of top scientists from around the world are starting to pay off. However, the answers they have found are *not* more expensive prescription drugs or high-tech surgeries.

Drugs have done very little to alleviate heart conditions. In fact, some drugs, such as calcium channel blockers, even increase the risk of heart attacks by 60 percent according to the American Heart Association.

Many high blood pressure drugs multiply your problems. Usually, the first drug prescribed dilates (expands) the blood vessels, thereby lowering pressure. However, it also causes the pulse rate to speed up, so the doctor prescribes a second drug to slow down the pulse. Often, this drug causes water retention, so the doctor gives you a prescription for a diuretic.

The *British Medical Journal* reported that 9 to 23 percent of men become impotent from these three drugs. Also, women and men get gout, diabetes, headaches, dizziness, depression and higher cholesterol levels as side effects.

The fourth group of drugs usually prescribed by doctors are beta-blockers, which are incredibly powerful. They block the effects of adrenaline on the heart, reduce the heart's output, inhibit some kidney functions, change the blood pressure control center in the brain and alter the sensitivity of nerves that monitor blood pressure.

On the other side of the coin, the side effects from beta-blockers are equally powerful: nausea, sexual dysfunction, drowsiness, dizziness, low blood sugar, loss of appetite, fatigue and depression.

Family members of patients taking these four drugs were interviewed by a group of researchers. Almost 98 percent of the families observed that the patients appeared much healthier *before* the drug treatment. This is a typical case of the treatment being worse than the ailment. Progressive doctors who are familar with the latest research believe that this drug system does more harm than good.

The *British Medical Journal* published a report on an

eight-year study of 117,534 people with high blood pressure. Half were taking hypertension drugs, and the other half were taking placebos. The number of deaths at the end of the eight years was about the same in each group, indicating that the drugs didn't lengthen the patients' lives. Considering the numerous side effects, those taking the drugs were probably more uncomfortable.

The success of heart surgery is even less appealing. The highly touted bypass surgery is a gold mine for doctors, but not for patients. Studies by Harvard Medical School researchers and the government's Office of Technology Assessment concluded that a whopping 85 percent of bypass surgeries were unnecessary.

Seven years after bypass surgery, more than 80 percent of patients are in the same shape they were before the surgery. In addition, 5 percent die during surgery; up to 19 percent have a heart attack, stroke or hemorrhage after surgery; and almost 30 percent have slight brain damage. Another 20 percent suffer severe depression, and many men become impotent.

The popular angioplasty is not much better. Within six months, over 40 percent of patients are back in the same condition.

Angiography, an X ray of the heart and main arteries with dye injected, is often used to determine if a person needs angioplasty. Unfortunately, angiography is inaccurate and overused. Researchers in Boston examined 171 patients who had been recommended for angioplasty following angiographs. They found that only about 50 percent of these patients could benefit from angioplasty. The prestigious *Journal of the American Medical Association* reported that only about 4 percent of the patients given angiographs really needed them.

Doctors rarely question other doctors' procedures publicly, but the editors of the monthly journal of the American College of Cardiologists chastised its members with this question: "Are you doing angioplasty for the money or the patient?"

A significant amount of scientific research has shown

that a multitude of conditions cause problems for the heart and vascular system. Therefore, it is patently unrealistic to think that a single drug or surgical technique is going to correct so many contributing influences. That would be like saying that replacing a spark plug will correct all the problems with your car engine. By studying each individual factor that contributes to heart problems, scientists have found twenty-seven natural substances that one by one help relieve those factors.

■ Breakthrough by Nobel Prize Winner

The most remarkable discovery in treating heart conditions was found by two-time Nobel Prize winner Dr. Linus Pauling. He knew that most animals get the same ailments as humans, with a few exceptions. (A notable exception is clogging of the arteries, which afflicts only a few animal species.)

In a roundabout way, he found out why. While examining the arteries of a young person killed in an accident, he noticed the arteries were beginning to develop arteriosclerosis. Dr. Pauling saw many lesions in the artery walls—small lines where the walls were thinner and weak. Some of the lesions were in the process of being covered with fibrin, a fibrous substance. The body was trying to repair the weakened lesions with fibrin. In other areas of the arteries, cholesterol was collecting in the meshlike fibrin.

Dr. Pauling was astounded and immediately believed that he knew the cause. There's a disease called scurvy that is caused by a deficiency of ascorbic acid (vitamin C). When a person dies of scurvy, the walls of their arteries literally crack open, and the person bleeds to death internally.

The interior artery walls are covered with collagen. The most important nutrient that builds collagen is ascorbic acid. Dr. Pauling's conclusion was that the lesions were being caused by a deficiency of ascorbic acid. His conclusion was logical, but he had yet to prove it.

Hamsters are one of the few animals that get arteriosclerosis (hardening of the arteries). Most animals produce ascorbic acid in their livers—human-sized animals produce about five grams a day. Some animals—hamsters, rabbits, primates (apes and humans) don't. They *must* get ascorbic acid either from the food they eat or from supplements.

Since normal life span of hamsters is only a couple of years, they are ideal for showing the results of experiments in a relatively short time period. So Dr. Pauling obtained fifty hamsters and split them into two groups of twenty-five each. He fed one group a diet lacking ascorbic acid. The second group received a substantial amount of ascorbic acid and lysine.

Lysine is an important nutrient that is so slippery it shares characteristics with liquid Teflon. Dr. Pauling added lysine to the hamsters' diets because he believed it could deter fibrin and cholesterol from adhering to the artery walls.

After one year, Dr. Pauling autopsied all the hamsters. All of those receiving a regular diet had arteriosclerosis. None of the hamsters that were given ascorbic acid and lysine had any sign of the affliction. The arteriosclerosis in hamsters was a result of a deficiency of ascorbic acid and lysine.

Knowing the condition could be avoided by correcting the deficiency of ascorbic acid and lysine, Dr. Pauling wondered if the same formula would reverse the affliction. So he obtained fifty middle-aged hamsters. He terminated twenty-five of them and examined their arteries. All had varying stages of arteriosclerosis. He assumed the other twenty-five had the same problem, so he added ascorbic acid and lysine to their diets.

At the end of a year, Dr. Pauling terminated the remaining hamsters, who were now very elderly, and examined their arteries. To his delight, most of them had no arterial plaque, and the ones that did had very little. Dr. Pauling had succeeded. On January 11, 1994, he was awarded U.S. Patent No. 5,278,189 for his awesome discovery. Several scientists around the world, such as Dr. Fred Bey at the University of Bern in Switzerland, confirmed in laboratory tests that Dr. Pauling was right.

The recommended supplement dosage is high. Start taking one thousand milligrams of ascorbic acid (vitamin C) morning and night. Take one thousand milligrams of lysine in the morning only. Increase the dosage of both by one thousand milligrams a day until you get loose bowels, then reduce the dosage by five hundred milligrams twice a day and maintain that level. Most people can take about three thousand to five thousand milligrams before they get loose bowels. Make sure the vitamin C you choose has flavonoids added to its formula. Vitamin C without flavonoids is only half as effective.

In addition, Dr. M. Yoshioka, a professor at a medical school in Japan, analyzed the blood of two groups of people: one group had high blood pressure and the other group didn't. He found that those with the lowest levels of ascorbic acid had high blood pressure.

Famous nutritional scientist and best-selling author Dr. Richard Passwater says that a deficiency of ascorbic acid deters the liver from converting cholesterol to bile, which could cause up to 30 percent more plaque deposits in the arteries.

■ Clogged Arteries Are Not the Only Heart Problem

Imagine moving your hand six inches up and down every second for an hour. Obviously, your arm would get tired quickly, but that's about the same exertion that your heart experiences every second of your life.

The heart is a highly complex muscle, pump and valve system that must respond quickly with exact precision to supply your bodily needs that vary tremendously from sleeping to climbing stairs and to experiencing stress and fear. Additionally, it must contend with foreign chemicals, such as alcohol, nicotine, sugar and drugs.

On a twenty-four-hour basis, your heart uses more physical energy than any other muscle in your body. Consequently, it demands and must have a variety of nutrients in order to maintain its energy and functional ability.

One of the most important substances that the heart needs, as well as your entire body, is magnesium. Magnesium is involved in over three hundred enzyme actions that affect glucose use, fat and protein production, muscle contractions and many other bodily functions.

Dr. Lloyd Iseri at the cardiology division of the medical school at University of California says that magnesium is nature's own calcium channel blocker. Calcium channel blockers are a new class of prescription drugs that relax artery and heart muscles, reducing their oxygen requirements. However, patients taking these blockers have to be monitored very closely because the drug can cause heart failure.

Many scientists believe the need for calcium channel blockers is the result of a magnesium deficiency. Magnesium naturally regulates the amount of calcium allowed to reach the heart and artery muscles. (The walls of all arteries have a fine layer of muscle behind the collagen.)

Dr. Iseri said that many dying heart patients have symptoms of magnesium deficiency. Clinical tests by Dr. Robert Lewis of heart patients in a Scottish hospital showed that most of the patients had magnesium deficiencies.

Dr. K. A. Chadda reported in the medical journal *Circulation* that animals deprived of magnesium had coronary spasms. French medical professor, Dr. Yves Raysignier reported in the *Journal of the American College of Nutrition* that his animal studies showed a deficiency of magnesium induces heart tissue damage.

Dr. Dan Roden of the Vanderbilt University School of Medicine conducted double-blind, placebo-controlled studies of patients with irregular heartbeats (arrhythmia). He reported in The *American Journal of Cardiology* that magnesium reduced arrhythmias significantly.

Studies at the University of Bordeaux in France showed that the supplementation of magnesium lowered bad cholesterol by 24 percent in only ten weeks. However, diuretics, anticholinergics, and alcohol force magnesium out of your body.

Your body can not metabolize magnesium without pyridoxine. Also, it is necessary for the metabolization of zinc, another important mineral. Women taking birth-control pills are usually deficient in pyridoxine because the pill forces it out of your system.

Another clue that indicates a pyridoxine deficiency is

skin lesions or cracks around the nose or mouth, although this condition doesn't show up in every case. Those that drink alcohol usually have a deficiency of pyridoxine, which worsens the more you drink. Those that experience depression, anxiety and a diminished sex drive, typically have symptoms of a pyridoxine deficiency according to studies by Dr. Pat Bermond at the medical clinic of the University of Reims in France.

Taurine, a protein building block, works hand-in-hand with magnesium in controlling calcium in the heart. Heart tissue contains over one hundred times more taurine than is found in the bloodstream, making it a critical nutrient for the heart. Taurine effects the heart muscle's ability to contract.

Dr. Junichi Azuma at the Osaka University Medical School in Japan found in a rigidly controlled laboratory test that animals fed a taurine-deficient diet developed serious heart problems. Yet, when their diets were supplemented with taurine, the heart condition was reversed. Dr. Azuma tried the same process on humans with heart conditions. In a double-blind, placebo-controlled study, up to 79 percent of those taking taurine significantly improved without any side effects.

Dr. H. Trachtman conducted double-blind, placebo-controlled tests on patients with hypertension. He reported in the *American Journal of Hypertension* that taurine supplementation lowered blood pressure by 24 percent in four to sixteen weeks. Other studies indicate that taurine helps normalize irregular heart beating.

Did you know that your body produces a substance that dissolves blood clots and deters cholesterol from adhering to artery lesions? It's called chondroitin sulfate A (CSA). Unfortunately, when you pass the age of about twenty-five, your body produces less and less of CSA.

Dr. Lester Morrison, a famous scientist and professor at the Institute of Arteriosclerosis Research at Loma Linda University School of Medicine in California did extensive tests on animals with CSA and found that it practically removed arteriosclerosis as a threat and even reversed the condition.

After the successful animal tests, Dr. Morrison put together a group of 120 human patients with chronic heart problems to participate in a test of CSA. In a double-blind, placebo-controlled environment, 60 patients were given CSA for an average of two years, and 60 were given a placebo.

At the end of the test period, those taking CSA had 83 percent less coronary incidents than those getting the placebos. Dr. Morrison said, "Probably a million heart attacks could be avoided every year if heart patients would take CSA daily." Dr. Morrison's work suggests that a deficiency of CSA may be a prime indicator of potential heart problems.

One of the conditions that makes clogged arteries more dangerous is the lack of flexibility of the layer of muscle in the artery walls. That danger is easily addressed because there are several natural substances that help improve the ability of arteries to flex and expand.

For years, scientists have wondered why the Greeks, Italians, Spaniards and Portuguese have fewer heart problems than Northern and Central Europeans. Recently, researchers found one of the reasons. There's a substance called oleuropein in olive tree leaves and, to a lesser extent, in olive oil, that is a vasodilator. In other words, oleuropein helps the arteries flex and expand. The Southern Europeans consume a lot of olives in their diets.

Animal studies at university medical research centers in Spain and Bulgaria found that oleuropein reduces blood pressure from 25 to 50 percent and also stabilizes irregular heartbeats.

An extract from the leaves and bark of the Hawthorn bush (*Crataegus*) has shown a similar effect in animal tests. The Bulgarian Academy of Sciences found that *Crataegus* raises blood flow up to 57 percent within minutes due to dilation of the blood vessels.

Tests on humans who had heart problems were reported by Dr. V. Schmidt in the journal *Phytomedicine*. *Crataegus* was given to 78 patients for fifty-six days. Their capacity for exercise was tested on an ergometer bicycle before and after the supplementation. At the end of the test period, their exercise capacity had increased over 500 percent, and there was a large drop in the average blood pressure. No side effects were observed.

Sometimes, the heart muscles are responsible for high blood pressure. Dr. M. B. Aqel tested an extract from the garlic plant called allicin and found that it relaxes cardiac muscle. Dr. B. Rietz, a scientist at the medical school of the University of Dusseldorf in Germany, found another valuable trait of allicin. In animal tests, it reduced arrhythmias by 88 percent.

The most amazing aspect of allicin is its ability to lower bad cholesterol. Researchers at University of California found that it lowered LDL cholesterol by 42 percent. Dr. Arun Bordia reported in the *American Journal of Clinical Nutrition* that he was able to achieve a 53 percent drop by experimenting with various dosage levels.

Niacin is a well-known nutrient that also helps lower bad LDL cholesterol and raise the good HDL. Niacin is even more effective when combined with chromium, which stops the flush feeling normally associated with niacin. Scientists at Auburn University and government researchers found that they could lower cholesterol by an average of 14 percent with just a tiny amount of niacin and chromium.

A deficiency of chromium is most prevalent in people with clogged arteries when compared with those not suffering that affliction, according to a test by Dr. H. A. Newman that was published in the *Journal of Clinical Chemistry.*

Chromium plays an important part in controlling your blood sugar and the insulin sensitivity of heart tissue. Dr. S. Yoneda at the University Medical School in Japan reported that chromium picolinate also decreases blood viscosity (thins the blood), making it flow easily to all extremities of the body.

Dr. V. M. Dilman reported in the journal *Gerontology* that chromium picolinate increased the life span of rats by an awesome 26 percent. Many scientists believe the reason is that it stimulates the production of one of the most important anti-aging hormones, DHEA. (Note that chromium picolinate and plain chromium aren't equivalent or interchangeable. Plain chromium is not easily absorbed by the body.)

If you are on a low-fat diet, you may not be getting another important heart nutrient, carnitine, which is found mainly in red meat. The primary function of carnitine is to escort fatty acids to the mitochondria (a kind of cellular furnace), where the fat is burned to produce energy. In doing so, it reduces the fat levels in the blood dramatically. Also, *Johns Hopkins Medical Journal* reported that carnitine lowers bad cholesterol and raises the good.

Dr. Carl Pepine of the Division of Cardiology at University of Florida Medical School reported that tests show carnitine increased blood flow in the heart by 60 percent and reduced vascular resistance by 25 percent. Also, he found that carnitine reduces arrhythmias from 58 to almost 90 percent in patients with chronic heart problems. Dr. A. Feller concurred with Dr. Pepine when he reported in the *Journal of Nutrition* that arrhythmias are usually a result of a carnitine deficiency.

Dr. Pepine stated in the journal *Clinical Therapeutics* that supplementation of carnitine reverses heart muscle ailments (cardiomyopathy) in patients who have a carnitine deficiency. In addition, he found that carnitine supplementation of heart patients increased their ability to walk further by 80 percent before discomfort set in.

■ The Heart Attacker—Free Radicals

Free radicals are wild electrons produced during the creation of energy and other biochemical functions in the body. They destroy cells or alter their DNA, causing malformed new cells. Since the heart is always pumping and using energy, a lot of free radicals are produced in and near the heart.

When you are young, your body produces a free radical destroyer or antioxidant called superoxide dismutase (SOD). However, the production of SOD begins to drop when you are about twenty-five years of age and production goes downhill from there. By fifty, you really notice the effects as many of the ailments common with aging begin to show.

Scientists have finally concluded that one of the major causes of afflictions of older people are free radicals. Oral supplementation of antioxidants (free radical destroyers) are a vital necessity. Dr. Richard Cutler, director of the government's anti-aging research department of the National Institute of Health, said, "The amount of antioxidants that you maintain in your body is directly proportional to how long you will live."

The most important antioxidants for maintaining heart health are ascorbic acid, beta-carotene, RRR-tocopheryl (a type of vitamin E), selenium and the flavonoids: Adoxynol or Pycnogenol, EGCG, quercetin and rutin.

Without flavonoids present, vitamin C is mostly oxidized and useless. If you are taking vitamin C without flavonoids, you are wasting your money. In addition to scavenging free radicals, flavonoids also protect the integrity of the capillary walls, reduce blood clots and inhibit the oxidation of LDL cholesterol. LDL must first be oxidized before it can become part of the plaque in the arteries, according to research conducted by Dr. Michael Herzog at the government's National Institute of Public Health.

The flavonoid EGCG, which is found in tea leaves, reduces the body's ability to absorb cholesterol from food according to research done by Dr. T. Chisaka at the Kyoto Pharmaceutical University in Japan.

Dr. Carl Herzog, an American scientist, participated in a study of over twelve thousand elderly men conducted by the public health divisions of seven European countries. This tremendous research project determined that those with a high intake of flavonoids had about 50 percent less risk of heart problems than those with a low intake.

The most powerful flavonoid and antioxidant is a proanthocyanidin that is distributed in this country under the names Adoxynol and Pycnogenol, which is obtained from grape seeds. It is fifty times more powerful than vitamin E and twenty times stronger than vitamin C.

Dr. David White, a researcher at the University of Nottingham in England, addressed a group of scientists at a symposium in Paris shortly after completing tests on the active ingredient in Adoxynol and made the following comment, "It may not reverse arteriosclerosis, but it is one of the best deterrents I've ever seen."

If you have varicose veins or edema (heaviness or swelling of the legs), Adoxynol and ascorbic acid could be very important to you. Varicose veins are actually leaking capillaries (the very fine blood vessels that branch out of the main arteries to deliver nutrients to your body). The capillaries leak because the collagen that forms the blood vessel walls has deteriorated. Ascorbic acid and Adoxynol are the main nutrients used in the body's repair of the capillaries. Edema is caused by the swelling up of the blood in the legs because the pumping action of the veins (which bring oxygen-depleted blood back to the heart) has diminished due to hardening.

Professor Henri Choussat of the medical school at the University of Bordeaux conducted two double-blind studies of people with varicose veins and edema. Within seventy-two hours, the patients taking Adoxynol had increased their capillary resistance to leaking by 140 percent. Within sixty days, those with edema had almost complete relief, and their legs felt invigorated.

Dr. Juan Duarte and medical experts from the National Institute of Public Health of the Netherlands conducted two separate studies on the active ingredients in Adoxynol to see the effect on blood clots. Their conclusion was that those ingredients improved the dilation mechanism of the aorta, thereby reducing blockage clots and the risk of heart problems.

Dr. Richard Passwater studied 17,894 people between the ages of fifty and ninety-eight. He found that those taking RRR-tocopheryl for nine years or more had 90 percent less heart problems than those not taking that nutrient. Dr. Fred Gey found that a deficiency of RRR-tocopheryl was an important risk factor in predicting heart conditions.

Dr. J. A. Manson of the Women's Hospital in Boston studied the diets of 87,245 nurses for eight years. She found that those taking 100 milligrams of RRR-tocopheryl had 36 percent fewer heart problems than those taking much less.

The American Heart Association reported that 100 milligrams is much more than one could get even from the most balanced diet.

Dr. Knut Haeger conducted a double-blind, placebo-controlled experiment with patients who had intermittent claudication (partially blocked arteries in the legs that cause pain in the calf muscle when walking). Half of the patients were given RRR-tocopheryl, and the other half were given placebos. Of those taking RRR-tocopheryl, 82 percent increased their walking distance up to 30 percent without pain, and 88 percent had improved blood flow in the legs.

Dr. Katalin Losonczy, at the government's National Institute on Aging, told USA Today reporters that 10,289 people over the age of sixty-seven were tracked for nine years. Those taking RRR-tocopheryl and ascorbic acid had a 53 percent lower risk of dying from heart problems and a 42 percent lower risk of dying from other ailments.

At the medical research laboratories of University of North Carolina, Dr. Dexter Morris and his research team followed the heart health of 1,899 men who had very high cholesterol. They examined the men's blood beta-carotene levels periodically for thirteen years. Those who maintained high levels had almost one-third less heart problems than those with the lowest levels even though their cholesterol levels stayed about the same.

Dr. Manson also found that those taking 25,000 IU of beta-carotene daily had 22 percent fewer heart problems and strokes than those taking less than 10,000 IU. Dr. Charles Henneken reported that beta-carotene reduces the incidence of heart problems by almost 50 percent in his double-blind, placebo-controlled clinical trial.

Dr. Monika Eichholzer, a scientist at the medical school at the University of Bern, Switzerland, studied the diets and heart health of 2,974 people for twelve years and found those with the lowest intake of beta-carotene had over 150 percent greater risk of heart problems than those with the highest intake.

Several studies have shown that patients with heart problems have very low levels of selenium in their bodies. Many scientists suspect that free radical attacks of delicate heart membranes may be one of the causes of heart conditions. Evidence from numerous clinical trials show that selenium is a key destroyer of free radicals in the heart.

The National Cancer Institute of the United States recently completed a nine-year study in Linxian County in China. This area has the highest death from heart problems and tumors of any place in the world. The average person only lives to the age of forty-five years.

Over thirty-five thousand Linxian residents participated in the study. Half were given selenium, beta-carotene and RRR-tocopheryl. The other half of the residents, a control group, were given placebos. At the conclusion of the study, those receiving the nutrients had 40 percent fewer heart problems and 19 percent less tumors than the control group.

Linxian County has practically no selenium in the soil. In the United States, all the states east of the Mississippi River and in the Pacific Northwest have very little or no selenium in their soil. In other states, commonly used sulfur-based fertilizers prevent plant uptake of selenium. Therefore, we get very little or no selenium from the foods we eat.

Dr. P. Suadicani studied the diets of 3,387 men from the ages of fifty-three to seventy-four and found that those who consumed the least selenium in their diet had a 70 percent higher incident of heart problems than those who ingested the most selenium.

Research scientists at the University of California fed one group of rats a diet deficient in selenium, beta-carotene and RRR-tocopheryl. They took an equal number of rats and fed them a diet rich in those antioxidants. After six weeks, they exposed all the rats to a flood of laboratory-created free radicals. On examining the rats for free radical damage, they found that those on the antioxidant diet had over 50 percent less free radical damage.

■ Most Heart Patients Have Dangerous Homocysteinia

If you leave even one small hole in a dam, the water is going to leak out. The same applies to maintaining heart health. If you don't address every one of the factors thought to cause heart problems, you may still develop problems.

In the past few years, scientists have been studying a phenomenon in the body called hyperhomocysteinia. They have come to realize that it is the culprit that kicks off a cascade of problems for the heart. Homocysteine (HCY) interferes with ascorbic acid's attempt to repair the artery walls by preventing collagen from knitting itself back together. Second, HCY creates occasional blood clots in the heart and arteries that can lead to attacks and strokes. Third, HCY generates enormous amounts of free radicals, which oxidize bad LDL cholesterol, allowing it to adhere to the fibrin and clog the arteries.

The Physicians Health Study, which was conducted by Harvard scientist Dr. Meir Stampfer and published in the prestigious *Journal of the American Medical Association*, concluded that people who have high HCY levels are at thirty times greater risk of heart problems than those with low levels.

As further proof of the danger of HCY, Dr. P. M. Leland injected baboons with HCY. Within three months, they had lesions on the artery walls. Baboons don't normally get arteriosclerosis.

At the government's Human Nutrition Research Center at Tufts University, Dr. Jacob Selhub confirmed that the relationship between high HCY levels and heart problems was consistent and should not be taken lightly. And not just the heart is endangered. Dr. J. B. Ubink found that HCY could contribute to osteoporosis because of its interference with collagen, a fibrous protein that keeps the bone structure strong.

Progressive doctors, who are aware of the extensive research on the HCY phenomena, are now testing patients for HCY levels as part of their annual physical procedures. They are doing this to determine potential heart problems that begin very subtly and advance slowly often for years before a problem is detected. Autopsies of young men killed in Vietnam showed that almost 40 percent had some arterial plaque, though most of them were in their early twenties.

The good news is the very strong evidence that HCY is caused by a deficiency in cobalamin, pyridoxine and folate—three very important nutrients. Since heart problems are very common, researchers believe the deficiencies of those nutrients are widespread.

Dr. Ubink found the reason for folate deficiency. He reported the results of extensive laboratory tests in the *American Journal of Clinical Nutrition*. He said that cooking destroys over 98 percent of the folate in food. Also, Dr. Ubink found that up to 50 percent of pyridoxine is lost in food processing.

The highest concentration of cobalamin is found in red meat. The current trend of not eating much red meat to avoid fat may be counterproductive by creating a cobalamin deficiency. Vegetarians are typically deficient in this nutrient.

Supplementation of folate, cobalamin and pyridoxine have been very successful in reversing HCY. Dr. Lars Brattstrom reported at the Tenth International Congress on Thrombosis that he reversed HCY with those nutrients in controlled studies of heart patients without any side effects.

Dr. Charles Lewis conducted similar studies at the Georgia Heart Clinic for the University of Alabama Medical School with the same results. Scientists in assorted medical research centers in the United States and Europe have confirmed these findings in numerous controlled clinical trials.

One factor that augments the dangers of arterial plaque is calcium. Oxidized cholesterol foam adheres to the porous fibrin. Then, calcium particles collect in the openings of the foam and harden. The fibrin, cholesterol foam and calcium form the body's equivalent of reinforced concrete. That's not an outrageous comparison either, because pathologists say that hardened arteries actually make a cracking sound when cut.

The clogging of the arteries forces the heart to work harder and harder to pump the blood through the narrowed opening until the heart muscles cramp. That's a heart attack.

■ Hot Heart Pills

In Richard Quinn's book, *Left for Dead*, Quinn tells about his experience of having a heart attack, followed by bypass surgery that was supposed "to make me as good as new but didn't." His cardiologist at the time said, "There is nothing more we can do."

Determined not to become a death-by-heart-attack statistic, he followed the advice of a friend and purchased cayenne pepper. He filled several capsules and swallowed them. He reported that the next morning he arose and shoveled four feet of wet snow off his twenty-eight-foot long porch roof.

Thirteen years later, Quinn was still healthy. He studied the medicinal properties of other well-known herbs and began a company called Heart Foods. He started helping people with his inexpensive, safe cayenne capsules. However, the Federal Drug Administration (FDA) began harassing businesses that were selling his products.

Cayenne capsules probably treat cardiovascular disease by acting as a general stimulant and reducing cholesterol buildup. Studies with albino rats show that capsaicin (which gives cayenne pepper its hotness) increases the change of cholesterol to bile acids. Cayenne lowers the blood cholesterol level by binding cholesterol and bile acids in the intestinal tract, which then is excreted. Bile, which aids in digestion, is the bitter yellow, or greenish fluid secreted by the liver and found in the gallbladder.

Cayenne capsules can also aid in the cure of gastric ulcers, depression, chronic fatigue or prostration. The strength of the cayenne pepper is measured in heat units. Taken in gelatin form, cayenne does not burn the mouth. Cayenne-based formulas are sold in health food and vitamin stores.

■ New Findings Question Aspirin

"Taking an aspirin every day to help cut your risk of heart disease is no longer the way to go for many people," reports the American Heart Association (AHA). According to the AHA statement, aspirin therapy should only begin with a doctor's recommendation.

A special report issued by Dr. Valentin Fuster of Harvard Medical School and Dr. Charles Hennekens, lead investigator of the Physicians' Health Study (a study to test the effects of aspirin on heart disease), examined the benefits and dangers of using aspirin therapy. This report concludes that only a small segment of the population should be taking aspirin daily to prevent heart attacks.

While aspirin does prevent platelets in the blood from clumping together to form clots, it only helps prevent clots which lodge in already narrowed arteries. According to the AHA, aspirin does not reverse the "hardening" caused by atherosclerosis. Dangerous side effects of using aspirin therapy affect patients with kidney disease, liver problems, peptic ulcers, gastrointestinal problems and bleeding disorders.

The AHA recommends prudent use of aspirin therapy in middle-aged or older men with obvious risk factors for heart attack. Other heart disease patients should seek their physician's advice regarding the use of aspirin therapy.

Clots formed in arteries are composed largely of protein. A protein mesh of fibrin encases each clot that includes fats and cholesterol. "Protease," or bromelain, is an enzyme extracted from the pineapple plant which breaks down those proteins. The new clot-busting drugs Streptokinase (or Streptase) and urokinase dissolve 70 percent of the clots in heart patients by breaking down fibrin.

Bromelain, a non-prescription nutrient, also breaks down the fibrin mesh encasing clots of fats and cholesterol as reported in several medical journals, including the *Archaeological International Pharmacodyn*, the *Medical Hypothesis* and *Journal of the International Academy of Preventive Medicine*.

Bromelain may also "clean" plaque from arteries before a problem occurs. In a study of the aortas of rabbits, bromelain broke down existing plaque. It also appears to keep clots from forming. This natural aspirin substitute prevents the production of prostaglandins. Some of these prostaglandins make cells sticky, which enhances clot formation.

Reported studies have shown the American diet is considerably low in omega-3 oil. Fish oil containing omega-3 fatty acid has been found to actually reduce the bad LDL cholesterol and raise the good HDL cholesterol. Abnormalities in heartbeat, kidney malfunction, fatty degeneration of the kidneys and liver, brain damage, elevated cholesterol, triglycerides and high blood pressure have all been shown to be caused by a deficiency in omega-3 oil. One or two tablespoonfuls of an oil rich in omega-3 can be an important part of a healthy diet, especially if fish is not a regular part of the diet.

Dr. Dattilo advised people to eat fish that have omega-3 in his article in the *Journal of Cardiopulmonary Rehabilitation*. Eicosapentaenoic acid (EPA) is an excellent source of omega-3 oil. EPA comes from cold-water marine fish such as halibut, salmon, mackeral and albacore tuna. EPA in the diet can result in a higher HDL-to-LDL ratio and much lower blood cholesterol and triglycerides. Fish oils may also keep blood cells from sticking together on the arterial wall, thereby reducing triglycerides.

■ Coenzyme Q-10 Strengthens Heart Muscle

In a six-year study of patients with cardiomyopathy (a severe form of heart disease), a 75-percent survival rate was achieved when patients took coenzyme Q-10 (CoQ10). In comparison, patients receiving conventional therapy achieved only a 25-percent survival rate. Heart disease patients often are deficient in CoQ10 and require more of it. CoQ10 may improve the strength of the heart muscle tissue, preventing congestive heart failure.

In his article, "Coenzyme Q-10: The Nutrient of the 90's," Dr. R. A. Passwater explains CoQ10's function in the production of energy in heart cells. He states that a number of heart attacks may result from a deficiency in CoQ10. According to Dr. Passwater, CoQ10 is present in most foods people eat, but it can't survive food processing and storage.

In 1957, CoQ10 was isolated by researchers who found it
was a necessary nutrient for the body's cells. Since then the
clinical value of CoQ10 has been demonstrated in the treatment of cardiovascular disease, angina, heart failure, hypertension and other serious disorders. Dr. Karl Folkers, the
researcher who first identified vitamin B_6 and the father of
CoQ research, believes CoQ deficiencies may be the major
cause of heart disease.

Several heart patients at the Methodist Hospital of Indiana, who were given only days to live with traditional medications, had CoQ supplements added to their diets. Seventy
percent survived for one year and 62 percent were alive after
two years. Their cardiac functions improved, and they
showed decreased difficulty in breathing and less fatigue.
The symptoms of congestive heart failure present before
using CoQ supplements disappeared afterward.

Other such studies have been conducted, with similar
results, at the following institutions: Scott and White Clinic;
Texas A & M; University at Temple, Texas; Kitasato University School of Medicine in Kanagawa, Japan; University of
Bonn in West Germany; Municipal Hospital in Aarhus, Denmark; plus many other institutions around the world. Dr. Folkers has studied patients with severe heart arrhythmias. He has
shown these irregular heartbeats were a direct result of a lack
of CoQ. His research showed that the use of CoQ reduced or
totally eliminated five of six patients' arrthythmias.

According to Dr. Passwater, millions of people worldwide take CoQ10 supplements to counter heart disease, high
blood pressure, aging and weakened immunity, as well as
other conditions. More than 12 million Japanese are taking
daily doses of CoQ10, prescribed by their physicians to prevent and treat heart and circulatory diseases, reports Dr. G.
L. Hunt in his article, "Coenzyme Q10: Miracle Nutrient?",
printed in *Omni* magazine.

Heart attack victims in a Belgian study at the Free University of Brussels increased cardiac output and heart muscle strength after taking 100 milligrams daily for twelve
weeks. Normally, heart muscle deterioration follows a heart

attack. Once withdrawn, cardiac output and muscle strength declined to pre-study levels.

■ Understanding Cholesterol

Cholesterol is actually a modified fat called a sterol, which is waxy, not oily or fatty. It doesn't dissolve easily in water or the bloodstream. Cholesterol is made by the liver and smaller amounts are manufactured by the small intestine and individual cells throughout the body. Cholesterol is important because it is used by every cell in the body to construct protective cell membranes. It acts as a barrier against substances trying to enter or leave the cell.

It also supplies a protective barrier for the skin. Cholesterol in the skin prevents certain liquids from penetrating the body and keeps water from leaving the body too quickly (dehydration). The body loses only 10 to 14 ounces of water per day through evaporation, thanks to cholesterol. Cholesterol helps provide the basis for steroid hormones produced by the adrenal glands, the ovaries and the testes. It also helps make vitamin D.

Between 1,500 and 1,800 milligrams of cholesterol are produced by the body every day. About 80 percent of it is used by the liver to help produce bile salts, which are stored in the gallbladder and used to aid in digestion and absorption of dietary fat. In addition, the average American consumes between 200 to 800 milligrams of cholesterol in their daily diet. The body produces cholesterol no matter whether we consume any or not.

In a Federal Proceedings Abstract, Dr. Slater reported that dietary cholesterol has only a slight effect on blood cholesterol levels in his article, "Effect of Dietary Cholesterol on Plasma Cholesterol, HDL Cholesterol and Triglycerides in Human Subjects." This study was further confirmed in the famous Farmington study of 437 men and 475 women as reported by Dr. Gordon in "High Density Lipoprotein as a Protective Factor Against Coronary Heart Disease: The Farmington Study," published in an issue of the *American Journal of Medicine. Dr. Gordon found no correlation*

*between dietary intake of cholesterol and blood serum cho-
lesterol.* There's a growing consensus among medical scientists that the amount of cholesterol in your blood is not the
problem, rather the oxydation of the LDL cholesterol, due to
homocysteinia is the culprit that causes clogging of the
arteries.

■ High Blood Pressure

The Surgeon General's Report on Nutrition and Health
stated that hypertension affects 20 to 30 percent of the adult
population, or approximately 40 million Americans. High
blood pressure causes heart failure and stroke. High blood
pressure is related to coronary heart disease and atherosclerosis as well as other disorders.

Blood pressure is read by expressing the systolic (measured when the heart is pumping the blood through a vein or
artery at its greatest speed and volume) and diastolic (measured when the heart is resting and no blood is being
pumped). Blood pressure is the ratio between these two
readings. Normal blood pressure readings range from 110
(systolic)/70 (diastolic) to 140/90. Readings of 140/90 to
160/95 indicate borderline hypertension. Any pressure reading over 180/115 is extremely dangerous.

Advanced signs of hypertension include headache,
sweating, rapid pulse, shortness of breath, dizziness and
vision disturbances. Another common precursor of hypertension is atherosclerosis. Atherosclerosis involves the
thickening and loss of elasticity in the walls of the arteries.
The arteries become obstructed with cholesterol and mineral
plaque, making circulation of blood through the vessels difficult.

Potassium is the chemical opposite of sodium (salt) and
aids in balancing the amount of salt in the body so that the
heart and blood pressure remain normal. Conditions known
to deplete potassium from the body include excessive salt
consumption, prolonged diarrhea or vomiting, use of diuretics, alcohol, coffee and sugar. Cortisone-like medications
and patients with digestive tract diseases may also register

low potassium levels. A recent study showed that taking 9,000 milligrams of potassium chloride a day could drop blood pressure five to twenty points.

Calcium has been found to lower blood pressure by relaxing the small muscles surrounding blood vessels and helping to excrete extra salt from the body. A University of Oregon study showed that taking 1,000 milligrams of calcium daily for eight weeks dropped blood pressure ten points in over 40 percent of the study participants.

Because high fiber diets (as opposed to high sugar diets) require less insulin to aid in digestion, blood pressure levels can be affected. Insulin makes the body retain salt, which can raise blood pressure. Eating or supplementing one's diet with increased amounts of fiber can lower blood pressure levels as much as ten to fifteen points. Studies at the University of Texas, and in Osaka, Japan, have shown that supplementing one's diet with 45 to 60 milligrams of CoQ10 could lower blood pressure levels as much as twelve to twenty-five points.

In a recent study of sixty-one older men, magnesium has been shown to result in lower blood pressure readings, according to an article in the *American Journal of Clinical Nutrition*. Normally magnesium is lost through normal body functions by perspiring. It also is lost because of stress, use of alcohol, diuretics and sugar.

The natural dietary sources of magnesium include fresh green vegetables, raw wheat germ, soybeans, figs, corn, apples and nuts rich in oil. Those whose diets are not rich in these natural foods may use magnesium supplements. Researchers recommend taking 500 milligrams daily. Also, injections of magnesium sulfate lower blood pressure safely. In one study, the incidence of second heart attacks was cut by 87 percent.

Vitamin E helps the heart muscle use oxygen, while iron increases the oxygen-carrying ability of the blood. This vitamin and mineral can aid in lowering blood pressure. Initial high doses of vitamin E may temporarily raise blood pressure; thus scientists recommend that you start with a low dose of 200 IU and gradually increase the dosage every week until you reach 1,600 IU daily. The dosage should be split and taken half in the morning after breakfast and half after the evening meal. Your body cannot store vitamin E or C, so they should be taken twice a day.

- ■ Sources of Substances Mentioned in this Chapter

Most of the substances mentioned in this chapter are available from local health food and vitamin stores.

Adoxynol (proanthocyanidin)
Allicin
Acorbic acid (vitamin C)
Beta-carotene
Bromelain
Capsaicin (cayenne)
Carnitine
Chondroitin sulfate A (CSA)
Chromium picolinate
Cobalamin
Coenzyeme Q-10 (CoQ10)
Crataegus
E vitamin
EGCG
Eicosapentaemoic acid (EPA)
Folate
Lysine
Magnesium
Niacin
Oleuropein
Potassium Chloride
Pycnogenol (proanthocyanidin)
Pyridoxine
Quercetin
RRR-tocopheryl (vitamin E)
Rutin
Selenium
Superoxide dismutase (SOD)
Taurine

The following are mail-order sources:

Vitamin Research Products
1044 Old Middlefield Way
Mountain View, CA 94043
(800) 877-2447

Gero Vita makes a product called HHF which contains all the nutrients mentioned in this chapter except Omega-3 fish oil, iron and CoQ10. The HHF formula should be supplemented with these nutrients and at least 1,000 milligrams each of vitamin C and lysine.

Gero Vita International
Dept. Z101
2255-B Queen Street East #820
Toronto, Ontario M4E 1G3, Canada
(800) 825-8482

16

■ ■ ■

A Strong Immune System Means Less Sickness, Less Doctors and Less Drugs

RESEARCHERS, HEALTH-CARE PROFESSIONALS and the public are asking the same question. Why are some people better able to resist illness than others? Ever since the bubonic plague in 1350, which killed over 50 percent of the people in Europe (over 25 million), scientists and doctors have wondered why some people survived and others died.

Finally, thanks to the advance of technology, scientists have concluded that most people succumb to disease and illness due to weakened immune systems. What weakens the immune system? Stress, poor nutrition, drugs (prescription or illegal), chemical pollution; but most of all *lack of particular enzymes*.

What are enzymes and why are they so important? If you removed all enzymes from the body, it would stop working and die! Enzymes are responsible for the healthy functioning of every organ. The body is a big, efficient chemical factory, and enzymes are needed for every chemical action and reaction.

Every gene's program is associated with the actions of

enzymes. Even vitamins and nutrients can't be used effectively without enzymes. The immune system's function is to fight off all foreign invaders in the body such as bacteria, viruses, carcinogens and other chemicals. It relies almost totally on enzymes to do its job.

A weakened immune system has a diminished volume of enzymes that includes those that are defective or worn out. Enzymes have a limited life and must be replaced regularly. Where do we get enzymes? Nine basic enzymes come from food, and the body takes these and certain proteins in the body and changes them into over three thousand varieties of enzymes needed for various purposes.

Unfortunately, if you cook food at temperatures exceeding 129 degrees Fahrenheit, all the enzymes are destroyed. So you must obtain enzymes from raw foods or special enzyme supplements. Some important enzymes are found only in meat, which most people won't eat raw. Today, the majority of food consumed is processed, so people get very few enzymes in their diets.

When you are young, your body is very efficient. It can take a very small amount of enzymes and proteins and manufacture large numbers for the body's needs. But as you get older, your body's ability to make sufficient quantities diminishes dramatically. Your immune system weakens, allowing disease and illness easy access.

Tests have shown that seventy-year-old people have about half the enzymes of twenty-year-olds. Once illness or infection have invaded, the older body works overtime struggling to produce enzymes the immune system needs to overcome the problem. Often it cannot produce enough, and chronic diseases, such as cancer, heart disease, and arthritis, set in.

Over two hundred other diseases result from worn out or defective gene-controlled enzymes such as: high blood pressure, hardening of the arteries, circulatory problems, diabetes, tuberculosis, psoriasis, dermatitis, prostatitis, cirrhosis, hepatitis, pruritis, cholecystitis, rheumatism, edema, varicose veins, sores, pancrcatitis and many more.

Extensive research at hundreds of the best medical centers in the world have proven that by taking supplements of the basic nine enzymes, you can help alleviate or prevent the majority of these and other diseases. Dr. R. Michael Williams, Professor of Medicine at Northwestern University, and Dr. David A. Lopez, Associate Clinical Professor of Medicine at the University of California, stated in their book, *Enzymes, the Fountain of Life,* "The therapeutic value of enzymes is enormous!"

American scientists have been so fascinated with genetic research that most of their efforts have gone toward that area recently. On the other hand, European and Japanese researchers, who are more inclined toward natural medicine, have concentrated on enzyme research and have made tremendous progress. Over fifteen million people in Europe and Japan have been given enzyme supplementation or therapy with enormous success—all with no important side effects! The reason there aren't any side effects is because enzymes are food forms—not drugs.

Dr. A. E. Leskovar reported that supplementation with enzymes increases the macrophages by 700 percent and killer cells by 1300 percent in a short time. Macrophages and killer cells are two of the immune systems' main defenses. European doctors have had significant success in stopping early-onset cancer with oral supplementation of enzymes and by injecting the enzymes directly into the tumor. If the cancer is in an organ where it can't be reached by injection, oral supplementation helps.

Extensive research has been done on oral enzyme treatment of inflammatory diseases—especially rheumatism and arthritis. Austrian Professor of Medicine, Dr. George Klein reported that enzymes were superior to gold as a treatment with no important side effects. In published reports in several medical journals, 141 physicians participated in multicenter controlled studies treating 1,004 patients with enzyme mixtures. Depending on the type of disorder, 76 to 96 percent were classified as considerably improved. The enzymes reduced stiffness, joint swelling, ability to bend and slowed down or completely halted the deterioration of the joints.

In 1964, Dr. Robert Dorrer of the Prien Hospital tested twenty-four patients suffering from shingles with oral enzymes. Within three days, the pain ceased and the blisters started healing. A German medical journal reported his impressive success.

Dr. Wilhelm Bartsch, the director of a cancer clinic in Germany took particular notice of his article because very often cancer patients—his patients—develop shingles. He began a double-blind study using enzymes and the then-current drug prescribed for shingles. Half way through the study, he abandoned the drug for ethical reasons because all those taking the enzymes were significantly improved in a short time.

Just recently, Dr. Michael Kleine did a double-blind study with oral enzymes and the now-current drug for shingles—acyclovir. He concluded that both were equally effective—but the enzymes prevented the recurrance of neuralgia, had no side effects and cost much less!

■ Olympic Athletes Use Enzymes

Injury is a common problem with all those that are athletic—especially professionals and Olympians. Sports medicine doctors know that they can't prevent injuries so they look for methods to heal players as quickly as possible.

Karate fighters experience considerable injuries so doctors chose them as a test group for a double-blind study testing oral enzymes against a placebo. Those taking enzymes three times a day in advance of the events healed 50 percent quicker than those taking the placebos. The German Olympic team doctors conducted similar tests with all types of athletes. The results were comparable for 82 percent of the players. Soreness from strenuous events was considerably less.

Professor Raas of the University of Innsbruck, who is responsible for the health of Austrian athletes in the Winter Olympic games, also confirmed those findings. He stated that, "a good portion of the success achieved by the athletes under his care would not have been possible without enzyme preparations."

He advises even casual athletes to take enzymes daily to lessen the effects of potential injury. Another benefit of enzymes is that they regulate your metabolism. The fewer enzymes in your body, the lower your energy level. Chronic fatigue sufferers take note and consider enzyme supplementation.

Doctors elsewhere have found that oral enzymes taken prior to surgery accelerates healing, allows patients to get out of hospitals quicker and resume their daily routines earlier.

■ Other Nutrients That Boost Immunity

Beta-carotene is processed by the body into vitamin A. Increased beta-carotene intake has been recommended to help prevent certain cancers. In the *American Journal of Clinical Nutrition*, Dr. R. R. Watson reported a study that demonstrated increased T-cell production in a group of ten men and ten women given 30 milligrams or more of beta-carotene per day for two months. Useful as an antioxidant, beta-carotene may possibly kill viruses, and has been shown to boost CD4 cell production. Vitamin A deficiencies are thought to result in increased vulnerability to infection.

A recent study by Dr. S. N. Meydani in the *American Journal of Clinical Nutrition* found that a group of people over age sixty showed increased immune system function when given 800 IU of vitamin E every day for thirty days. In this study, the subjects were also found to have increased production of Interleukin-II, which stimulates T-cell production. Vitamin E is under investigation for AIDS treatment.

At the U.S. Department of Agriculture's Human Nutrition Research Center on Aging at Tufts University, studies proved that supplementing the diets of elderly people with vitamin E for one month strengthened their immune systems.

Arginine is an amino acid that has been shown to increase the production of human growth hormone in the pituitary gland. Human growth hormone stimulates the thymus gland, which manufactures the T-cells so vital to immune function.

Levels of this hormone decline in the normal course of aging, and decreased amounts have been linked to the development of cancer, stroke and heart disease. When combined with lysine, another amino acid—researchers at the Italian National Research Centers on Aging in Acona, Italy, observed enhanced thymus functioning and noted that thymus function can be stimulated to a "younger" level.

Natural killer cell development was observed in a group of young men, ages twenty-one to thirty-four who took 30 milligrams of arginine per day, according to a study published in the British medical journal *Lancet*. Natural killer cells are not manufactured in either the bone marrow or the thymus, but they can destroy tumor and viral cells. This finding is significant in AIDS and cancer treatment, since T-cells increased as well. Another study in the *Canadian Medical Association Journal* noted that patients given arginine in conjunction with omega-3 fatty acids and RNA supplements had less postsurgical infection and shorter hospital stays.

In an effort to combat age-related immune system decline, researchers studied the effects of another amino acid, dimethylglycine (DMG). Reporting in the *Journal of Infectious Diseases*, Dr. C. D. Graber noted that DMG improved human immune response by enabling various substances to be circulated through the bloodstream more quickly. An additional study by Dr. E. A. Reap in the *Journal of Laboratory and Clinical Medicine* documented that "immunologic aberrations are well-known consequences of aging," and that "immune function in these various states might profit by treatment with a non-toxic immunomodulator, such as DMG."

Selenium was found to increase lymphocyte production in a study of elderly nursing home residents by Dr. A. M. Peretz of the Department of Rheumatology and Physical Medicine at St. Pierre Hospital, Brussels, Belgium, in 1990.

Zinc encourages wound healing, aids thymus function and hormone activity. Dr. Castillo-Duran reported in the *American Journal of Clinical Nutrition* that giving zinc supplements to infants benefitted their immune defense ability.

Adequate iron is needed for red blood cell production and

copper is required to manufacture blood cells in the bone marrow—both vital functions in resisting disease processes. In addition, iron, copper and zinc deficiencies can weaken immune system functioning. Dr. R. K. Chandra wrote in the *Journal of Dentistry for Children* that a lack of any of these minerals limits immunity.

First discovered in 1922 in Japan, alkylglycerols are three natural substances produced in the liver. They also occur in breast milk, thus providing protection to newborns until their own immune systems develop.

In 1952 a Swedish physician, Astrid Brohult, M.D., discovered that children with leukemia increased their white cell counts when given bone marrow from newly slaughtered calves. Apparently, the marrow contained alkylglycerols. Later, Dr. Brohult found that patients with uterine or cervical cancer survived longer when given alkylglycerols.

Another potent and better-known source of alkylglycerols is shark liver oil, which has been used in Chinese medicine for over two thousand years to treat a variety of illnesses. Liver oil from certain species of sharks can contain up to a 90 percent concentration of alklyglycerols.

Alkylglycerols increase white blood cell (leukocyte) production. These cells contain antibodies, which are vital in warding off illness. Alkylglycerols have also been shown to slow white blood cell reduction during chemotherapy, to stimulate the immune system in viral infections and inhibit tumor growth in laboratory studies.

Echinacea has an antibiotic effect and increases the white blood cell count, thus strengthening the immune system. As D. Marley noted in *The Scientific Validation of Herbal Medicine*, "The herb acts effectively to close down one of the major routes of bug-invasion" by working with the hyaluronic acid found in human tissue to enable it to "stick together" and resist infection.

CoQ10 has been shown to improve the immune function of existing cells. Unlike many drugs used today to fight immune system disorders, CoQ10 is relatively free of side effects and has been used along with conventional cancer chemotherapy. Treatment with CoQ10 requires doses ranging from 30 to 100 milligrams per day. It is also an important heart nutrient and free radical scavenger.

■ Sources of Substances Mentioned in this Chapter

The following items discussed in this chapter are available at health food and vitamin stores:

Arginine
Beta-carotene
Copper
CoQ10
DMB
E vitamin
Echinacea
Iron
Selenium
Shark liver oil (alkylglycerol)
zinc

A good mail-order source is:

The Vitamin Shoppe
4700 Westside Ave.
North Bergen, NJ 07047
(800) 223-1216

Multienzyme formulas are found in some vitamin and health food stores, but you must read the label. Buy only those that have at least eight different enzymes. A good brand is Phytozyme. If you want to order by mail or phone, order Medi-zyme N from

Gero Vita International
2255B Queen's Street East, #820, Dept. Z101
Toronto, Ontario M4E 1G3, Canada
(800) 825-8482, Ext. Z101

■ ■ ■

17

Everyone Has Cancer Cells—Normally!

CANCER IS UNCONTROLLED multiplication of cells that crowd out healthy tissue, eventually shutting down vital body organs. Three medical school professors, Dr. R. Michael Williams at Northwestern University Medical School, Dr. David A. Lopez at University of California Medical School and Dr. Klaus Michlke at the University of Mainz in Germany say in their book, *Enzymes, the Fountain of Life,* everyone has from a hundred to ten thousand cancer cells floating around in their bodies at all times. However, enzyme-stimulated antibodies destroy them quickly. But if your immune system weakens sufficiently, the cancer cells attach themselves to an organ and build a covering of fibrin so antibodies can't find them. Then you're in trouble!

We know from ancient burial excavations and historical records that cancer has always been with us, although the incidence of cancer has been increasing with the industrial era, coinciding with extended longevity and an increasingly toxic environment. Cancer is second only to heart and circulatory failures as a leading cause of death.

Some people are genetically prone to get cancer, but they represent a small percentage of the number who succumb to this disease. Scientists have explored every conceivable avenue of cause without success, but their research has created a basic conclusion; the immune system kills potential cancer cells when we are young, but as we grow older and the immune system weakens, cancer can get the upper hand.

The obvious key to avoiding cancer is to keep the immune system in optimum health and avoid the chemicals that strain the system such as cigarette smoke and industrial pollutants. For example, the chronic cigarette smoker is constantly damaging lung tissue, which means the immune system must support a large force of fighters in that area. If you are injured or get sick, some of those fighters must leave the lungs to do battle in another part of your body. That's when cancer cells can establish themselves beyond the ability of the immune system to destroy them.

Of course, new technology has provided some of the means to identify and combat the effects of cancer by means of radiation, surgery and chemotherapy. In most cases, these methods are the last resort and only effective in 23 percent of cases.

Analyses of the blood of cancer patients always shows deficiencies of one or more nutrients. This is to be expected because the immune system needs a constant supply of nutrients. If you want to avoid cancer, you better maintain a healthy balanced diet. As you get older, the body's efficiency in processing food declines, which means fewer nutrients are obtained from food and absorbed into the system. Our suggestion is that everyone over forty should be taking a multivitamin/mineral formula daily.

Research has shown that certain nutrients inhibit, prevent, or even kill cancer cells. Scientists have discovered there are two varieties of estrogen—a good kind and a bad one. They've found that the bad one may cause breast cancer. Fortunately, there is some good news. Researchers have found a minute substance in broccoli that breaks down the dangerous form of estrogen into a harmless chemical.

Don't rush out and buy broccoli though. You would have to eat a huge amount of broccoli every day to get enough of the particular phytochemical needed to protect you from breast cancer. Thankfully, this phytochemical is being extracted from broccoli and is available without a prescription in pills sold in vitamin and health food stores. Since it comes from a common food source, there are no side effects.

According to Dr. D. L. Davis, senior science advisor at the U.S. Public Health Service, "Phytochemicals can take tumors and defuse them. They can turn off the proliferative process of cancer."

Dr. Paul Taladay of Johns Hopkins Medical Institute says that a phytochemical found in broccoli (sulforaphane) kept cancer-prone animals from getting cancer even when excessively exposed to cancer-causing chemicals. Several other studies have found that sulforaphane-type phytochemicals actually *block* the development of cancer cells *before* they are formed.

Dr. John Potter, an epidemologist at University of Minnesota told *Newsweek* magazine, "At almost every step along the pathway to cancer, phytochemicals slow up or reverse the process."

Dr. Joseph Hotchkiss of Cornell University said that the phytochemicals, courmaric acid and chlorogenic acid eliminate many cancer-causing substances. The National Cancer Institute directors are so excited about the success and potential of phytochemicals that they've committed a substantial portion of their multimillion dollar budget to more extensive research.

The University of Illinois created a new department specifically for phytochemical research with sixty-three professors and scientists involved. The reason: It's apparent that phytochemicals are one of the most promising disease preventives to come along in many decades—and their use has produced no side effects!

The seventh most common cancer is that of the esophagus, to which smokers and drinkers often succumb. Dr. Mark Morse and other scientists at Ohio State University's Cancer Prevention Laboratory found that sulforaphane reduced esophageal tumors multiplicity by 90 percent and incidence by 40 percent.

Dr. Gary Stoner of University of Ohio reported that isothiocyanates, found in cabbage, inhibit lung cancer caused by chemicals such as those found in smoke. Cigarette smoke contains a tremendous number of free radicals, which are strongly implicated in causing cancer and other diseases. A phytochemical found in garlic specifically attacks cigarette smoke free radicals according to Dr. B. Torok's clinical tests at the University of Tubingen in Germany.

Scientists at Roswell Park Cancer Institute were able to reduce the number of tumors in cancer-prone rats by up to 75 percent with a garlic phytochemical. A study conducted by Johns Hopkins Medical School of 41,837 women for five years showed that those who consumed garlic regularly had 50 percent less incidence of colon cancer.

Dr. T. Tanaka reported in the medical journal, *Cancer Research,* that curcumin obtained from the tumeric spice plant reduced the frequency of tumors in cancer-prone animals by 41 to 91 percent.

Dr. H. Fujiki proved in tests at the National Cancer Research Institute that epigallocatechin gallate (EGCG), found in green tea leaves, seals cancer cells, preventing their growth and spread. The doctor was able to reduce the number of tumors by 73 percent in animals that had cancer. He concluded that EGCG is one of the best cancer preventives available. Researchers at University Hospital of Cleveland said that EGCG is an exceptionally powerful antioxidant. Their clinical tests showed that it prevents skin, colon and stomach cancer.

Dr. Edward Giovannucci of Harvard Medical School reported that the phytochemical lycopene is particularly attracted to the prostate gland. His research team also dis-

covered that men consuming lycopene had a much lower
risk of prostate cancer.

A phytochemical from the spice plant rosemary has been
proven in several tests to be a powerful antioxidant and cancer preventive. Dr. Keith Singletary of the University of Illinois reported that tests of cancer-prone animals treated with
a rosemary extract had 47 percent fewer tumors. Rose-
marinic acid, a part of the extract, also stimulates regular
beating of the heart.

Phytochemicals protect plants from disease, injuries,
insects, poisons or pollutants in the air or soil, drought,
excessive heat and ultraviolet rays. They form the plants'
immune systems. Since humans are programmed to eat vegetables, it is not surprising that Mother Nature passed the
protection of phytochemicals to humans. And that protection is not limited to cancer.

Phytochemicals lower cholesterol, reduce blood pressure, stimulate regular heartbeats, detoxify blood and
rebuild the liver, heal ulcers and skin sores, relieve allergies
and arthritis, improve memory, reduce deafness and ringing
in the ears, alleviate depression and impotency, and are powerful antioxidants in the immune system that even help prevent the flu.

■ Enzymatic Cancer Inhibitors

European scientists have found that enzymes can prevent
as well as kill cancer cells. Much of the serious scientific
interest in enzymes began when Dr. Ernst Freund noticed
that most cancer patients get thrombolysis (blood clots that
cause heart attacks), and most thrombolysis patients get cancer. He suspected that the common connection might be
enzymes. On testing their blood, he found both patient
groups to be lacking three important enzymes.

Recently researchers found that two of those enzymes
destroy blood clots while the third creates macrophages,
which break down fibrin. Cancer cells hide under a coating
of fibrin. Once the fibrin cover is removed, our bodies' killer
cells destroy them.

Macrophages and killer cells are two of the most important players on the immune system team. Dr. A. E. Leskovar reported that supplementation with enzymes increases the macrophages by 700 percent and killer cells by 1300 percent in a short time. That's why people with healthy immune systems don't get cancer.

European doctors have had significant success in stopping early-onset cancer with oral supplementation of enzymes and by injecting enzymes directly into tumors. If the cancer is in an organ where it can't be reached by injection, oral supplementation helps.

Dr. Chin Po Kim, a highly respected scientist and internationally recognized immunologist, cited a 23 percent overall mortality rate in cancer patients who took oral enzymes—about the same rate achieved by standard chemotherapy and radiation treatments but with none of the awful side effects!

Also, several studies conducted by European scientists show that oral enzymes taken with chemotherapy and radiation improves the response rate and reduces the side effects significantly.

■ Sharks Don't Get Cancer!

Research has shown that most animals and fish get cancer just like humans. Sharks are an exception to the rule. Considerable research has been done on sharks to determine why they are immune to cancer without any definite conclusions. However, various components of the shark's physiology have been tested as cancer inhibitors. The most promising part is shark cartilage. Sharks' skeletons are not ossified bone but made instead of cartilage. Cartilage has no blood vessels. In fact, it contains a protein that inhibits the development of blood vessels.

The rapid growth of cancerous masses requires that they have a matching growth in blood supply. A research team at Children's Hospital in Boston headed by Dr. Judah Folkman, working with various inhibitors, tried shark cartilage. They discovered that a tumor will stop growing at one to two millimeters when cut off from a blood supply.

The effectiveness of shark cartilage has been confirmed

on laboratory animals at Massachusetts Institute of Technology (MIT), reported by Dr. Robert Langner in the *Journal of Biological Response Modifiers*. Dr. G. Atassi of the Institute Jules Bordet in Belgium, had the same results. The application of shark cartilage was by oral administration of dried cartilage.

Terminal cancer patients at the Centro Medico del Mar in Tijuana, Mexico, showed great improvement—40 to 100 percent reduction in tumor size—within the first sixty days of the study. In this case, the shark cartilage extract was administered in solutions, rectally and vaginally.

Shark cartilage has been processed into a standardized form for research and therapy by Dr. William Lane. The cartilage is a by-product of sharks harvested for food in Costa Rica, where the product Cartilade is manufactured.

Although shark cartilage is not toxic and can be taken at the same time as any other cancer treatment, there are conditions under which it shouldn't be administered such as after a heart attack or stroke, during pregnancy, or in cases of lesions that won't heal.

■ Ginseng and Melatonin

There are several kinds of ginseng, which have been used in numerous human and animal studies. In test tube studies in Japan, ginseng is said to have caused liver cancer cells to revert to normal form.

Melatonin, an inexpensive, nontoxic and nonprescription drug, has had a favorable effect on the immune system of laboratory animals. It appears to halt the progress of breast cancer, and even to cause tumors to regress. It is the subject of several current studies.

There is general agreement, based on observation, that a diet rich in fruits, leafy vegetables and fiber protects against colorectal disease. To further refine this information, a group of researchers at Harvard Medical School, directed by Dr. Edward Giovannucci, found that folate (a B vitamin in leafy vegetables) and methionine (an amino acid found in high protein foods like fish and chicken) protect against colon polyps. Folate supplements (folic acid) give even greater protection, according to the *Journal of the National Cancer Institute*.

The head of the Cancer Research Institute at the University of Vienna, Dr. Heinrich Wrbe, has concluded that "dietary supplements can cut your risk of cancer by 50 percent." The exceptional health benefits of vitamin and mineral supplements have also been put forward in *Lancet*, the prestigious British medical journal.

The Harvard Medical School study, previously mentioned, queried 1,439 female nurses who developed breast cancer, and found no link to dietary intake of fat, according to the *Journal of the American Medical Association*. However, it is established that carcinogenic poisons such as DDT are stored in body fat for decades.

An extensive comparison of the lifestyles of Japanese and American women points to a vast difference in fat intake. Body fat increases the level of estrogen, and high levels of estrogen are associated with breast cancer.

The Japanese diet, unlike ours, is rich in fish, fiber, soy products and various seaweeds. The following substances, prominent in the Japanese diet, have been found to inhibit the growth of tumors in laboratory tests with animals.

Seaweed, especially Laminaria, was explored by Dr. Ichiro Yamamoto, because it is an ancient Chinese remedy. Extract of Laminaria appeared to cause regression of tumors in mice. The active ingredient is a polysaccharide that helps the body dissolve certain fatty substances and it is a powerful antibiotic, according to the *Japanese Journal of Experimental Medicine*.

People living in the southwestern seashore district of Okinawa, Japan, have the longest life spans and lowest incidence of cancer. They eat a high fat diet that includes a lot of pork, but Laminaria is served at practically every meal in one form or another. It is the staple of their diet.

Eskimos also consume a lot of fat, but Laminaria-type seaweed is their main vegetable. Dr. O. Shafer reported in the *Journal of the Canadian Medical Association* that the rates of breast cancer among Eskimo women is also one of the lowest in the world.

A well-known Japanese scientist, Dr. Hiroko Maruyama confirmed the effectiveness of Laminaria in clinical tests of Sprague-Dawley rats. These rats get breast tumors easily when given a cancer-causing chemical called DMBA. All of the rats were given DMBA, but half of the rats were also given Laminaria in their food. At the end of seven months, all of the rats were autopsied. Those with Laminaria in their diets had almost 50 percent fewer tumors.

Dr. I. Yamamoto did a similar study but in reverse. He took rats that had extensive tumors and added Laminaria to their diets. After six months, 67 percent of the rats had complete tumor remission, and the tumors stopped progressing in 95 percent of the others.

Soybeans inhibit a protein digesting enzyme (protease) that is more abundant when there is a breast malignancy. Laboratory experiments showed that animals exposed to carcinogens developed tumors at nearly half the rate of the control group when they were fed soybean products.

The Japanese diet abounds in soybean dishes, such as miso soup and tofu. Selenium, an essential mineral, is four times more abundant in the Japanese diet than in ours, and it is believed to be effective in preventing and reducing breast tumors.

Japanese women living in Japan have a fraction of the rate of breast cancer (about 75 percent less) that prevails in the United States. When they come here to live, their rate of breast cancer approaches ours.

Japanese studies have demonstrated that selenium, with other minerals and vitamins such as magnesium and ascorbic acid (vitamin C), inhibit the growth of breast cancer in laboratory rats. These studies were reported by Dr. A. Remesha in the *Japanese Journal of Cancer Research*.

■ Free Radical and Antioxidants

Free radicals damage cells and may alter the DNA, allowing the cell to mutate into a cancer cell. Antioxidants prevent free radicals from inflicting damage. Certain antioxidants, when combined, enhance each other's potency, in an effect called "synergy"—working together for a result that each alone could not achieve. For example, vitamins B_{12} and C together entirely prevented the growth of transplanted mouse tumors, in a study reported in *Experimental Cell Biology* by Dr. Poydock.

The National Cancer Institute is funding dozens of studies exploring the efficacy of nutrients in cancer prevention. Among the antioxidants now recommended are beta-carotene and selenium plus vitamins C and E. Vitamin C has long been promoted by Nobel laureate Dr. Linus Pauling as a cancer and arteriosclerosis preventive.

"Cured" foods such as ham and bacon and many others contain nitrates and nitrites for preservation. These combine, in the process of digestion, with amino acids to form nitrosamines, which are carcinogens. Vitamin C neutralizes the nitrates and nitrites.

Vitamin E has a similar effect and is thought to reduce the level of substances that cause mutation of cells. Two separate studies of human subjects showed that in breast cancer patients and lung cancer patients, lower levels of vitamin E were present than in matched control subjects. These studies were reported in the *British Journal of Cancer* and in the *New England Journal of Medicine*.

Many elements that occur naturally in food are being studied because they have an observable connection with lowering cancer risk or growth, though their processes may not be fully understood. Some examples are:

Folic acid, a B vitamin, was observed to reduce lung injury from smoking by Dr. Douglas Hamburger of the University of Alabama.

Glutathione appears to bind with cancer-causing toxins. In one study, this substance reversed liver cancer in rats, reported in *Science* magazine.

The amino acid cysteine neutralizes the chemicals that are produced by smoking cigarettes and that damage the immune system, according to Dr. Richard Passwater.

Fish oil appears to prevent or stop the growth of some of the most common cancers: breast, pancreatic and prostate.

Quercetin (a flavonoid found in broccoli, onion and squash) appears to protect against colon cancer and enhances the strength of cell walls.

Lactobacillus acidophilus, found in acidophilus milk and yogurt, inhibits the formation of carcinogenic substances in the colon. This was reported by Dr. B. R. Goldin in *Clinical Nutrition*.

Epigallocatechin gallate (EGCG), abundant in Asian diets, especially green tea, seems to be a factor in combating several specific types of cancer: colon, skin and lung. As reported during the proceedings of the American Chemical Society in 1991, EGCG reduces the rate of lung cancer in smokers.

Phycotene is extracted from a combination of spirulina and dunaliella algae. In research studies at Harvard University, oral cancers in laboratory hamsters showed total remission in 30 percent of the animals tested, and partial remission in the remaining 70 percent. Joel Schwartz, M.D., of Harvard, observed that phycocyanin-C (a component of phycotene) slowed tumor growth by creating a hostile environment around the tumor. In addition, phycotene increases TNF (a substance which destroys tumor cells) production, which, when combined with interferon (another natural substance in the body that combats viral infections), tremendously increases immune system functioning.

Dehydroepiandrosterone (DHEA) is a hormone secreted by our adrenal glands. We secrete less as we grow older. One of the principal investigators of DHEA, Dr. Arthur Schwartz of the Fels Research Institute of Temple University, has been working with mice. He found that DHEA helps burn off body fat and inhibit the growth of cancer cells. Other researchers have examined the effects of DHEA. Dr. Roger Loria of the Medical College of Richmond, Virginia, has demonstrated that it increases immune functions and helps fight viral infections.

There are many theories about how DHEA works to inhibit cancer growth. It appears to block the effect of carcinogens. It may slow the production of free radicals that are involved in the aging process and formation of abnormal cells. Another theory is that DHEA works like diet restriction, by inhibiting utilization of glucose, which is known to prolong life of laboratory animals.

It has been observed that DHEA levels fall during serious illness and rise during exercise, which tends to confirm its association with well-being. Among those who have made this observation are Dr. E. D. Lephart, in the *Journal of Clinical Endocrinology Metabolism* and Dr. P. Diamond, reporting in the *European Journal of Applied Physiology*.

■ If You Have Cancer Now

Infections after cancer surgery are the major cause of death in those patients, not cancer itself, according to Dr. G. P. Brodey. His study of over a hundred patients was published in the medical journal, *Cancer Treatment Review.* However, Dr. V. Cangemi followed one hundred eighteen patients taking thymic extracts after cancer surgery and found that none of them got infections. Tests showed that their immune systems were substantially bolstered by the thymic extracts.

Even patients undergoing chemotherapy lived longer if given thymic extracts along with the therapy. Dr. Massimo Fedrico guided a double-blind clinical trial of one hundred thirty-four people undergoing chemotherapy. Half of the patients were given thymic extracts, and they lived 49 percent longer than those taking a placebo.

Spleen extracts have been used successfully to prevent as well as kill tumor cells. The most powerful substance found in spleen extracts is an enzyme called tuftsin. Dr. I. Florentin reported in the journal *Cancer Immunology* , that laboratory animals given tuftsin showed an increase of disease-fighting cells by over 300 percent.

Dr. M. S. Wleklik found that even the tiniest amount of tuftsin *in vitro* stimulated the production of TNF lymphokines. These lymphokines are killers of tumor cells.

- **Sources of Substances Mentioned in this Chapter**

The following are usually available from vitamin and health food stores:

Beta-carotene
Cysteine
DHEA (take pregnenolone)
Fish oil
Folate supplements (folic acid)
Ginseng
Melatonin
Quercetin
Seaweed (Laminaria)
Shark cartilage
Soybean products (including miso and tofu)

Glutathione pills that are sold in stores are not effective because glutathione can't be absorbed through the stomach. Instead, take glutamic acid and cysteine, which are converted into glutathione in the body.

Epigallocatechin gallate (EGCG) is only for professional experimental use at this time, but it may be obtained by drinking Oriental green teas, which are available in some health food stores and in Japanese or Chinese neighborhoods.

Multiphytochemical formulas are available in vitamin and health food stores, but be sure the formula has at least six different phytochemicals. The best one is Phytoplex, which is only available by mail or phone order from Gero Vita International. Gero Vita also makes a excellent multienzyme formula called Medi-zyme n. Their address is:

2255-B Queen Street East, #820, Dept. Z101
Toronto, Ontario M4E 1G3, Canada
(800) 825-8482, Ext. Z101

Multienzymes are also available in vitamin and health food stores, but read the label carefully. You want one that contains at least the following enzymes: amylase, protease, lipase, cellulase, lactase, invertase, maltase, bromelain and pectinase. A popular brand is Phytozyme.

Thymic and spleen extracts may be found occasionally in vitamin and health food stores. The best source is Gero Vita International, which has a product called Bioactive Cell Complex. Their address is shown above.

18

■ ■ ■

Answers to Ulcers, Digestion and Colon Problems

IF YOU WERE asked to name the group of related diseases for which the largest number of Americans are hospitalized each year, what would your answer be? Surely, most people are admitted into the hospital due to heart and lung ailments, you might answer. Or perhaps, you are certain that diseases related to the body's immune system are the cause for most hospitalizations.

Surprisingly, according to Bio/Tech News, diseases of the digestive tract head the list of ailments that put Americans in the hospital. The statistics are particularly staggering. Nearly 100 million of us experience some form of recurring digestive disease, with 200 thousand of us missing work per day. These huge numbers point to an obvious problem. We are a nation ruled by its stomach (and other digestive organs), and apparently that battle is being won by the other side. A good strategist would tell you that the enemy must be studied to learn its strengths and weaknesses. After long years of study, scientists and doctors have found that the war we've been waging with prescription drugs may be better fought with natural supplements as our allies.

Two of the largest and most menacing of the players in

the war are cancer and various ailments of the colon, rectum and digestive system, which include constipation, appendicitis, diverticular disease, hemorrhoids, irritable bowel disease, ulcerative colitis, Crohn's disease, benign tumors and stomach ulcers. Evidence of these diseases hardly existed in the Western world a hundred years ago. This becomes even more telling when we look at certain non-Westernized cultures, like pre–World War II Japan and some parts of modern-day Africa. These cultures show almost no evidence of the digestive diseases mentioned. The culprits do show up as soon as these societies become "Westernized," that is, take on our diets.

A handful of doctors in the United States, Great Britain and the Third World nations began to make the connection between a low fiber diet and the upsurge of digestive diseases as early as the 1920s. British physicians Dr. Arthur Rendle-Short, Dr. Robert McCarrison and Dr. Arbuthnot Lane all drew attention to the need for a high fiber diet for a healthy digestive system. In the 1930s, American doctors Cowgill, Anderson and Dimmock supported the studies of those British doctors, promoting high fiber diets as wonderful aids in keeping digestive disorders at bay.

In the post–World War II years, three physicians delved further into the "Fiber Hypothesis." Dr. T. L. Cleave, Dr. Hugh Trowell and Dr. A. Walker did studies in the British Isles and in Third World countries, comparing digestive ailments in Great Britain to those in India and Africa. They found that the digestive illnesses common in Great Britain were almost nonexistent in those countries. High fiber was one thing found in Third World diets that was missing in diets in the "modern" countries. Those supposedly progressive countries had refined and processed all of the roughage out of their food, and, as a result, they suffered from digestive diseases that ranged from constipation to ulcerative colitis, stomach ulcers and colorectal cancer.

It seems with all of this scientific information showing the need for high fiber to combat digestive disease, the problem would be easy to correct by simply eating better. Unfortunately, this involves a commitment to diet change that most of us would find daunting. We would have to replace the foods that contain ultra-refined flours and sugars with whole grains; eliminate fried foods and those containing animal fat and tropical oils; and eat many more raw vegetables and fruits. This might read more easily than it actually is. Look at the ingredients of the foods stored in your pantry and refrigerator, and you will see how difficult a challenge it is. What is the answer? The best way to add high fiber to our diets without drastically changing our lifestyles is to take dietary fiber supplements.

In this hectic, fast paced society, pressures of job, family, finances, and a multitude of other stressors often manifest themselves in physical ways in our bodies. When the pressures become too great, our bodies break down. Two common, interconnected signs our bodies show when stressed are digestive problems and stomach ulcers. If we haven't had these problems ourselves yet, we probably know someone who has. Do you have a friend who, when in a stressful situation, reaches into his or her pocket or bag, takes out a familiar brown prescription bottle and pops a few tiny pills into their mouth?

Most likely what your friend has just done is take the drug Tagamet. A recent study shows that, over the last three years, doctors in the United States have prescribed more than $3 billion worth of the drug to ulcer sufferers. Tagamet is very effective. Unfortunately, it also has some side effects. One of the most disturbing for men taking the drug is gynomastia, or breast enlargement. According to Tagamet manufacturers, only 4 percent of the drug's users encounter this problem, and they feel that the percentage is so small that there should be no concern. Of course, if you were among those affected, you would probably be looking for an alternative treatment.

What doctors often do not tell ulcer sufferers is that there are options to Tagamet that are both nonprescription and produce no such side effect. One such treatment is deglycyrrhizinated licorice root (DGL). Doctors may tell you that licorice root does have side effects, like headaches and high blood pressure, especially when taken in large doses. Plain licorice root does contain a component called glycyrrhizinic acid, which can cause these side effects. Fortunately, with DGL, scientists have found a way to remove 97 percent of the glycyrrhizinic acid and still keep the excellent antiulcerative properties.

While Tagamet and prescription ulcer drugs work by decreasing acid secretion in the stomach, DGL aids your intestines and stomach in producing protective mucus. In the case of ulcer patients who must take aspirin, cortisone, or anti-inflammatory drugs (which can produce or promote ulcer), this extra production of protective mucus can be extremely beneficial. It should be noted that scientific studies have proven that DGL tablets perform better in the treatment and maintenance of ulcers if they are chewed before swallowing.

Although stress can play a large part in promoting ulcers or digestive problems, such as chronic stomach irritation (gastritis), scientists have recently linked these digestive disorders to the growth in the digestive tract of a germ called Helicobacter pylori. Researchers say, that our chances of being infected with the germ increases by 1 percent with each year that we live. In other words, by the time we're fifty, we will have a 50 percent chance of being infected with H. pylori.

Luckily, there is a simple test used to detect H. pylori that has proven 100 percent accurate. It's called enzyme-linked immunosorbent assay (ELISA). It can be done in your doctor's office, and in seven minutes you will know if you have H. pylori. Once this is determined, a treatment of antibiotics and Pepto Bismol can eliminate it. Tests of ulcer patients have shown that the treatment seems to heal ulcers permanently. Research physicians are also studying the possibility of using vitamin C and beta-carotene to kill the bacteria.

Even if ulcers do not plague you, it is probable that some form of digestive distress has touched you. How often have you reached for that little roll of antacids, or mixed up that bubbling concoction to help soothe your aching stomach and calm your "heartburn"? Although they can be effective, these over-the-counter antacids can hardly be called natural.

A natural digestive aid is available called bromelain. It is an extract of pineapple juice, that has been used for centuries to help in soothing indigestion. Bromelain is quite safe and shows no known side effects.

■ Constipation

One of the simplest and most natural ways to correct constipation is with vitamin C. Begin with 1,000 milligrams taken morning and evening. Increase the dosage by 1,000 milligrams each day until you are relieved. Maintain that dosage daily and you'll probably never be constipated again.

■ Sources of Substances Mentioned in this Chapter

Most of the products discussed in this chapter are available at health food and vitamin stores:

Beta-carotene
Bromelain
C vitamin
Deglycyrrhizinated licorice root
Fiber supplements

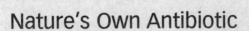

19

Nature's Own Antibiotic

TODAY, DUE TO hundreds of thousands of people traveling every day in airplanes, infectious diseases can spread around the world overnight. A woman infected with a new, powerful flu virus gets on an airplane in southeast Asia. She sits in the front row aisle seat. Flu viruses, as well as many infectious bacteria, travel in the air—on your breath. Almost everyone getting on the plane walks past her and is exposed.

The airplane lands in Los Angeles. Some of the people stay in California, while others board airplanes to other parts of the country. Many of them will be infected and may pass the germs on to passengers on the next plane or in crowded airports, or wherever they go.

As you can see, one woman (or man) could cause an epidemic. In 1918, a super strong flu virus killed 20 million people in America and Europe before a vaccine was developed. Most were children or adults with weakened immune systems. Sailors on merchant ships from Asia were believed to have been the culprits who brought the virus to the United States and Europe.

Vaccines may protect you from *known* flu bugs, but there is little to protect you if you are already infected; only the strength of your immune system can eventually destroy the virus. Modern antibiotics only kill some bacteria and fungi—*not viruses, such as flu and common cold viruses.*

Every day in our crowded cities, we're exposed to infectious bacteria, viruses and fungi—on our jobs, in stores and shopping malls, in schools, on trains, buses and airplanes. If your immune system is strong, you may fight off the bugs, but if your system is slightly weak at the moment of exposure, you're in trouble.

Recently, a cruise ship left Los Angeles for a trip to the Mexican resort, Cabo San Lucas. It never arrived in Cabo. Less than two days out to sea, over half of the passengers (over 400) came down with an unidentified intestinal ailment, so the captain turned the ship around and went back to Los Angeles. One man died.

In Bermuda, 1,200 passengers were evacuated from a cruise ship because of a Legionnaires' disease outbreak. The bacteria that cause Legionnaires' disease proliferate in air-conditioning systems.

■ Antibiotics Are Not Working Anymore

In 1969, the Surgeon General of the United States declared, "We can close the book on infectious diseases caused by bacteria." Little did he know that those bacteria were apparently smarter than the chemists who created the antibiotics. Most disease-causing bacteria are resistant or have developed resistance or immunity to antibiotics through normal evolutionary processes.

Now, worldwide, the occurrence of infectious diseases is rising dramatically—not just in Third World countries, but here in the good old United States. Medical scientists are getting very worried that we won't find new chemicals to fight them.

For example, there are several tuberculosis (TB) strains that are resistant to *all* antibiotics. Last year in Cincinnati, there was an 838 percent increase (over the yearly average) in whooping cough among children *who had been vaccinated.*

Even hospitals have become unsafe because *staphylococ-*

cus (staph) and *streptococcus* (strep) flourish in that environment. They've become resistant to *every* antibiotic except one—vancomycin. Infectious disease specialist, Dr. Thomas Beam told *Newsweek* magazine, "We know at some point staph and strep bacteria will become resistant to vancomycin."

We've become complacent about diseases such as staph and strep and should be reminded that before antibiotics were available almost 80 percent of hospital patients that contracted those diseases *died.* The *Muppets* creator, Jim Henson, was killed in 1990 by strep A, a very dangerous form of the bacteria.

Medical scientists say that some doctors hand out antibiotics like candy to people regardless of whether they're likely to help the person or not. Some prescribe them for preventing colds. *Antibiotics absolutely will not prevent a cold.* Approximately one-fifth of the antibiotic prescriptions are unnecessary or won't work. Dr. Steve Waterman, chief of epidemiology at the California Department of Health Services told reporters, "It's sloppy medical practice, but it's very common."

Dr. Peter Duesberg, a professor of molecular and cell biology at University of California reported in his book, *Inventing the AIDS Virus,* that sexually active homosexuals who took antibiotics as preventives of sexually transmitted diseases *actually destroyed their immune systems* and became afflicted with AIDS-related diseases.

■ The Forgotten Natural Antibiotic

You'll probably be surprised to learn that prior to World War II, the most powerful antibiotic, antibacterial and antifungal substance was *silver*! Yes, the same kind of silver that your jewelry or silverware is made from, but it was ground up into small particles and suspended in a fluid. It is called colloidal silver (CS).

It was doctors' most useful potion because it killed over six-hundred-fifty different illness-causing organisms—bacteria, *viruses* and fungi. But, there were problems with it.

Back then, CS cost about $400 per treatment (in today's dollars) making it very expensive. Health insurance was practically nonexistent, so only the wealthy could afford it.

Also, no one could grind up the silver into small enough particles that would be absorbed by the stomach, so it had to be injected by needle, making it inconvenient to use at home, as well as painful. After a month or so of sitting in the bottle, the silver particles would stick and clump together, making it unusable.

In 1928, Dr. Alexander Fleming discovered that *penicillum*, taken from a green mold, could kill certain bacteria. However, chemists couldn't grow enough of the mold to make it commercially viable. During World War II, they found a way to make it synthetically out of chemicals, and penicillin was born. It became the rage among doctors, much to the delight of the drug companies.

From the beginning, the supposedly wonderful penicillin had problems. Many people were allergic to it and suffered from shock, rashes, hives and some even died. That's why doctors still ask, "Are you allergic to penicillin?"

Since the 1940s, chemists have created numerous penicillin-type antibiotics. Initially their motivation was avoiding allergy problems, but there was another difficulty: Each antibiotic only killed certain organisms. In other words, you can't use the same antibiotic to kill a throat infection on someone who has a skin infection.

In the meantime, technology has come to the rescue of the forgotten colloidal silver. Instead of grinding up the silver into hard-to-use large particles, scientists found they could use electricity to break down the particles to as small as $\frac{1}{10,000}$th of an inch—much smaller than you can see with the naked eye.

Also, the electricity gave the tiny particles identical electric charges, which causes them to repel each other. There suddenly were no more clumping problems. Shelf-life increased to up to five years. This new silver is called "Electrically Generated Colloidal Silver" or EGCS.

EGCS can now be taken orally or sprayed on a wound,

burn or rash, and no shots are necessary. Also, the dosage costs dropped from four hundred dollars to as little as twenty-five cents each. Scientists found that using a tiny bit of EGCS worked better than the large amounts given in the early part of the century.

Silver has been known for its health values since before the time of Julius Caesar. The Greeks lined water and wine urns with silver to kill bacteria. The Romans discovered that a poultice of silver helped heal burns, cuts and sores.

■ Doctors Advised Wealthy to Eat with Silver

Did you know that silverware became popular almost 1,900 years ago for health reasons. Physicians advised their wealthy patients to only eat with silver if they wanted to stay healthy.

During the fourteenth century, about 25 percent of the people in Europe died from the bubonic plague, which swept through the continent. Wealthy people gave their children silver spoons to suck on to forestall the plague. That's where the expression, "Born with a silver spoon in your mouth," came from.

Because so few of the wealthy died from the plague, silverware and silver pacifiers became popular. Silver pacifiers are still given to babies in many countries. In the United States, people have forgotten that heritage and use plastic pacifiers today. If people are wise, they will return to using silver because babies are very susceptible to all kinds of bacteria, viruses and fungi.

American settlers knew the value of silver both as wealth and for their health. They often put silver dollars in milk to deter its spoilage in warm weather.

In 1884, Dr. K. S. Crede, a German obstetrician, discovered that a mild silver solution, put into a babies eyes at birth, dramatically reduced eye infections, which are common in babies.

Shortly thereafter, laws were created in the United States, Canada, Norway and Denmark requiring all physicians and hospitals to put a silver solution in the eyes of every baby born in their care. It is still done today in most countries, and undoubtedly, you experienced it as a baby.

Chinese folklore advised families to always have a silver item in their houses in case someone was bitten by a dog with rabies. They were instructed to rub the silver into the wound.

Dr. Jerome Alexander, in his book, *Colloid Chemistry*, said that he tested the concept and found that silver ions were rubbed off the metal and did indeed destroy harmful bacteria. History texts show that serious medical study of CS began in the late 1880s when it was used to treat typhoid and anthrax bacterial infections successfully.

Dr. Henry Crookes is credited for the wide use of silver in the early 1900s. He used it for subduing gonorrhea, tuberculosis, and staphylococcus, as well as many other infectious organisms. His scientific reports concluded that *there wasn't any known microbe that could not be killed* in the laboratory with CS within six minutes.

In 1915, Dr. A. Leggeroe found that CS was not only good for protecting babies' eyes, but it worked for adults as well. He said that it was "the most useful opthalmic remedy" he had ever encountered for eye infections. He claimed there was never any side effects or visual impairment as a result of using CS.

Dr. Malcomb Morris reported in 1917 that CS was a powerful remedy for inflamed and enlarged prostates or infected bladders. He also found that infected hemorrhoids responded well to the substance. Later he proved it was useful in ameliorating eczema.

By 1925, many dairy farms and cattle and sheep ranches were substantial in size. Often infections or viruses wiped out an entire herd. The best weapon veterinarians had was CS, and they used it extensively with great success.

Diphtheria and tetanus were a scourge for humanity in the first quarter of this century, and scientists were infecting animals with these bacillus toxins in laboratories in order to find an answer. In 1919, Dr. Alfred Searle succeeded. He found that CS could protect rabbits from lethal dose of those toxins.

CS not only killed bacteria, viruses and bacillus toxins, it bolstered the immune system, according to studies published in a 1916 issue of *Transactions of the American Association of Obstetricians and Gynecologists.* The author reported that CS actually doubled the white blood cell counts—our bodies' major germ fighters.

Dr. J. Mark Hovel reported in the *British Medical Journal* that CS was especially useful in controlling viruses. His studies covered shingles, pyorrhea, whooping cough, throat and nasal infections. The common cold retreated much quicker in the presence of CS, according to his report.

Medical research on silver dropped by the wayside during the forties and fifties due to widespread use of penicillin-type drugs. But, in 1963, doctors found that CS was best for destroying yeast infections and fungi. New interest in CS research began in 1970 when Dr. Carl Moyer, chairman of the Washington University Department of Surgery and his chief biochemists, Dr. L. Bretano and Dr. H. Margarf, received a federal grant to find better treatments for burn victims.

Most of the antiseptics used for this purpose created more severe problems due to their poisonous nature. Antibiotics worked only for a while before the bacteria on the burnt skin developed an immunity to the drugs. In addition, no antibiotic or antiseptic killed the most powerful bacteria known as *Pseudomonas aeruginosa.*

After reading some old medical research from the 1900s, Dr. Margarf decided to try CS. He found that just a tiny amount of silver killed the *Pseudomonas* bacteria and allowed the burnt tissue to heal.

One of the problems found with silver in the early 1900s was that large amounts colored the skin a blue-gray, a condition known as "argyria." This was due to the huge amounts doctors used, and because the size of the silver particles was much too large due to hand-ground silver in the solution.

Using a very small amount of ultra-fine silver particles, Dr. Bretano found it was the best burn antiseptic; no matter how often it was used, it did not discolor the skin. Also, the bacteria did not develop an immunity to the silver as they did to antibiotics, according to the results published in the journal, *Surgical Forum*. Dr. Moyer's team is responsible for developing the ultra-fine, low dose, electrically generated colloidal silver (EGCS) being used today.

Clinical researchers at the VA hospital in Syracuse, New York, confirmed that the new EGCS was ten to one hundred times stronger than the drugs formerly used for killing bacteria.

Fungi can create major aggravations in life when they infect finger and toenails, skin, scalp and feet. The most common fungus is athlete's foot. In 1976, Dr. T. J. Berger found that EGCS was a powerful antifungal agent. One application of EGCS could stop fungi, such as athlete's foot, in its tracks.

In 1977, Dr. William Foye showed that EGCS was great for dealing with tonsillitis, rhinitis (stuffy or runny nose) and conjunctivitis (pinkeye and related eye infections.) In the next year, researchers used EGCS to kill syphilis and malaria bacteria. Doctors in hospitals soothed varicose ulcers and bedsores with EGCS.

■ Our Mightiest Germ Fighter

In 1978, Dr. Jim Powell wrote an article in *Science Digest* entitled, "Our Mightiest Germ Fighter," pointing out how much more powerful EGCS was than antibiotics.

The greatest progress EGCS has made in the last decade is the result of a prominent doctor getting a seemingly incurable disease. That doctor, Paul Farber, is one of the most educated medical scientists in the country, holding seven degrees in various health fields.

In 1992, after a hunting trip in Texas, Dr. Farber found he couldn't get out of bed. He was paralyzed from the chest down. He was in excruciating pain with severely swollen joints. Overnight, the middle-aged doctor was like a crippled ninety-year-old who had been suffering from rheumatoid arthritis for decades. His condition puzzled specialist after specialist. Their guesses ranged from multiple sclerosis to the rare Guillian-Barré syndrome—a multiple neuritis-type of affliction.

Confined to his bed, able to move only his arms and head, one day Dr. Farber felt a tiny lump in the scalp above his forehead. He suspected a tick was imbedded there, and summoned an intern.

The intern carefully removed the tick and sent it to Dr. Thomas Craig, a professor of veterinary medicine at Texas A & M University. After examining the tick, Dr. Craig suggested that Dr. Farber had Lyme Disease, commonly carried by the type of tick removed from Dr. Farber's scalp. Blood tests confirmed it was the terrible Lyme Disease (LD), which is named after a small town in Connecticut where an outbreak crippled over fifty people in 1972.

Antibiotics, such as penicillin and Rocephin, are the first line of defense against LD, but they are not cures because they only repress it. Continuous use of the antibiotics causes a severe form of yeast infection. The drugs have to be stopped until the yeast infection clears up, but shortly after the drugs are withdrawn, the horrible LD symptoms return, and the whole process starts over again.

Dr. Farber searched medical literature for something that could possibly destroy the bacteria that was making his life so miserable. Dr. Farber found what he calls "the Dead Sea Scrolls of medicine" in early 1900s' research on colloidal silver. Dr. Crookes' comments about it killing any microbe in six minutes got his attention. Then he found doctors Moyer, Bretano and Margarf's research and development of EGCS.

He immediately began taking EGCS. The results were nothing short of spectacular. Within a short time, tests at the Neurological Department of Parkland Hospital in Texas showed that the bacteria was no longer in his body. Clinical research has since shown that the LD bacteria simply hides from the antibiotics; however, recent testing at Fox Chase Cancer Center in Philadelphia proved that EGCS actually destroys the LD bacteria.

Because EGCS literally saved his life, Dr. Farber has devoted the last few years experimenting with its powerful effects. He wrote a book entitled, *The Micro Silver Bullet*, and regularly treats patients at his Mountain Health Retreat in Colorado.

One of his most interesting cases was a man named Jack, who worked for a private construction company in Kuwait during the Gulf War. Shortly after returning to the United States, Jack developed aching joints, insomnia, persistent high fevers, loss of balance and a total lack of energy. He couldn't work, and even the famous Mayo Clinic couldn't determine the cause of his affliction. He saw specialist after specialist, from cardiologists to oncologists, but none could pinpoint the cause of his problems. Typical of scalpel-happy surgeons, they took out his gallbladder, and then his spleen. Nothing helped.

Finally, Jack heard about Dr. Farber and visited him. The doctor put Jack on EGCS for eight weeks. Soon, Jack was back working ten hours a day, six days a week as if nothing had ever happened.

In his book, Dr. Farber tells about a patient named Yvonne, who had a persistent eye infection that wouldn't go away. Her opthalmalogist gave her antibiotic eyedrops, which would help for about two weeks, and then the infection would return again.

After cycling through this routine several times, Yvonne visited Dr. Farber. He told her that it was once standard practice to put a silver solution in a baby's eyes at birth to ward off eye infections. Yvonne began using EGCS as eyedrops, and within 24 hours her infection was gone and hasn't returned since.

Dr. Farber also tells about a woman who suffered from cystic acne since she was eleven years old. Dermatologists had given her many antibiotics and Accutane, but nothing worked for very long. At twenty-four, she was planning to get married and wanted to look her best at the wedding. She visited Dr. Farber, who gave her EGCS a month before the big day. Within three weeks, the acne had totally cleared up.

Psoriasis is another skin disorder that doctors find most difficult to subdue because it seems to come back regularly after treatment, accompanied by annoying, itching and scaly skin.

A patient of Dr. Farber's named Susan from Glassport, Pennsylvania, suffered from psoriasis and joint pain called fibromyalgia. Doctors had tried everything from antibiotics to methyltrexate (a form of chemotherapy) with no luck. In fact, most of the drugs made Susan feel worse. After three months of using EGCS, the joint pain was completely gone, and 90 percent of her psoriasis symptoms had disappeared.

A lady named Patrice from West Milfin, Pennsylvania, read Dr. Farber's book and decided to try EGCS on her asthma problem. At the time, she was enrolled in a special program at the medical research center of University of Pittsburgh, where new asthma remedies were being tested.

After two weeks of taking EGCS, her asthma symptoms cleared up. She dutifully called the university to cancel her involvement, and the doctor asked her why. When she told him about EGCS, he showed no interest in it, and quickly excused himself from the phone call. Perhaps they were worried about losing their drug company grant for testing its medicines.

Dr. Robert O. Becker, an orthopedic surgeon and a medical professor at both State University of New York and Louisiana State University, is the author of two popular books, *Body Electric* and *Cross Currents*. He discovered that a silver impregnated nylon dressing attached to a small battery would cause previously untreatable osteomyelitis (bones that refuse to knit) to heal quickly. This combination of silver and tiny electric currents worked so well that today, when broken bones refuse to knit, it is standard practice to use Dr. Becker's electrified silver process.

Dr. Alex Duarte reported a personal experience in his newletter, *Health Breakthroughs*. His daughter was in a near-fatal auto accident that punctured her heart when she was eighteen. An artificial ring had to be put around one of the heart valves to save her.

She knew that some time in the future, she would have to undergo surgery to replace the ring. Years later while waiting for surgery, her heart muscle was attacked by the Coxsackie virus. Doctors were able to subdue the virus and perform the surgery, but six months later, her heart became re-infected with the virus.

In the meantime, Dr. Duarte had learned about EGCS

from Dr. Farber and administered EGCS to his daughter to ward off the virus. Within a month's time, she recovered and is healthier than ever before.

Dr. John Barltrop of the University of Toronto conducted toxicity tests on rats, giving them enormous amounts of EGCS. He found there were absolutely no toxic effects. The amount he gave the rats (1cc of a solution of 300,000 ppm of EGCS) was equivalent to 7,500 times the amount Dr. Farber and other scientists found was the proper dose (40 ppm).

According to the Environmental Protection Agency (EPA) Poison Control Center, EGCS is considered harmless. Dr. Samuel Etris, a senior consultant at the Silver Institute, says there has never been any allergenic, toxic or cancerous reactions to silver. The government's Center for Disease Control confirmed that fact in 1995.

In 1966, Dr. I. H. Tipton reported in the journal, *Health Physics,* that the ideal daily intake of silver was between 50 and 100 micrograms (mcg). It's an important trace mineral used by the body like chromium and selenium.

Bacteria, fungi and viruses cause a great majority of minor illnesses we have today from runny noses or colds to minor food poisoning. We catch many of these illnesses from being exposed to people as we go through our daily routines. At the end of the day, a quick spritz of EGCS into your nose and mouth could stop dangerous germs you've picked up at work, school, or the store from doing any damage. This is especially important with children and the elderly, who don't have strong immune systems. Also, burns, scrapes, cuts and rashes open the door, allowing harmful organisms to enter the body.

Knowing that EGCS kills over 650 kinds of disease-causing microbes, it is ideal to have around the house to use when you feel something coming on or you get a cut, burn or rash.

In 1982, Dr. J. Cowlishaw demonstrated that EGCS would kill a bacteria called *Escherichia coli* or *E. coli.* In 1993, *E. coli* infested hamburgers at a few Jack-In-The-Box fast-food restaurants on the West Coast and killed several people.

Other bacteria can contaminate food and cause minor food poisoning that millions of people experience every year. Usually, this type of food poisoning only makes your stomach uncomfortable, but over five hundred people die from food poisoning every year. EGCS may be handy to have around when you eat something that makes you sick.

■ Sources of Substances Mentioned in this Chapter

Colliodial silver is available in many vitamin and health food stores, but usually it contains only 3 to 5 parts per million (ppm) and has an eyedropper-type top. According to most clinical studies, 40 ppm is a more effective dose. Also, most germs enter your body through your nose and mouth. Doctors suggest that spraying EGCS into your nose or throat can stop cold and flu bugs, as well as relieve nasal infections and asthma. The best way to disinfect cuts and rashes is with a spray.

The only company that we found that makes EGCS with a spray top is Gero Vita International. They have a solution of 40 ppm of EGCS called "EGCS-40". To take it orally, remove the top and use it by the spoonful. EGCS-40 is available only by mail or phone order. Place phone orders at (800) 825-8482, Ext. Z101. Their address is 2255-B Queen Street East #820, Toronto, Ontario M4E 1G3, Canada.

20

∎ ∎ ∎

Live Cell Therapy for Liver Problems, Colds, Infections, Allergies, Headaches or Fatigue

WEALTHY PEOPLE FROM around the world take annual trips to Switzerland, not to check on their bank accounts, but to visit Clinique La Prairie for live cell therapy! This is not a new phenomenon. It has been going on since the 1940s.

Winston Churchill attributed his physical endurance to live cell therapy. French Prime Minister Charles De Gaulle claimed while in his seventies that his tremendous energy and power of concentration was due to live cell therapy. German Prime Minister Adenauer, although in his nineties, was the backbone of the rebuilding of Germany after World War II. He too made annual trips to Clinique La Prairie.

Charlie Chaplin fathered a child in his seventies. He told the press that live cell therapy made it possible because the therapy had increased his potency and virility. It is rumored that Cary Grant, George Burns, Bob Hope, Gloria Swanson and a host of other famous stars were regulars at Clinique La Prairie.

Pope Pius XII underwent live cell therapy and found the

results so remarkable that he inducted the discoverer, Dr. Paul Niehans, into the Papal Academy of Science.

■ What Is Live Cell Therapy?

Over twenty-four hundred years ago, Hippocrates, the father of medicine, theorized that if you had liver problems, the answer would be found in the healthy liver of a young animal because the livers of both man and animals operate almost exactly the same way. His theory applied to all organs and glands of the body: heart, lung, thymus, adrenals, spleen, etc. Needless to say, most modern doctors and scientists scoff at Hippocrates' theory.

In the 1930s, Dr. Niehans found a way to extract the valuable constituents from organs and glands. But, his success in curing patients with those extracts didn't impress most doctors and scientists. The mode of thinking in the medical field at the time was that if the cure wasn't a high-tech prescription drug, it wasn't any good. This attitude still persists today in the United States and to a large degree, but much less so, in Europe and Asia.

Although news of Dr. Niehans' success with live cell therapy spread throughout the world, it wasn't until the 1960s that scientists were forced to pay attention. At that time new technology made it possible for scientists to tag any substance with a radioactive isotope and then follow its path through your body.

Separate studies at two of Europe's most distinguished research centers, the University of Vienna and the University of Heidelberg, showed unquestionably that the vital constituents of a calf's gland or organ, when given to a human, went directly to the same gland or organ.

As scientists analyzed what was happening, it became very obvious why Dr. Niehans' live cell therapy was so successful. The calf's body had processed and converted food into not only selected vitamins and minerals, but also into unusual biochemicals specifically needed by particular glands or organs. *Some of these biochemicals were unattainable elsewhere*!

Dr. Niehans felt that the constituents of the gland or organ had to be extracted before the gland or organ began to deteriorate. He had his own cattle ranch next to Clinique La Prairie and butchered calves the same day he planned to use them. So, the gland or organ was still warm or "live" when he processed it.

Even though scientists had recognized the value of live cell therapy, there was still a big problem to overcome. Extracting the important substances was excruciatingly slow. That's why treatment at Clinique is so expensive.

Only recently has the progress in technology made it possible to do the extraction inexpensively and quickly. The cattle organs are processed while still fresh and then freeze-dried to retain their valuable nutrients. This caused the cost to drop steeply and now even the average person can afford this extremely beneficial therapy. You'll be amazed at what it is doing for people and what it can do for you.

Although your liver has several functions, it is the most important organ for metabolism. An improved metabolism creates a higher level of energy and a greater feeling of well-being. If you often feel tired, poor liver function is usually the culprit.

One of the most important nutrients needed by the liver is iron; however, the usual iron supplements may not be the answer. Less than 3 percent of iron supplements are absorbed by the body, and they often cause side effects, such as nausea, flatulence or diarrhea. Too much of those iron supplements can cause heart problems. The safest iron comes from animal liver and is called "heme" iron. Almost 35 percent ingested is absorbed, and there are no side effects.

Anemia is caused by a deficiency of iron and makes you very susceptible to infections. About 30 percent of the population is anemic. A double-blind study published in the *American Journal of Diseases in Children* by Dr. H. J. Kraitman showed that when iron was given regularly to children, the incident of infections dropped by almost 50 percent.

Dr. S. S. Basta reported in the *American Journal of Clinical Nutrition* that factory workers given iron had 33 percent fewer episodes of flu than those not taking it. He also found that those taking iron had 37 percent more stamina and endurance.

Several scientists have found that animal liver extracts are very helpful in ameliorating liver ailments. Liver extracts have much more than just iron in them; they also contain important liver enzymes, specific amino acids, and peptides. Dr. W. Boecker directed a double-blind clinical trial on one hunded forty-six patients with cirrhosis. Half were given a placebo and half took a liver extract. In a short period of time, 67 percent of those taking the liver extract showed significant improvement in liver function.

The liver is the only organ that can regenerate itself after damage by alcohol, disease or chemicals. However, the rebuilding process is normally slow. Had Dr. Boecker's trial proceeded for a longer period, many think the results would have been even better.

The same thinking applies to another double-blind study of 600 patients suffering from hepatitis. It was conducted by Dr. Kiyoshi Fujisawa at the Jikei University School of Medicine in Tokyo. In only twelve weeks, 35 percent of the patients taking a liver extract showed substantial improvement.

If you ever notice someone who likes to eat ice, it's a sure sign of liver problems or iron deficiency, according to British scientist, Dr. P. C. Elwood. In fact, anyone who likes to chew on nonfood items usually has the same problem. Pregnant women often have similar cravings due to additional nutrition demands of the growing fetus.

■ Allergies, Headaches and Many Other Ailments

Rarely does one see an article in magazines and newspapers about the thymus gland, though it probably affects our health more than any other gland. The thymus determines the health of your immune system and controls production of the disease-fighting cells—our prime protectors against illness.

If you suffer from any one of the following, your thymus may be responsible: chronic infections, eczema, dermatitis, asthma, hay fever, food or other allergies, chronic runny nose, headaches, yeast infections, herpes, arthritis, hepatitis, Epstein-Barr and chronic fatigue.

With today's technology, immunological defects are quite easy to detect, but thymus gland extracts are very helpful in restoring the immune system. Dr. Pietro Cazzola conducted a study of 130 patients with malfunctions of the immune system. He reported in a medical journal that treating those patients with thymic extracts effectively corrected the malfunctions.

The older you get, the less efficient your thymus becomes. However, several studies have shown that thymic extracts can substantially improve its function, according to Dr. D. M. Kouttab of the Roger Williams Hospital and Brown University.

Dr. Franco Pandolfi of the medical school at the University of Rome directed a double-blind clinical trial on elderly hospitalized patients. Half of the patients were given a thymic extract and half took a placebo. Those taking the extract had 86 percent fewer infections over a six-month period than those receiving the placebo.

If you get several colds or other respiratory ailments each year, your immune system is definitely weak. Dr. Alec Fiocchi led a double-blind clinical trial on patients with chronic respiratory infections. Half of the patients were given thymic extracts, and the other half received placebos. In only three months (but not during the winter cold season) those taking the thymic extracts had 31 percent fewer infections than the placebo group.

Scientists call rheumatoid arthritis an "autoimmune" disease because the body's own disease fighters (antibodies) actually attack and destroy some of the cartilage in the joints. Dr. Michael Murray, a well-known expert on natural medicine, says that clinical tests have shown that thymic extracts restore normal functioning to the affected joints by reducing the number of antibodies in that area. In other words, the extracts help keep this progressive ailment from getting worse, while allowing the body to do whatever repair it can.

Another overlooked organ is the spleen. It is located behind the lower portion of your rib cage on the left side. Its primary purposes are to produce white blood cells and destroy bacteria in the blood. Of course, white blood cells are your infantry or first line of defense against disease. If your spleen is not functioning well, you are probably going to be sick.

The most powerful substance found in spleen extracts is an enzyme called tuftsin. Dr. I. Florentin reported in the journal *Cancer Immunology* that laboratory animals given tuftsin showed an increase of disease-fighting cells by over 300 percent.

Your immune system becomes less and less efficient as you grow older. The most amazing attribute of tuftsin is its ability to reverse aging of the immune system. Dr. M. Bruley-Rosset gave elderly mice tuftsin for a few months. She reported in the journal *Annals of the New York Academy of Sciences* that the capacity of disease-fighting macrophages in these old mice was restored to the level of much younger mice.

Dr. M. Fridkin found that a deficiency of tuftsin is commonly found in people who get frequent infections as well as in cancer patients. AIDS patients also have very little tuftsin in their systems.

Many older people find even the simple chore of driving to the local supermarket extremely stressful. Years of handling the day-to-day stresses of life have caused the adrenal gland to skrink. This shrinkage means it operates less effectively.

Hundreds of thousands of people take the prescription drug, prednisone. It makes handling stress much more difficult, causes fatigue and reduces resistance to disease. There is a way to combat this problem. An extract from calf adrenal glands seems to revitalize human adrenal glands and make stress less noticeable. In fact, Dr. R. Bernardini found that adrenal extracts are more helpful than prescription drugs designed to reduce stress.

■ Heart to Heart

One of the most incredible sources of nutrients for the human heart is the heart tissue from cattle or sheep. Calf heart extracts have seventeen amino acids, five B vitamins, folic acid, calcium, iron, heparin, coenzyme Q10, cytochrome C and mesoglycan.

Folic acid helps stop the oxidation of "bad" cholesterol. Heparin's main function is to keep the blood from clotting. Coenzyme Q10 assists the heart muscle in energy production. Cytochrome C helps all cells in the body (including the heart) convert oxygen and nutrients to energy. The more cytochrome C in your body, the more energy you'll have.

The aorta is a large tubular chamber where blood leaves to fuel the body with oxygen-rich blood. This portion of the heart is composed mostly of an amazing substance called mesoglycan. In fact, all blood vessels are constructed with mesoglycan because it functions as structural support and much more.

Dr. G. Laurora and researchers from the Cardiovascular Institute conducted double-blind trials on patients with early stages of arteriosclerosis (clogged arteries). Half of the patients received mesoglycan, and half took a placebo.

A small section of one artery was scanned with a high-resolution ultrasound machine before and after the trials. At the end of eighteen months, the occlusion (clogging) of the arteries of the patients taking the placebo had increased seven times more than those taking mesoglycan. Several clinical trials have shown that mesoglycan also deters blood clots and reduces the risk of strokes—even for people who have severely clogged arteries.

■ More Help for the Liver

The liver helps regulate blood sugar levels and simultaneously breaks down fat through the secretion of bile, which helps absorb fat soluble vitamins A, D, E, F, and K. It filters over a liter of blood per minute, screening and purifying toxins out of the blood and removing them from the system. It's a four-pound miracle machine and the undisputed champ in the breakdown and metabolism of food and drugs.

The bad news is that the liver is an embattled gland, constantly under attack by a variety of damaging agents. High fat diets, drugs, dangerous chemical compounds, industrial pollutants, viruses and alcohol all cripple its ability to function smoothly.

If the liver becomes infected through viruses from contaminated food, syringes, needles, sexual secretions, or blood transfusions, it becomes inflamed and enlarged, releasing toxins into the bloodstream that produce fever, fatigue and yellow jaundice. If the liver becomes damaged by fat deposits from too much alcohol, then its hardened cells become impervious to cell regeneration, causing scarring or cirrhosis of the liver. It eventually becomes unable to process and filter blood. In short, if it's not properly treated, our body's chemical treatment plant becomes its own toxic waste site.

Working against the ravages of liver disease, a long list of scientific studies have confirmed what the Chinese and many European cultures have recognized for centuries—that there's a botanical garden of protecting compounds and substances that have a natural affinity to the liver. These compounds and substances act like blood brothers in preventing and alleviating liver disease. And some, like Taraxacum officinale, a.k.a. the dandelion, are literally in your own backyard.

This plant's seeds, stems and tooth-like leaves are rich in vitamins, minerals, protein, pectins and other catalytic substances that help the liver purify the blood of toxins. Containing enzyme-like agents that aid in cell metabolism, dandelions also stimulate the secretion of bile in the liver and gallstones. As a result, the dandelion root alleviates bile duct inflammation, hepatitis and jaundice, as reported by Dr. D. B. Mowery in the Scientific Validation of Herbal Medicine.

Other studies show that the dandelion has antiinflammatory properties and protects against liver enlargement. Dr. H. Santillo in *Natural Healing With Herbs,* confirms that dandelions have a high mineral content, which helps cure anemia.

The Encyclopedia of Common Natural Ingredients Used in Food, Drugs and Cosmetics reports that dandelions contain more vitamin A than carrots, explaining its therapeutic value in curing a variety of liver disorders. Additionally, dandelions contain the chemical choline, which plays a catalytic role in the breakup of fatty acid deposits. And while choline has not been shown to have a lipotropic or fat-removing effect in treating this condition in humans, it has a remarkable affinity to another amino acid that does—methionine.

This catalytic compound is the liver's best protection against alcohol-induced fatty liver. Methionine is a sulfur-containing amino acid that stimulates the body's production of lipotropic, or fat removing, agents and helps metabolize fatty acids, according to Dr. R. Montgomery in "Biochemistry: A Case Oriented Approach."

Methionine also guards against the depletion of glutathione in the body, essential to the metabolism of alcohol. Glutathione is a sulfur-containing protein that combines with toxic agents like alcohol and converts them into water-soluble compounds that are then eliminated from the body by way of the kidneys. By restoring high levels of glutathione to sustain this metabolic process, methionine has become the weapon of choice in defending the liver against alcohol-induced liver damage.

Extracts from the milk thistle plant have profound effects on treating all types of liver disease, from acute viral hepatitis to cirrhosis. The fruit, seeds and leaves of this plant, a member of the daisy family, contain the principle substance silymarin, which is more potent than vitamin E, as reported by Dr. R. F. Weiss in *Herbal Medicine*.

Silymarin, a flavonol, helps prevent liver tissue damage by scavenging free radical agents that are the offspring of fatty acid metabolism, according to Dr. H. Hikino in the journal *Planta Medica*. Dr. Hikino also found that silymarin stimulates the liver to synthesize its own chemical scavengers, which ingest these toxic particles and eliminate them from the system.

Its therapeutic effects have been confirmed by a wide range of studies, which showed that silymarin protects against such damaging chemicals as carbon tetrachloride in animals. It also produces none of the debilitating side effects common in other liver medications. What's more, silymarin even helps synthesize proteins in the liver that produce new liver cells, according to Dr. H. Wagner in *Natural Products as Medicinal Agents*. Like methionine, silymarin also prevents the depletion of glutathione, offering drinkers double protection against alcohol-induced fatty liver.

If you're a drinker and want to protect against fatty acid deposits which could lead to cirrhosis, Dr. Jane Heimlich, a noted nutritional authority, recommends a liver detoxification program two or three times a year that calls for taking 200 to 250 milligrams of silymarin daily for a month.

Carnitine is another substance that causes the breakup of these fatty acid villains. Manufactured in our own bodies and also obtained from red meat, this vitamin-like compound facilitates the conversion of fatty acids into energy, neutralizing their damaging effects on the liver. A 1984 study by Dr. D. S. Sachan appearing in the *American Journal of Clinical Nutrition* suggests that alcohol impairs the body's ability to synthesize carnitine and, thus, its ability to convert fatty acids into energy.

Dr. Sachan asserts that higher levels of carnitine in the body are necessary to handle the toxic overload from alcohol and high fat diets. By supplementing the liver with carnitine, those levels are restored, preventing fatty acid deposits from building up in the liver.

Extracts from the plant, *Cynara scolymum*, have an impressive track record in treating liver disorders. The active ingredient, cynarin, aids in the excretion of cholesterol and also stimulates the liver's ability to regenerate cells, according to Dr. H. Wagner in "Plant Flavonoids in Medicine." With over twenty million Americans diagnosed with gallstones attributed to high fat/low fiber diets and alcohol, maintaining the liver's ability to manufacture and transport bile is crucial.

Another plant, *Curcuma longa*, helps stimulate bile flow. Because of this ability it is specifically prescribed for gallbladder disorders in preventing the formation of gallstones, according to Dr. A. Y. Leung.

Artemisia capillaris and *Canna indica* are two more

botanicals that help stimulate bile flow. Additionally, *Canna indica* also protects the liver against viral hepatitis. As reported by Dr. H. M. Chang in *Pharmacology and Application of Chinese Materia Medica*, virtually a hundred out of a hundred cases of viral hepatitis were cured with mixtures of *Canna indica*, which made symptoms disappear.

While millions of Americans are courting hepatitis through indiscriminate sex and contaminated needles, millions more are unintentionally exposing themselves through contaminated food. Public health officials in Colorado recently reported an outbreak of hepatitis among thirty school children who became infected when a food server negligently failed to wash his hands. Barely escaping an epidemic, the conclusion is obvious. Everyone is at risk.

Like uninvited guests at a party, eliminating viral hepatitis from the system isn't easy. But a number of investigative studies have confirmed that many natural substances have a profound therapeutic effect in treating the disease. *Uncaria Gambier*, also known as catechin, is a flavonoid that significantly reduced serum bilirubin levels in patients suffering from acute viral hepatitis. The increased presence of bilirubin toxins in the blood lead to jaundice, a sickly pale yellowing of the skin.

In a double-blind study reported by Dr. H. Suzuki in the medical journal *Liver*, catechin improved liver blood tests two times faster than the control group. In another double-blind study, the control group experienced a return of appetite and more rapidly overcame symptoms of nausea, weakness, and stomach pain; skin color returned to normal in a short period of time.

Angelic sinensis (gentian root) is another natural substance shown to inhibit viral reproduction in forty cases studied. It also improves immune system functions and increases red blood cell count, and is effective in treating anemia. The gentian root is effective in treating jaundice. Clinical studies, according to Dr. H. M. Chang, revealed that it had healing effects on twenty-seven out of thirty-two patients suffering from hepatitis.

Extracts of the plant, *Glycyrrhiza glabra*, is yet another

in the long line of natural substances that inhibit viral reproduction in chronic hepatitis, according to Dr. Suzuki. It has also been shown to protect the liver against damage from toxic chemicals.

The beneficial role of vitamin C in promoting liver health has been well documented in several studies. Dr. F. R. Klenner, in the *Journal of Applied Nutrition* confirmed that daily doses of 40 to 100 grams of vitamin C, administered to patients with viral hepatitis, significantly relieved symptoms in two to four days and cleared up jaundice within six days. Although with this high dosage of vitamin C, the patients experienced severe diarrhea.

A double-blind study concluded that 2 grams or more of vitamin C each day prevented all participants in a controlled group of hospitalized patients from developing hepatitis B. Other studies report that vitamin C protects the liver from tissue damage by helping eliminate free radical agents often formed after the metabolic breakdown of fatty acids.

Longevity, say nutritional experts, is directly related to the health of your liver. In a toxic environment where exposure to liver-damaging agents has never been greater, scientists emphasize the importance of liver protectant therapies to ensure longer, healthier lives.

■ Sources of Substances Mentioned in this Chapter

Most of the products listed below are available at health food and vitamin stores. You might also locate some in Chinese herb shops.

Angelica sinensis (gentian root)
Artemisia capillaris
C vitamin
Canna indica
Carnitine
Catechin (Uncaria Gambier)
Choline
Curcuma Longa
Cynarin
Glycyrrhiza glabra

    Liver extracts
    Methionine
    Silymarin (mild thistle)
    Taraxacum officinale (dandelion root)
    Thymic extracts

Mail-order sources for these substances are available through:

Ethical Nutrients (800-692-9400) and L & H Vitamins (800-221-1152).

A product called D-Tox contains many of these substances, such as: carnitine, silymarin, cynarin, methionine, artemisia, liver extract, taraxacum, angelica and glutathione. D-Tox is available from:

    Gero Vita International
    2255-B Queen Street East #820, Dept. Z101
    Toronto, Ontario M4E 1G3, Canada
    (800) 825-8482, Ext. Z101

Gero Vita also manufactures one of the only multiglandular extracts called Bioactive Cell Complex, which contains pharmaceutical-grade extracts from the thymus, spleen, heart, liver, adrenals and lung tissue of healthy, young beef cattle. Gero Vita has added threonine, an amino acid that works in conjunction with tuftsin and *Laminaria* extract, which enhances the digestion and absorption of this product.

■ ■ ■

21

Hair Loss May Be Reversed—and Not with Rogaine (Minoxidil)

CAN ELEMENTS WITHIN our lifestyles play a role in helping accelerating or decelerating hair growth? Dietary deficiencies can contribute to gradual hair thinning. Serious disorders of the endocrine glands, such as the thyroid or pituitary, can result in hair loss. Exposure to nuclear radiation or the anticancer drugs are well known for the unfortunate baldness they produce as a common side effect.

Baldness is an inherited trait that is found with higher frequency among males. It's that male hormone, testosterone, that is the culprit here. In fact, hormonal imbalance may in part produce early baldness.

It is well known that a more sudden type of baldness can be produced by stress factors. Sometimes hair will turn gray almost overnight. Other times it will actually fall out. Illnesses such as the flu, typhoid fever or pneumonia—even excessive stress—all can play a role.

There is one pharmaceutical drug on the market that has been shown to produce hair in balding men. After all the hullabaloo, the problem with Rogaine is that you have to keep using it forever! Stop taking Rogaine and hair growth stops. Even worse, the hair that had been growing in falls out!

Besides the relatively high cost factor, it has been found to be most effective on younger men who have male pattern baldness who have only recently begun to lose some of their hair. Another unfortunate aspect of Rogaine is that sometimes it produces hair where the recipient might prefer it not appear! So be careful where you apply it.

The life of each hair on your head has a beginning and an end. But contrary to popular belief, hair growth is not continuous. If allowed to grow unchecked (never cut), a hair might reach three feet in length. That strand could sit on your head for three, four or even five years! But that doesn't mean hair growth is continuous.

There are three phases of hair growth. The anagen phase is when the hair is actively growing. A chemical compound, PDG, is known to stimulate hair production. Dr. D. Adachi, in 1987 at the World Congress of Dermatology, discussed the mechanism of this hair growth compound, which in scientific circles is called glucose "6" phosphate dehydrogenase, or PDG.

When hair growth slows down, it enters the catagen phase. During this period, there is a tapering of the growth pattern. Finally the hair stops growing altogether and eventually falls off the scalp. The latter represents the telogen phase. Obviously if we could shorten the catagen and prevent the telogen phases there would be many fewer scalps showing!

Under normal conditions, 90 percent of the hair found on a person's head is in the anagen phase. Only 10 percent, therefore, has stopped growing or will be coming out in the shower or onto the hairbrush and comb. If one could help the hair follicle switch back into the anagen phase, then perhaps hair loss could be prevented!

This provided the path for hundreds of researchers around the world to begin the search for substances which could switch hair follicles out of the catagen or telogen phases and back into the anagen phase.

Where did the path lead to? Odd-numbered fatty acids. After evaluations of almost three hundred different substances, Japanese researchers led by Dr. Kenkichi Oba demonstrated that application of a high energy-related substance found in actively growing hair, such as 3-carbon compound of pentadecanoic acid glyceride caused a 350 percent increase in the production of ATP in animal tests.

Dr. Oba has written about different products that stimulate hair growth. Helping the energy level during the anagen phase can prolong hair growth, he points out. Apparently, where baldness sets in, there is a reduction in the energy metabolism in the follicle.

Dr. Oba has shown that PDG (the same as G6PHD) even outperforms Rogaine. It seems to increase the metabolism of the hair roots and counteracts the androgenic hormone which hails the telogen (or falling-off-the-skull phase). Using PDG with 253 volunteers, men ranging in age from twenty-seven to sixty-two, were then evaluated by nineteen dermatologists in a double-blind clinical test. The PDG solution won over the falling hairs! Both men and women can take comfort in knowing it is permanent help.

Dr. Oba did not observe any harsh side effects in blood analyses, liver functions or in urine samples. Now PDG has a big following in Japan and Germany.

Perhaps the best known nutrient for healthy hair is biotin. This coenzyme assists carboxylation reactions (introducing carbon dioxide into a compound with resultant formation of carboxylic acid). In the case of the follicular energy cycle, empirical data have been gathered that show its power to renew hair growth when applied topically. This process can reverse thinning and depigmentation of the hair.

Ginseng roots have been used medicinally for thousands of years in China. Dr. John Chang reported in *Cosmetics and Toiletries* magazine on the use of ginseng for prevention of hair loss. Apparently it offers protection to hair and prevents brittleness.

It has been found that it is possible to extract and refine hinokitiol oil from a Japanese tree, called hiba. Also a similar oil from the western red cedar can be extracted as well. The result is (b-Thujaplicin), which was discovered in Formosa by Dr. Zozao. Hinokitiol has a very rare seven-membered organic ring compound, or carbocyclic chemical.

When hinokitiol copper salt was mixed into a tonic used to treat areas deprived of hair, Japanese studies showed that thicker hair growth occurred. Then, at the University of Nihon's Department of Dermatology, a study was done with eleven patients, both male and female. Downy hair growth occurred between seven and sixty days.

Another study using hinokitiol was conducted at Chiba University's Department of Dermatology. This time ten patients were treated for alopecia areata. Here, 60 percent effectiveness was noted, with downy hair growing within two months. Another study performed in a Tokyo hospital on fifty patients yielded similar results (68 percent effective in growing downy hair).

Other remedies include Orizanol, a derivative from rice oil, which stimulates microcirculation and acts as an antioxidant. There is a Japanese botanical that is applied topically to stimulate hair roots to hasten growth, called swertia (toyaku in China).

Another Japanese product, Takanal, demonstrated in a clinical study 92 percent effectiveness in growing downy and, eventually, coarser hair. It has been approved for use in cosmetic preparations by the Japanese Ministry of Health and Welfare.

In one study published by Dr. Takashima in the 1985 *Journal of Clinical Therapeutics and Medicine*, a placental extract was used on the scalps of twenty-seven balding men. Over 70 percent were noted to have a reduction in hair loss. The explanation was that the placental extract was a kind of cell enhancer or activator. The application of the extract led to additional oxygen being provided to the cells from the blood; hence, hair rejuvenation.

Three amino acids are known to offer nutritional support to hair. These are cysteine, serine and glutamic acid. Dr. Nishimjima, from Japan, added takanol to the amino compound that he applied topically to the scalp. In his work, the addition of Takanol brought an ample supply of these amino acids, which are not easily available through diet, and the result was accelerated, thicker hair growth.

There are trichopeptides (amino acids directly affecting

the hair) that stimulate the receptors that enhance cell growth. Dr. Mendes and Dr. Taub, two scientists from Europe, tested sixty people with trichopeptides, both men and women, who suffered from alopecia. They were successful in the majority of cases and noted that the women had a 100 percent improvement!

Double-blind tests show that a compound called Tri-Genesis produced a 227 percent increase of vellus hair count within six months. AMA Laboratories, an independent certified testing laboratory in New York, performed a clinical study using the standard double-blind methods over a six-month period. Dr. Martin Schulman directed this study of Tri-Genesis, which was reviewed by a board-certified dermatologist.

In addition to the remarkable increase in hair count, this study showed that 78 percent of the people studied had a successful outcome. More than three-quarters of the subjects who participated in this study benefited with improved hair growth. Clearly, such success might be worth investigating before resorting to more drastic procedures such as surgery.

This essential component of the product is a naturally occurring source of a unique, uneven-chained (odd-numbered) fatty acid, a-angelica lactone. It has been found that this ingredient dramatically reduces the resting stage of hair follicles and actually gives each hair a tremendous burst of energy.

Dr. Oba discovered what a specific odd-numbered fatty acid was doing to cause hair growth. Science Forum 2000, reported, "His team found biological evidence how uneven-chained fatty acids increased the amount of ATP (energy) to the hair follicles. In 1987, governments in Japan and Germany approved the sale of products containing these active agents."

Another scientist, this time from China, developed an herbal formula to prevent hair loss. When the skeptical Japanese examined Dr. Zhao's formula, they found safflower extract, ginko and ginseng, all excellent vasodilators.

The action of a vasodilator is to enhance blood flow.

Rogaine (minoxidil) is a vasodilator. In the case of hair, when there is a more abundant supply of blood to the hair follicles, this nourishment seems to enhance hair growth. Those who experience hair loss, including those who lose hair prematurely may not be receiving ample blood supply to the roots of their hair.

The Tri-Genesis formula contains many of those substances that have been found to be effective in hair growth stimulation. The innovative contribution by those who created this product, however, is that the various active ingredients can now all be found within the same formula. To summarize, these ingredients are:

TRF or Tissue Respiratory Factors in the liposomal delivery system helps cells use oxygen. The critical phase of oxygen uptake, before the anagen phase, is when these factors come into play, just before the changes occur that result in enhanced hair growth.

B-Glycyrrhetinic acid, also in the liposomal delivery system, acts as an anti-inflammatory agent and is a reductase (an enzyme) inhibitor.

Biotin is a coenzyme for carboxylation reactions (introduction of oxygen) in the follicular energy cycle. Topical application has resulted in rejuvenated hair.

Oleum serenoa repens liosterolic is an extract that counteracts the conversion of testosterone to dihydrostestosterone (DHT) and inhibits DHT binding to cellular and nuclear receptor sites, thereby increasing DHT breakdown.

Swertia and Dangui are sources of 5-hydroxygenteopicroside (Swertianmarin), and has been shown to activate ATP, DNA and G6PDH activity.

Pregnenolone acetate exercises dermatographic activity similar to B-estradiol with no hormonal side effects. A-Angelical actone derived from 15-hydroxypentadecanoic acid, increases follicular metabolism. Sodium undecylenate-NA, (salt of undecylenic acid) is a fatty acid that occurs in sweat and may contribute to increased follicular metabolism.

Undecylenamid DEA, an undecylenic acid diethanolamide, has anti-fungal and anti-dandruff activity. Tocopheryl acetate enzymatically bioconverts in the skin into an active form which activates ATP, DNA and G6PDH in hair follicles. Tocopheryl nicotinate improves blood flow. Niacin improves blood flow and accelerates function.

■ Sources of Substances Mentioned in this Chapter

A number of the products mentioned in this chapter can be located in health food and vitamin stores, such as:

biotin
ginseng root
swertia.

Further information about Tri-Genesis is available by writing to Tri-Genesis Corp., 520 Washington Boulevard, Suite 385, Marina del Rey, California 90291; or call (800) 654-0456.

Products listed below may be found in Japanese or Chinese pharmacies or herb shops in the major cities in the country.

Hinokitiol
Orizanol
Takanal

There are herbal preparations which can be found in local health food stores that will contain one or more of the ingredients listed in this chapter, although not necessarily specifically prepared for purposes of hair regeneration. Check with your local merchant.

22

■ ■ ■

Stop Insomnia, Jet Lag, Breast Cancer and Live Longer

SLEEP PATTERNS VARY from person to person and are affected by such factors as age, chronic pain, breathing problems, or emotional disturbances like anxiety or depression. As people age, they require less sleep. Although this change may be described as insomnia, it is a normal phenomenon and can be managed by increasing exercise during the day and using various relaxation techniques.

When sleeplessness often stems from anxiety, it is usually temporary and is resolved as the troublesome situation is solved. Breathing problems such as sleep apnea can be treated with surgery, weight loss or medication.

Although various medications are prescribed for insomnia, prolonged use is associated with the risk of addiction, overdose and increased tolerance, which leads to the need for higher doses in order to fall asleep. In addition, sleep patterns can be disturbed once the drugs are discontinued, creating a cycle of dependency. This also results in confusion, anxiety and symptoms of dementia, especially in the elderly. Therefore, sleep experts discourage long-term use of sedative medication and recommend natural methods to induce sleep once other causes of insomnia are ruled out.

A natural sleeping aid is an extract from the valerian root. As Dr. Olov Lindahl reported in a study published in *Pharmacology, Biochemistry and Behavior*, "Valerian has been used as a medication for as long as historical information has been available."

Dr. Peter Leathwood conducted a double-blind, placebo-controlled study of valerian, which was also documented in *Pharmacology, Biochemistry and Behavior*. The one hundred and sixty-six subjects taking valerian reported improved sleep, without the usual "hangover" feeling associated with conventional sleep medications. In addition, smokers in the study found that they slept more soundly.

Valerian is nonaddictive, and its effects are not amplified by alcohol intake, thus eliminating two of the risks of narcotic sleep medications. As Dr. Andrew Weill noted in his book *Natural Health, Natural Medicine*, "Valerian is a safe and effective sleeping aid, more powerful than l-tryptophan or such sedative herbs as hops and skullcap."

In addition, it provides relief from such stress-related symptoms as headaches, irritability and fatigue. Valerian is commonly used in Europe. In France, for example, over one million people take valerian capsules regularly.

The pineal gland in the brain controls our sleep processes. When it receives information from the optic nerves that the sun has gone down, it causes serotonin in the brain to be converted into melatonin. As melatonin levels rise in the bloodstream, a sedative effect is obtained, thus inducing sleep. At dawn, the process is reversed.

When you are young and have insomnia, it is usually due to anxiety. As you get older, a lowered production of serotonin due to aging or lack of sufficient brain nutrients, reduces the available melatonin, which makes it more difficult for you to go to sleep.

A study in the journal *Biologic Psychiatry* demonstrated that when persons with insomnia took melatonin before bedtime, they slept for longer periods, without impairing their daytime alertness. Additional research described in *Psychopharmacology* indicated that melatonin helped patients fall asleep faster, stay asleep longer, and have heightened energy levels upon awakening.

Melatonin is responsible for controlling our circadian or biorhythmic cycles. In other words, our body clock. Dr. Al Lewy, of the Oregon Health Sciences University in Portland, has conducted numerous successful experiments with low doses of melatonin, enabling adults to shift their body clocks forward and backward. Dr. Lewy believes that these findings can be applied to those who must work varying shifts, so that they can adjust to their changing schedules more easily and avoid the health problems caused by lack of sleep.

Traveling across the country or continents and crossing multiple time zones in a short time is a fact of life for many people today. Unfortunately, air travel can cause a phenomenon known as circadian dysrhythmia, or "jet lag." It is a strange phenomena because some people feel jet lag more in one direction than in the other.

Characterized by fatigue, disturbed sleep patterns, impaired concentration and various other symptoms, jet lag usually requires twenty-four to forty-eight hours before the body adjusts to local time.

It is also thought that the effects of jet lag can be diminished by gradually adjusting sleep patterns to the destination time a few days before departure and avoiding alcohol while in flight. In addition to its ability to safely induce sleep, melatonin has also been found to alleviate the symptoms of jet lag in many travelers.

A double-blind, placebo-controlled study published in the *British Journal of Medicine* reported that male and female subjects of varying ages were given 5 milligrams of melatonin for two days before, during and two days after a round-trip flight between London, England and Auckland, New Zealand. When compared to the group that was given a placebo, those who received melatonin were able to adapt their sleep patterns more readily to the new time zone and had increased energy.

It is important to note that the melatonin *must* be taken at a time equivalent to dusk in the proposed destination before you leave, during the flight at dusk and again at dusk when you arrive at your destination. Otherwise, it doesn't seem to have much effect. Apparently, the timed doses help set up a new dawn-dusk cycle in your body.

■ Slow the Aging Process

In addition to its other properties, melatonin has also shown the potential to delay the aging process. At the Institute of Integrative Bio-Medical Research in Switzerland, Dr. Walter Pierpaoli noted that mice lived for the equivalent of twenty additional human years when given melatonin, and that many symptoms related to aging were delayed or even reversed.

As Dr. Keith Kelley reported in *Medical Hypotheses*, "Melatonin deficiency syndrome is perhaps the basic mechanism through which aging changes can be explained in a simple causative action. This may require replacement of melatonin in order to achieve a more youthful endocrine balance . . . and subsequently repair the body as a whole."

Since melatonin controls our daily body clocks, scientists believe it may also control our aging clocks. Decreased levels of melatonin are thought to adversely affect all body systems, causing them to operate less efficiently and creating changes commonly associated with aging. Most twenty-five-year-olds have four times the level of melatonin in their bodies as sixty-year-olds. As a result, Dr. Pierpaoli suggests that daily melatonin supplements be taken after age fifty, and believes that by doing so, ninety- to one hundred-year life spans are possible.

Melatonin has also been found to lower cholesterol, according to Dr. Georges Maestroni of the Institute of Pathology in Locarno, Switzerland. In his study, subjects with elevated cholesterol who were given melatonin experienced a 15 to 30 percent decrease in LDL (artery-clogging) cholesterol, while those with normal cholesterol levels were not affected.

Seasonal affective disorder (SAD) is a form of depression that occurs in some people during the winter months when there is less daylight. Clinical tests have shown that patients suffering from SAD can be relieved by exposure to bright lights for two hours a day. They believe that this process causes increased melatonin production during the night, thus lessening or eliminating depressive symptoms.

■ Sources of Substances Mentioned in this Chapter

Melatonin and valerian are available in many health food and vitamin stores.

23

You Can Live Longer, Healthier, No Matter How Old You Are Now

UNTIL RECENTLY, MEDICAL science has been more concerned with the treatment of diseases associated with old age than with aging. Scientists have only seriously begun to look at the causes of aging in the last decade. In 1900 the average life expectancy for a man living in the U.S. was 49.5 years; in 1955 the average rose to 68.5 years. Today the average life span in America is about 72.1 years for the males and 79 years for females, a 46 percent increase since the turn of the century!

The *Wall Street Journal* reported that in 1950 the probability of a sixty-five-year-old American reaching age ninety was 7 percent, but forty years later it was 25 percent. According to *USA Today,* in the past decade the number of Americans a hundred years or older doubled to 35,800. The *Wall Street Journal* predicted that by 2050 the number of centenarians would number in the millions.

After the age of maturity, usually around twenty-five to thirty years, the body begins to deteriorate at the rate of .7 percent a year. The average weight for an adult human brain is 1,500 grams. At the age of seventy, the brain's mass is reduced to 1,000 grams. One third of the brain is no longer there! Along with the brain, every major organ in the body is affected by this slow process. This self-destruction process has been confirmed by Dr. Roy Walford, one of the nation's leading anti-aging researchers and founder of the immunological theory of aging.

Although serious research on the aging process is fairly new, there have been a number of discoveries that not only promise to increase average life span, but the quality of life will be immeasurably increased as we grow older! "What drives most of this research is not the desire to be immortal, it's the desire not to die in a nursing home," says Dr. Richard Sprotta, biologist with the National Institute of Aging. "I think most of us would trade dying at age eighty-five rather than one hundred and five if we knew we could be healthy up to eighty-five, then we could have one last cigar or bourbon and kick off."

Dr. Michael West, a molecular biologist at the University of Texas Southwestern Medical Center in Dallas, discovered that two mortality genes, M-1 and M-2, can speed aging or reverse the aging process, depending on whether they are turned "on" or "off." Aging cells normally have the M-1 turned in the "on" position. In an experiment reported in the *Chicago Tribune*, Dr. West successfully turned the M-1 gene "off." The aging cells reversed their aging, becoming younger and increasing the number of times they could divide. By turning the M-2 gene off, cells appeared to go on agelessly, dividing indefinitely.

Dr. West told *Chicago Tribune* reporters, "There is no turning back, for the first time in history we have the power to manipulate aging on a very profound level." He went on to speculate that by controlling these genes, life expectancy would eventually extend to two hundred, four hundred or even five hundred years.

Dr. Michael R. Rose, at the University of California at Irvine, has successfully bred a strain of fruit fly that is able to live twice as long as the ordinary fruit fly. The super flies are also far more robust than their ordinary counterparts.

They produce a more effective form of the cellular antioxidant, superoxide dismutase. Dr. Rose told *Scientific American*, "The work on drosophila is trial-run stuff for doing the same thing in mice. If we can create long-lived mice, specific genes, enzymes and cell processes involved in longevity should be revealed."

Dr. Thomas Johnson, a biologist with the Institute for Behavioral Genetics at the University of Colorado in Boulder, discovered that the life span of roundworms can be doubled by altering a single gene. This was the first successful attempt to significantly increase an animal's life span through manipulation of genetic controls. *Scientific American* reported, "Strikingly, the mutant worms produce elevated levels of antioxidants (both cytoplasmic superoxide dismutase and an enzyme called catalase) and are more resistant to the toxic effects of paraquat, a herbicide that leads to generation of the superoxide radical."

Based on research by molecular biologist Dr. Thomas Maciag of the American Red Cross's Jerome Holland Laboratory for the Biosciences, it was discovered that the life span of skin cells is doubled by switching off a gene that controls production of the protein called interleukin 1. The technique used by Maciag to turn off the gene is called antisense. Antisense is currently used to create ageless tomatoes that stay ripe indefinitely.

Dr. W. Wright and Dr. J. Shay, from the University of Texas Medical Center, have found a genetic mechanism that causes cells to die. The researchers discovered a way to deactivate this "death" mechanism. Cells with the deactivated mechanism live indefinitely without aging.

Dr. Richard Cutler of the National Institute on Aging Gerontology Research Center in Baltimore says that the human life span is not set in stone. He sees no reason why our descendants won't achieve an average life expectancy of two hundred years.

There are theories—other than the genetic cause of aging—that are receiving attention from prominent scientists the world over. The free radical theory of aging has received the most attention and positive results achieved through antioxidant treatments have been well established. The free radical theory of aging is based on importance of oxygen. Dr. Denham Harmon is considered the discoverer of the free radical theory of aging. Beginning in 1954, he formed one of the most important theories on life extension developed in the twentieth century. Harmon asserts that oxygen-based compounds (oxygen free radicals) in the human body are primary causes of aging. "Chances are 99 percent that free radicals are the basis of aging," says Harman.

In an article written for the *Chicago Tribune*, Dr. R. Kotulak amplified, "Aging is the ever-increasing accumulation of changes caused or contributed to by free radicals."

Dr. Earl Stadman, chief of the laboratory of biochemistry of the National Heart, Lung and Blood Institute in Bethesda, Maryland, agrees that damage from oxygen free radicals contributes heavily to accelerating the aging process. The free radical theory is more important than science was previously willing to accept. Life span is dependent on cellular damage caused by oxygen free radicals. The body's cells do resist some oxygen damage, but eventually these cells become so damaged that they can no longer function. Studies suggest that oxygen free radical reactions cause the age-related deterioration of the cardiovascular and central nervous systems. Dr. Harmon says that free radical reactions may also be significantly involved in the formation of the neurotic plaques associated with senile dementia of the Alzheimer type. Senile people showed higher levels of plaques than those found in healthy people.

Time magazine describes free radicals as " . . . great white sharks in the biochemical sea. Cellular renegades wreaking havoc by damaging DNA, altering biochemical compounds, corroding cell membranes and killing cells outright, scientists believe such molecular mayhem plays a major role in the development of ailments like cancer, heart or lung disease, and cataracts. The cumulative effects of free radicals also underlie the gradual deterioration that is the hallmark of aging in all individuals."

Oxygen free radicals differ from stable oxygen molecules—the electronically charged particles (electrons) that make up free radicals are unpaired and unbalanced. The chemical process for creating energy in the human body is an imperfect process. It often strips an electron from an oxygen atom, creating an unpaired electron and a very unstable molecule. This alone sets the free radical apart. Their action against cells is called oxidation.

Did you ever notice metal rusting or an apple turning brown? These are common examples that we see occurring every day caused by the process of oxidation. Eventually the metal and the apple will slowly disintegrate to nothing. Free radicals are elusive and extremely difficult to study, as they live only a millionth of a second. Yet many respected scientists believe that oxygen free radicals are responsible for numerous ailments affecting the human body. These illnesses include: atherosclerosis, Alzheimer's disease, cancer, Parkinson's disease, Down's syndrome, stroke, paralysis, cataracts, arthritis, emphysema, wrinkling and memory loss. The list is increasing daily.

A simple way to understand free radicals is that they are sparks. If you've ever had a spark hit your skin and felt it burn, you can imagine the damage a free radical does when it hits a delicate cell.

Helen Brody, a sixty-five-year-old retired State Department employee, is blessed with a double dose of "Methuselah" genes—named after the biblical character who lived for nine hundred sixty-nine years, according to the *Bible*. Scientists don't expect Helen to live for nine hundred sixty-nine years, but an excess of one hundred years is a reasonable estimate.

Helen's physician, Dr. William Harris, head of the lipid laboratory at the University of Kansas Medical Center, says, "She's preventing free radical damage like crazy. Her arteries are probably squeaky clean."

Dr. Michael Rose, an experimental biologist at the University of California, inserted extra Methuselah genes in fruit flies and doubled their lives. Probably, in a couple of decades, we will be able to do this for humans.

We all have one Methusaleh gene, which is responsible for producing a substance in our bodies called "superoxide dismutase" or SOD. It is found in the mucus surrounding *every* cell in your body. SOD's sole function is to destroy free radicals (oxidants) before they hit the cells. It is *the most powerful antioxidant known to scientists.*

Your body is a chemical factory. You eat food, drink liquids and breathe air to keep it running. In the process of converting food and liquids to the chemicals the body needs, free radicals are created. It's SOD's job to destroy them.

From birth to about twenty-five years of age, your body produces enough SOD to destroy most of the free radicals created in the process of breaking down food. Each year after twenty-five, the body produces less and less SOD, but the quantity of free radicals never drops. Consequently, every part of the body is eventually damaged as cells are destroyed or their DNA mutated by oxidation.

As you get older, with less SOD to protect the cells, the free radicals kill cells faster than they can reproduce. The result is that each organ either shrinks in size, or its ability to function properly diminishes. As your brain is reduced in size, you have decreased memory, slower mental response, reduced alertness and a diminished ability to handle stress.

Livers and kidneys, excessively damaged by free radicals, can't remove toxins and waste efficiently. The damage to cells in the lungs prevents them from putting enough oxygen into the bloodstream; you tire faster.

The skin becomes thinner, losing its smoothness, and wrinkles form. The eyes develop cataracts. Joints lose their ability to lubricate properly, bringing pain and stiffness. Muscles become thinner, losing their strength. The pancreas doesn't produce enough digestive juices, causing indigestion and bowel problems.

Aging of the central control of the body, the brain, causes more health problems than any other area. Norepinephrine is a key compound that maintains primary brain functions. A reduction in this substance usually brings on accelerated aging and depression. Dr. C. Cohen of the Mount Sinai School of Medicine in New York showed in clinical tests that free radicals quickly destroy norepinephrine, while SOD and some other antioxidants try to deter the destruction. The devestating Lou Gehrig's disease occurs when SOD production in the brain stops altogether.

One of the food products that results in the greatest production of free radicals in our bodies is polyunsaturated fats! This is ironic because millions of people have switched from saturated fats to polyunsaturated for cooking with the hope of reducing their chances of heart disease. Animals fed polyunsaturated fats in their diets showed a dramatic increase in free radicals and an increase in tumors, while those fed saturated fats had much lower free radical counts and fewer tumors.

The polyunsaturated fat users are actually accelerating the aging of their cells. Dr. Harry Demopoulos, the world-famous professor at the New York University School of Medicine, said, "If I were forced to choose between the two, high cholesterol is a lesser hazard to health."

He is probably right, because heart disease researchers say that cholesterol is not the problem, but that it is the *oxidation* of the cholesterol that causes arteriosclerosis. Free radicals cause the oxidization.

Researchers at Duke University's Department of Medicine and Biochemistry have demonstrated the immense power of SOD. They took white blood cells and split them into two groups. SOD was introduced into one group. Then they created free radicals in both groups. The SOD-protected cells remained alive, while the other group died.

They took some more white blood cells and split them into two groups. SOD was introduced into one group. Then they put carcinogens (cancer-causing material) into both groups. The SOD-protected culture remained healthy, while the other group became cancerous.

Dr. Richard Cutler, former director of the government's National Institute of Aging commented that numerous studies have shown that in virtually all species, *those that live the longest have the highest levels of SOD!*

Anyone exposed directly to nuclear radiation dies because an incredible amount of free radicals are immediately created in the body. No amount of SOD can be introduced quickly enough to stop the mass destruction of the cells. Eventually, those exposed to such intense radiation die. One scientist said the process is like each cell is electrocuted individually. The few that survive become mutated and are unlikely to reproduce healthy cells.

Bacteria grow everywhere—but would you believe that there is even a bacteria that lives inside nuclear reactors? It is called a "radiodurans," and there is no living thing on earth that has more SOD in it per gram of body weight. Obviously, that is why it can survive in the reactor.

SOD was discovered in 1968 by Dr. Irwin Fridovich at Duke University. Since then, a multitude of scientists worldwide have found that even though the Methusaleh gene is programmed to make SOD, it can't be produced unless three nutrients are present—copper, zinc and manganese. Biochemists have synthesized SOD and you can find it in stores, but don't buy it. It is destroyed in the stomach. The only way you can increase the levels of SOD in your body is to take zinc, copper and manganese.

A study conducted at Pennsylvania State University showed that the recommended portions of the four basic food groups do not provide adequate amounts of the minerals copper, zinc and manganese. The reason for the deficiency of these minerals in our foods is simple. If the minerals don't exist in sufficient quantities in the soil, the plants can't extract them.

Years of farming with chemical fertilizers that commonly don't contain zinc, copper or manganese has almost totally depleted our farm and ranch soils of these minerals and of many others.

Dr. Denham Harmon, professor emeritus of the University of Nebraska School of Medicine and the discoverer of the free radical aging connection, said, "Over 90 percent of the people in North America have a zinc deficiency."

Dr. Mireille Dardenne, a prominent French scientist, found that as we age, our bodies' ability to process zinc diminishes, and the function of our very important thymus glands decline because of zinc deficiencies. The thymus glands are often called the "youth glands." However, Dr.

Dardenne said that zinc " . . . can be restored to youthful levels with only six months of zinc supplementation."

Dr. A. S. Prasad assembled 180 elderly people who appeared to be healthy to determine the amount of zinc in their bodies. He found that exactly 20 percent had severe zinc deficiencies, and almost 70 percent had mild deficiences. Supplementation corrected their deficiencies. If your taste buds don't seem to be operating very well and food tastes bland, that is a sure sign of an *extreme* deficiency of zinc.

The National Cancer Institute reported that the tissues surrounding tumors are almost always low in zinc as well as copper and manganese. If you have a zinc deficiency, you will have a copper deficiency automatically because copper can't be metabolized (used) by the body without zinc. Although copper is necessary for the body's production of SOD, copper by itself has SOD-like qualities as an antioxidant. Dr. Ludovit Bergendi found that copper has anti-inflammatory actions that are important to arthritis and back pain sufferers.

The third mineral in the SOD family, manganese, also operates as an antioxidant throughout the body, and specifically protects heart muscle cells from free radicals, according to studies by Dr. Elise Malecki at the University of Wisconsin Nutritional Research Center. Dr. C. D. Davis of the same research group proved with a double-blind, placebo-controlled trial that manganese alone could increase the SOD levels in the blood.

Recently, scientists discovered that an enzyme called glutathione (GT) is actually a powerful assistant to SOD in fighting free radicals. It appears that GT joins SOD in the brain, eyes, liver, kidneys, heart, ears and joints to destroy free radicals. To simplify how it works technically, you might say that SOD takes one side of the street in an organ while GT takes the other to keep free radicals at bay.

Although most free radicals are a result of oxygen combustion in the cells, there are other types of free radicals. The most common one is the hydrogen peroxide free radical. GT simply reduces it to water.

GT is created by the body from other nutrients, although a few foods have small amounts; and, just like SOD, its production by the body continually drops as we get older. Autopsies of the brains of people who have died of Parkinson's disease show deficient levels of GT. Dr. J. D. Adams and Dr. I. N. Odunse of the University of California found that proper levels of GT are important in deterring the onset of Parkinson's disease.

Dr. M. L. Torres found that when GT levels were increased in the brains of elderly mice, they lived 46 to 91 percent longer if the supplementation continued for at least fourteen months.

A study conducted at the University of Louisville School of Medicine showed that the GT content in red blood cells decreases with age. Dr. George Hazelton, one of the scientists, stated, " . . . the present evidence suggests that a low GT content may be a general phenomenom in all aging tissue."

Dr. C. M. Farber and Dr. D. N. Kanganis of the New York University School of Medicine reported that " . . . several disease processes have been associated with decreased GT levels."

Dr. L. W. Oberley of the University of Iowa Radiation Research Laboratory reported in the medical journal, *Molecular and Cellular Biochemistry,* "GT appears to be the most important antioxidant enzyme in animal and human cells [after SOD]."

Dr. Roger Williams of the University of Texas found that GT is a very powerful anti-tumor agent, and an aid in the treatment of allergies, cataracts, diabetes, hypoglycemia and arthritis, as well as a protector against tobacco smoke and alcohol.

Harvard Medical School scientist, Dr. Gareth Green says that a study has shown that GT is intimately related to phagocytic activity of lung cells. The phagocytes gobble up harmful bacteria, dust particles and tobacco smoke.

Dr. Robert Atkins, author of the bestselling book, *Dr. Atkins' Diet Revolution,* said on a recent radio show, "GT disarms the toxicity of fats in our diets and expels them in urine. GT is a wonder drug even though it is a nutrient—one which can be used in a good tumor deterrence program."

Dr. Atkins was joined on the show by another famous scientist, Dr. Harry Demopolis. They went on to say that German scientists have given GT to rats with liver cancer in a double-blind, placebo-controlled study. Afterward, the animals were examined, and the tumors had completely regressed, leaving only a small scar where the tumor had been.

The primary reason HIV causes AIDS is that HIV depletes all the GT in the body, which allows massive destruction of the disease-fighting cells by free radicals. Anyone with any type of disease, such as diabetes, arthritis, heart or artery problems, osteoporosis, asthma, kidney malfunctions, lupus, allergies, chronic fatigue and even people who are chronically cranky, will have low levels of GT.

It is a major nutrient for the brain and helps produce GABA, which is a calming agent. The liver can't do its job without GT. And through its actions in the brain and liver, GT controls craving for alcohol and sometimes sweets. Dr. A. Wendel states in his book, *Functions of Glutathione,* that many scientists believe GT will help protect against alcohol-induced liver damage.

Dr. R. Greco and Dr. G. Menecacci of the University of Siena, Italy, found that people with cataracts had 60 percent less GT in their blood than those with normal vision. Other scientists have confirmed that the GT antioxidant activity in the eyes is more intense than that of any other free radical fighter. Free radicals are the prime suspect in the formation of cataracts.

In a double-blind, placebo-controlled study of GT on laboratory animals, Dr. M. L. Torres found that those getting GT in their diets lived from 46 to 91 percent longer than the placebo-fed animals, if the supplementation continued for at least fourteen months. That study suggests that the longer you take GT, the more effective it becomes.

Although health food and vitamin stores promote and sell synthetic GT, don't buy it. Numerous clinical tests have shown that *the body simply will not absorb it.* The body makes its own GT from the amino acids cysteine and glutamic acid, which should be taken daily.

All of us need to get sunshine because it stimulates the production of vitamin D. However, everyone knows the danger of ultraviolet rays (UV) to the skin. Recently, Dr. Donald Darr at the Duke University Medical Center found that both vitamin C and GT are destroyed in the skin during even mild exposure to UV. Anyone who spends hours a day in the sun should be aware of this and supplement their diets after UV exposure.

GT works in synergy with vitamins C and E, the most well-known antioxidants. Actually, GT protects them from oxidation, making those antioxidants last longer in the body before they are depleted. However, GT can't be used in any way without selenium being present. Selenium, another powerful antioxidant, is needed for the metabolism of GT.

Every state east of the Mississippi River, as well as Oregon, Washington and Idaho have soils with little or no selenium. Common fertilizers don't contain selenium, so food and animals grown in these areas are deficient in it.

The most potent outside sources of free radicals are noxious gases from cars, industrial fumes and cigarette smoke. Those gases cause what is called "respiratory burst reactions" (RBR) in your lungs, which are bursts of free radicals attacking lung membranes. Dr. Jorgen Clausen published a study in the journal *Biological Trace Element Research,* showing that smokers have almost 33 percent less vitamin E in their bodies than non-smokers because the nutrient is used in fighting excess free radicals. Dr. Clausen also found that heavy supplementation of vitamin E and selenium reduced free radicals by up to 75 percent. (You must take selenium with vitamin E because the vitamin can't be metabolized without selenium).

▪ The World's Oldest and Most Powerful Antioxidant

In the winter of 1534 French explorer, Jacques Cartier landed his ship on the shores of the St. Lawrence River in Quebec, Canada. Tragedy stuck however, when the river froze over, stranding the ship. Cartier and his crew had been living for three months on salted meat and biscuits. Shortly after his arrival in Canada, twenty-five men in his one hundred and ten-man crew died of scurvy and fifty more were seriously ill.

In desperation, Cartier approached a friendly Indian tribe and asked to see their medicine man. The medicine man told Cartier to make a tea for the men from the bark and needles of the Anneda pine tree. Within a week most of his crew had miraculously recovered. When the spring thaw came, Cartier's ship left for Europe with several chests filled with Anneda pine bark and needles.

Recently scientists discovered that vitamin C by itself cured scurvy very slowly, but when a citrus bioflavonoid was added, the cure was quick. Analysis showed that much of vitamin C is destroyed in the body by oxidation. The bioflavonoid prevented vitamin C's oxidation and was a potent vitamin C helper. So if you are taking vitamin C without bioflavonoids, you are wasting your money.

More than four hundred years later, Professor Jacques Masquelier, dean emeritus of the medical school at the University of Bordeaux in France, made a special trip to Quebec to investigate the Anneda pine tree. He knew that pine needles commonly contain vitamin C, but he also wanted samples of the bark to see if there was a medicinal substance in it. When Professor Masquelier examined the Anneda bark in his laboratory, he discovered that it contained a rare and very powerful bioflavonoid. It turned out to be much stronger than any citrus bioflavonoid, in fact it proved fifty times more powerful than vitamin E and twenty times stronger than vitamin C!

Soon scientists worldwide heard about Dr. Masquelier's discovery and began experimenting with this remarkable substance. They made an astounding finding that it not only protected and helped vitamin C work better, but it was one of the most powerful antioxidants ever discovered.

But there was a problem. To make this bioflavonoid available to the world, stripping the bark from the trees and extracting it would be quite expensive—and the trees would die. So Dr. Masquelier began tedious search for another source. After several years, he finally found an even stronger source in grape seeds. Now it is commercially available under the trade names, Adoxynol (ADN) and Pycnogenol.

Dr. Richard Cutler, director of the government's anti-aging research department at the National Institute of Health said, "The amount of antioxidants that you maintain in your body is directly proportional to how long you will live!"

Thanks to the progress of science, we can now dramatically lengthen our lives, and experience fewer illnesses and debilitating diseases in our older years. The answer is to maintain a full spectrum of antioxidants in our bodies to fight off the killer free radicals.

▪ Seven Antioxidants with Different Jobs!

It is important to understand that each of the seven antioxidants work in different parts of the body. Vitamin A and beta-carotene do their best free-radical fighting in the mucus membranes of the body. Vitamin C works best in the water soluble tissues. Vitamin E and selenium extinguish free radicals in the fats and oils of the body—including the heart. Cysteine protects the bladder, lungs and eyes. Zinc watches over the prostate and the hormonal system.

Scientists radioactively tagged ADN so they could follow it through the body. They found that it went to every part of the body, except bones, with the largest concentration in the aorta—the main trunk of the artery system. Dr. David White of the University of Nottingham in England, found that ADN reduces oxidized LDL cholesterol and foam cell formation. From his extensive clinical tests, he concluded that ADN was the best protection from atherosclerosis.

If you have varicose veins or edema (heaviness or swelling of the legs), ADN could be very important to you. Varicose veins are actually leaking capillaries (the very fine blood vessels that deliver nutrients to your body and pick up the waste). The capillaries leak because the collagen that forms the blood vessel walls has deteriorated and lost its flexibility. Edema is caused by the welling up of the blood in the legs because the pumping action of the veins has diminished due to the stiffness of the collagen.

Professor Henri Choussat of the medical school at the University of Bordeaux conducted two double-blind studies of people with varicose veins and edema. Within seventy-two hours, the patients taking ADN had increased capillary resistance to leaking by 140 percent. Sixty days later, all those taking ADN no longer had edema and their legs felt invigorated; 75 percent of the varicose veins had disappeared. Dr. G. F. Haake, a German scientist confirmed the results with a similar study. He also found that 93 percent of those taking ADN had much fewer legs cramps.

The collagen which makes up the blood vessels is the same collagen that gives your skin its smoothness, elasticity and strength. Studies at Baylor University showed that ADN attaches itself to damaged collagen, reactivates it and protects it from free radical invaders.

Dr. A. H. Arstila, professor of a Finnish medical school found that ADN (taken orally) actually prevents about 85 percent of the potential damage from ultraviolet light. That means ADN is one of the first oral cosmetics that will improve the appearance of your skin and protect it at the same time.

ADN is one of the few antioxidants that can cross the blood/brain barrier to protect brain cells from free radicals. Loss of brain cells means loss of memory. To test ADN's stroke prevention ability, scientists genetically bred a variety of laboratory rats that are prone to early death from strokes. However, when ADN is added to their diets, they live almost twice as long.

ADN apparently strengthens blood vessels and prevents them from bursting, which is often the cause of stroke-causing clots. Since the major concentration of ADN is in the aorta, it has also been explored as a heart attack preventive.

Dr. Juan Duarte, a Spanish scientist and a Dutch medical expert from their National Institute of Public Health concluded in separate studies that ADN improved the dilation mechanism of the aorta, thereby reducing blockage clots and the risk of heart attacks.

Recently, ADN and Pycnogenol lost their titles as the most powerful antioxidants. Lycopenes, obtained from tomatoes, are about 20 percent more powerful.

■ Another Little Known but Powerful Antioxidant!

N-acetyl cysteine, a modified form of the amino acid, cysteine, is not only a powerful antioxidant, but it is crucial to many functions in the body. Various studies indicate that it helps prevent breast cancer. In the bladder, it destroys nitrosamines, commonly found in animal fats, cigarette smoke and alcohol. Nitrosamines are strongly suspected as cancer-causing elements.

Cysteine is extensively given to patients who are undergoing chemotherapy treatment for cancer. It counteracts many of the awful side effects of cancer-fighting drugs. Cysteine aids in the treatment of allergies, diabetes, hypoglycemia, arthritis and may prevent kidney and gallstones from forming. It assists selenium in being metabolized and works synergistically with vitamin C and E making them more powerful.

A 1991 study, published in the journal *Experimental Eye Research,* showed that as your eyes age the amount of cysteine diminishes. The researchers concluded that regular supplementation of this amino acid could prevent cataracts in later years.

Dr. Eric Braverman reported that at his medical center he uses cysteine in treating patients with bronchial disease, asthma and bronchitis. Four asthmatics were able to stop using bronchodilating drugs and inhalers within sixty days after beginning supplementation of cysteine. They had been on these drugs for up to ten years before they began taking the nutrient.

With all the hoopla in the press about the value of antioxidants, a lot of drug companies have brought out antioxidant formulas—and some are questionable. For example, tests have shown that 36 percent more of natural vitamin E (d-alpha-tocopheryl) is absorbed by the body than the synthetic form, dl-alpha-tocopheryl. The "l" behind the "d" indicates that this formulation is synthetic.

- **Other Answers to Slowing Down Aging**

Dr. Ana Aslan, Romania's first female physician, cardiologist and head of the Geriatric Institute of Romania, learned from the *Journal of Physiology* that there is an enzyme in our bodies called monoamine oxidase (MAO). The journal reported that the level of MAO stays at about the same level until our mid-thirties, then increases dramatically as we grow older. People suffering from debilitating diseases such as arthritis, neuritis, arteriosclerosis, senility and depression were found to have much higher levels of MAO than the norm.

Using 920 aged white rats, Dr. Aslan conducted a series of experiments to see if she could lower MAO levels using various formulas. Dr. Aslan discovered a combination which lowered the rats' MAO by 85 percent within a two-week time frame. The rats with lowered levels of MAO lived 21.2 percent longer than normal. Dr. Aslan considered testing her formula on a patient who had been admitted to the hospital with arthritis so severe he could not move his leg. After agreeing to volunteer for the experimental treatment, the man found he could move his leg within a day after Dr. Aslan began the treatment. Two days later the man was released. He walked out of the hospital as if he had never had arthritis!

Later, police brought a homeless, elderly man to the hospital. The dirty and disheveled cripple suffered from depression and loss of memory. He could not speak and was in a terminal stage of senility. Within a year, Dr. Aslan's treatment rejuvenated and restored many of the old man's lost or eroded functions. He was vigorous, alert, very mobile, and had much of his memory restored. The publicity surrounding Dr. Aslan's success with the old man attracted the attention of a woman who recognized the rejuvenated man as her father. The woman brought in documents verifying the old man's true age as one hundred and nine years. He was an Armenian named Parsh Margosian.

Dr. Aslan's formula was named Gerovital H3 and primarily contains procaine, which is often used as an anesthetic. Over the next fifteen years, Dr. Aslan kept meticulous records on 111 patients who were taking her treatment. On the average, the test group lived approximately 29 percent longer than the average life expectancy. Throughout the years, thousands of Dr. Aslan's patients reported improved or alleviated problems connected with aging, such as arthritis, neuritis, impotence, mental deterioration, memory loss, psoriasis, asthma, angina pectoris, ulcers, arteriosclerosis, depression, bad skin and muscle tone, no sexual drive, loss of energy, osteoporosis, and hearing loss. Some patients' hair also darkened.

Dr. Aslan's research did not go unnoticed by the scientific community or high profile patients. Nikita Kruschev, Cary Grant, Kirk Douglas, Aristotle Onassis, Marlene Dietrich, Prince Ranier, Somerset Maugham, Charles De Gaulle, Sukarno, Imeldo and Ferdinand Marcos, Stalin, and Chairman Mao all benefited from Dr. Aslan's treatment.

Dr. Joseph P. Hrachovac of the University of Southern California (USC) found that Dr. Aslan's formula, Gerovital H3, reduced the MAO level in the body by as much as 87 percent. Dr. David MacFarlane of USC confirmed Dr. Hrachovac's research.

Dr. Arnold Abrams of the Chicago Medical School performed double-blind tests of GH3 that resulted in very positive findings. Based on these results, the enthusiastic Dr. Abrams visited Romania in order to obtain more information.

East German physician Dr. Fritz Wiederman treated over 600 patients with Gerovital H3 and remarked that "The results were stunning and happened very fast." To illustrate his findings, he gave reporters a file on a sixty-seven-year-old female subject who was experiencing frequent bouts of crying. The woman also suffered from arthritis and a total inability to work. After undergoing treatment with Gerovital H3 for only one week, the woman was able to return to work. Less than three months after beginning the treatment, her swollen hands were restored to their former size and her arthritis pains disappeared. After five months, her hair regained its former color and began to grow in where it had fallen out. The most surprising result of the treatment was that, in her sixty-eighth year, the woman's wisdom teeth appeared, " . . . proving how extensive regeneration had occurred in her case," Dr. Wiederman remarked.

In a report to the Gerontological Society, Dr. Keith Ditman, medical director of Vista Hill Psychiatric Foundation in San Diego and Dr. Sidney Cohen, professor of Psychiatry at UCLA stated that they found 89 percent of aging patients suffered less depression after taking Gerovital H3. Doctors Cohen and Ditman reported that the majority of patients who took the drug " . . . felt a greater sense of well-being and relaxation, slept better at night, obtained relief from depression and the discomforts of chronic inflammation or degeneration disease."

At the annual meeting of the American Geriatrics Society in 1975, Dr. William Zung, professor of psychiatry at Duke University and associate professor Dr. H. S. Wang, reported that their double-blind test with Gerovital H3 and a placebo showed significant improvement of mental conditions for those taking Gerovital H3. Dr. Leonard Cramor of the New York Medical College conducted his own double-blind test and later concurred with the findings of Dr. Zung and Dr. Wang.

Dr. Albert Semord, a prestigious member of the American Medical Association, the New York County Medical Society, the American Geriatrics Society and the New York Academy of Sciences, tested Gerovital H3 on fifty patients and on himself for several months. He said, "Every month I'm more stupefied with the results—not only physically, but mentally and emotionally."

Dr. Semord said, "All my patients feel the same as I do. I don't look my age (seventy-eight). I fish, I hunt, I ski. I make love twice a week. I feel extremely well." He reported that Gerovital H3 had " . . . an astonishing effect on his patients' mental clarity and emotional stability."

A number of MAO inhibitors are being marketed in the United States as antidepressants. Gerovital H3 proved to be a better inhibitor of MAO than prescription drugs, which produced liver damage, hypertension, chest pain and headaches as side effects. Gerovital has demonstrated no side effects.

Dr. Hochschild says, "By its very nature, this substance cannot be compared with any other . . . it neither stimulates or depresses in its many actions, but rather regulates and normalizes." Dr. Aslan concurred, "If you are tense, it will relax you. If you are listless, it will revive you."

Dr. Aslan confirmed procaine's ability to correct problems of the circulatory system. Procaine has been found therapeutic for the heart and the vascular system and is a natural vasodilator.

Several years ago, scientists discovered that procaine breaks down in the body to paraaminobenzoic acid (PABA) and 2-dimethyl aminoethanol bitartrate (DMAE). DMAE and PABA are well-known substances contained in minute amounts in foods we eat. They compared procaine to the DMAE/PABA mixture and found the same positive results for the DMAE/PABA mixture as for procaine itself.

Until recently, the only way a person could benefit from procaine was by injection in a doctor's office. American scientists have developed an improved version of Gerovital H3 that does not require a prescription. A combination of DMAE and PABA is now marketed as Gero Vita GH3.

- Growth Hormone Reverses Aging!

The body's production of growth hormone slows when people reach their thirties. In about one-third of the population, production virtually stops at around age sixty. Dr. Daniel Rudman, of the Medical College of Wisconsin, published his findings of a study of the human growth hormone (GH) in the *New England Journal of Medicine*. The study examined the effects of GH on twenty-one healthy men between sixty-one and eighty-one years old. "What we saw over six months was that several of the body composition changes (of aging) were reversed," said Dr. Rudman. "These represented the reversal of one or two decades of aging with regard to these factors."

Dr. Rudman's research demonstrated GH's ability to rebuild muscle mass in the aged. Scientists are of the opinion that the benefits are more wide-ranging and rejuvenating. GH treatment increased the men's lean body mass (muscle) by 9 percent and fat tissue decreased 14 percent. Their skin thickened by 7 percent. Dr. Mary Lee Vance of the University of Virginia, in an accompanying editorial to the GH double-blind study, commented that the work is "an important beginning."

The only nutritional supplements that are known currently to increase the growth hormone are methionine, melatonin and arginine. The men in Dr. Rudman's study group were given shots of bovine GH. You can get these shots from some natural medicine doctors at a cost of about $12,000 a year.

For centuries, ginseng and ginger have been known as "anti-aging" herbs in China. People knew that ginseng could be used to calm nerves, heal ulcers, and increase potency. Western researchers have recently confirmed what the Chinese have known for thousands of years.

Current research has shown that ginseng helps strengthen the immune system. Dr. Tsung isolated the immunostimulating polysacchrides within the ginseng in 1986. Dr. Ruriko Haranaka discovered that ginseng has powerful antioxidant qualities. The saponins inherent in ginseng's makeup have been shown to lower cholesterol levels.

The journal *Modern Research* states, "Ginseng does not appear to possess any specific, well-defined pharmacological action, but rather exhibits a large number of different pharmacological activities, all of which contribute toward its total therapeutic effect."

The scientific community believes that the malfunction of the pineal and thymus glands contributes to the start of the aging process in the body. Failure of these two glands to function properly causes a decreased ability to handle stress. Every organ in the body is affected, physical and mental abilities decrease, and a person's appearance degenerates.

Scientists have discovered that serotonin in the brain is converted to a neurohormone called melatonin at night. According to the medical journal, *Medical Hypotheses*, "The Melatonin Deficiency syndrome is perhaps the basic mechanism through which aging changes can be explained in a single causative action. This may require replacement of melatonin in order to achieve a more youthful endocrine balance, and consequently repair the body as a whole."

Melatonin is pretty amazing because it is the brain's most powerful free radical fighter, and it dramatically boosts our immunity to diseases. Melatonin does that by stimulating our natural killer cells, which destroy tumors and viruses. Also, it increases the production of our all important growth hormones. They keep the body in a more youthful physical condition.

A clinical test was done on elderly laboratory animals. Half of the animals had melatonin added to their diets. While the group not getting melatonin showed the increasing effects of aging by moving slower, limping, losing fur and their interest in sex, the melatonin-treated group grew more energetic, sexually active and their fur became glossy and healthy looking. They also lived over 20 percent longer. Scientists surmise that because melatonin controls our internal daily clocks, it must also regulate our aging clocks.

With respect to the thymus gland, Dr. N. Fabris reported that, "Decline in thymic activity is not an irreversible event, and some nutritional intervention, such as amino acid treatment, may reactivate the production in the thymus. Recently, it has been shown that arginine accelerates wound healing and increases thymus weight. Some aspects of immunological decline with advancing age can be corrected with arginine and lysine."

Probably sometime in your life you've been given a shot of cortisone (or predisone), or you've heard other people say they've gotten cortisone shots for back problems, arthritis or a variety of other ills. Usually, a doctor will tell the patient that he or she can only have one or two shots, and then they must wait for several months before getting additional treatment.

If asked why, the doctor probably will say that too much cortisone is not good for you. Cortisone may indeed temporarily relieve your pain, but it's worse than "not good for you." *It can destroy you!*

Cortisone or prednisone is converted in your body to a hormone called cortisol. Cortisol is known as the "death hormone." (The average person thinks of hormones as only "sex hormones," but the body produces a variety of other hormones for numerous purposes. Hormones help you handle stress, produce gastric juices, modulate the pancreas, help in bone formation and repair, stimulate the adrenal glands, process phosphorus and calcium, pigmentate the skin, activate the thyroid, and maintain muscular stability.) What will surprise you even more is that your body produces cortisol on demand from the moment of birth until death.

In small amounts, cortisol has a defined purpose in your body. Following an injury or very stressful event, cortisol is automatically produced to boost your energy, and increase your blood flow, while slowing down other functions so your body can concentrate on fighting infections and healing damaged tissue. In non-emergencies, cortisol controls inflammation and the rate at which you metabolize nutrients—both very important jobs.

In a way, cortisol is like an aggressive, unruly child. If you keep the child busy, usually he or she will not be a problem, but let them have some idle time and look out. The old saying, "The idle mind is the devil's playground," certainly applies to the unruly child, cortisol. If the body produces a little more than is necessary for its normal functions, the extra cortisol literally wrecks havoc.

The cortisol your body produces is not usually a problem until you pass the age of about thirty. The reason is that your body also produces a regulator that controls how much cortisol is produced. That regulator goes by the name dehydroepiandrosterone (DHEA).

Between the ages of twenty-five to thirty, DHEA levels in the body start dropping at the rate of 1 to 2 percent per year, yet cortisol production doesn't ever drop. By the time you hit the age of fifty, there isn't enough DHEA to stop an excess of cortisol from damaging your body. By the age of seventy, you have only about 25 percent of the DHEA you had as a thirty year-old.

Dr. Alfred Sapse, a famous specialist in cortisol research, said, "Cortisol is the most violent immunodepressant there is."

That means excess cortisol destroys white blood cells, and T-cells, which fight bacteria, viruses and other disease-causing agents. It also interferes with the building of new cells throughout your body. This interference causes muscles and bones to get weaker; artery walls are damaged and become catchers of cholesterol (atheriosclerosis); blood pressure goes up; your memory is reduced, and your glucose and insulin balance is offset. In very extreme cases, cortisol can shut down your adrenal glands, leading to shock and even death.

As you get older and DHEA levels continue to drop, the continual cortisol damage over the years steadily weakens every organ until eventually you die. Although the death certificate may list the cause of death as heart disease, or cancer, accumulated damage caused by cortisol—the death hormone—is always a contributing factor. Autopsies of the elderly always show high cortisol and very low DHEA levels (5 percent or less).

There are several things that increase your cortisol levels even when you are young. Smokers and heavy drinkers always have more cortisol in their systems. Poor diets raise cortisol levels. A deficiency of chromium raised cortisol 45.6 percent in a test group. Hypoglycemics and diabetics have excess cortisol.

An analysis of the blood of a group of women suffering from depression showed their cortisol levels 39 percent higher on average than normal for their ages, which may be the reason why depressed people heal much more slowly than mentally healthy peers when injured.

Literally, thousands of clinical tests have been done on DHEA. It was not surprising that the results show that people suffering from practically any disease had low DHEA levels: arthritis, asthma, cancer, diabetes, heart disease, Alzheimer's, Parkinson's, Huntington's, osteoporosis, varicose veins, emphysema, lupus, AIDS, high blood pressure, infections, etc. Even women on estrogen replacement therapy and those with chronic fatigue and high cholesterol had low DHEA levels.

Dr. Laura Mitchell at Washington University Medical School conducted tests of men who recently had heart attacks. Their DHEA levels were much lower than men of the same age without heart problems.

Over 5,000 women in England had their DHEA levels monitored for nine years. The majority of those with the lowest levels got breast cancer.

Dr. Sonia Lupien, a professor at University of Montreal Medical School, found that when elderly patients were supplemented with DHEA to lower their cortisol levels, their memory and mental ability increased almost to that of much younger people.

Animals fed DHEA didn't develop tumors when exposed to a cancer-causing drug, according to Dr. Arthur Schwartz of Temple University Medical School. It also deterred artery clogging in animals on a high fat diet.

DHEA has had a dramatic effect on everyone who has participated in clinical tests. Cholesterol drops; there are less clots in their blood; tumor growth stalls; energy and stamina increase as fatigue fades—even for people suffering multiple sclerosis; bones grow stronger; people with thyroid deficiencies dramatically improve, and the incidence of minor infections and colds decrease.

A double-blind, placebo-controlled study of overweight men was conducted at the Medical College of Virginia. Half of the men were given DHEA daily for three months, while the other half took a placebo. The fat thickness on the bodies of those taking DHEA decreased 31 percent, and their cholesterol dropped 7 percent.

DHEA stimulates the fat burning mechanism and reduces the desire for fatty foods. According to Dr. S. C. Yen of the University of California Medical School, muscle strength increased by 16 percent for men and 11 percent for women when they took DHEA daily. Also, Dr. Yen said the participants' disease fighters, white cells and lymphocytes, almost doubled in twenty weeks of taking DHEA.

A double-blind study of elderly folks getting flu shots

was done in Florida. Half of the group were give DHEA two days before getting the shots. A week later, their blood was tested for flu antibodies. Those taking DHEA had four times more antibodies, which means they had four times more resistance against catching the flu.

Pregnenolone (PN) (not to be confused with predisone or predisolone, which are synthetic cortisone) and DHEA control the production of the sexual hormones in men and women. It isn't surprising that both sexes report increased sexual interest and ability after taking PN or DHEA.

Dr. Eugene Roberts said that he had a male patient who had *not* had an erection in five years. After two weeks of taking DHEA, the man told the doctor that he was astounded by the erections he was getting during the day.

Dr. Joseph Mortola of Harvard reported that many postmenopausal women have been able to decrease their hormone replacement after taking DHEA for a while.

Our hormones often affect the condition of our skin, hair and nails, according to Dr. Owen Wolkowitz of the University of California. He said that those who take DHEA regularly will have softer, more radiant hair and skin, and any brittleness of the nails will usually disappear.

DHEA is a powerful antioxidant and the most abundant hormone in the body. Dr. Gregory Fahy at the research laboratories of the American Red Cross said, "We've identified the hormones as a major key to why we age. When they dwindle, our bodies deteriorate."

Dr. Schwartz of Temple University proved that the quantity of DHEA that you maintain in your body determines how healthy you will be in later years, as well as how long you will live. He took one hundred young laboratory animals and divided them into two groups. Both groups received identical diets, except DHEA was added to the food of one group. That group lived over 50 percent longer.

▪ Problems with DHEA Supplements

A few years ago, a book was released that promoted DHEA as the best thing since sliced bread. It became one of the biggest best-sellers of the year, and newspapers, magazines, radio and TV shows everywhere started hyping the benefits of taking DHEA. Naturally, drug companies jumped on the bandwagon and rushed two forms of DHEA to the stores and mail-order companies.

The "natural" form was an extract from the wild Mexican yam (no relation to the yams sold in grocery stores). It contains what the drug companies call "a precursor to DHEA," diosgenin. There's a small amount of research that indicates that a little diosgenin will convert to DHEA.

Most scientists say the research indicates that you would have to take an enormous amount of wild yam extract to get enough DHEA to help you. There's another problem with diosgenin. It was the base for the first birth-control pill. It converts to progesterone (a female hormone), which upsets the hormonal balance of some women. If men take it for a while, their testicles and penis begin shrinking, and their breasts enlarge.

The other DHEA, which is most commonly sold in stores today, is a synthetic crystal DHEA. It is coarsely ground and packed into a pill or capsule. The drug industry calls it "plain DHEA."

What the author of the book and that news media didn't say, if they knew, was that the DHEA, used in *all* clinical tests, was an expensive "micronized" pharmaceutical grade of DHEA.

There's a big difference between the micronized and the plain DHEA. The particles of DHEA in the miconized formulation are incredibly small, and the plain DHEA particles are large. In the stomach, the micronized DHEA goes directly into the bloodstream and travels throughout the body. The plain DHEA goes to the liver so it can be broken down.

Only a small portion of the plain DHEA gets into the blood system from the liver because the liver is unaccustomed to receiving DHEA in that form and flushes most of it out of the body.

Although the micronized DHEA is superior, recent studies show that *it is not the best way to increase your DHEA levels.* In fact, it can upset your whole hormonal system because it bypasses an important control in the body. In doing so, it increases the androgens, which cause facial hair in women and prostate disorders in men, according to Dr. J. F. Mortola of Harvard. He also says his clinical tests show that taking synthetic DHEA *causes your body to stop producing natural DHEA!* (If you have been taking DHEA, your hormonal system may be out of balance. If you are healthy your body will fight to correct it, so the effects you will notice are very subtle. However, if you are not well, it could be making your condition worse or creating other problems.)

Dr. Eugene Roberts of the famous Beckman Research Center at the City of Hope says his studies show that it gets even worse. Supplementation of DHEA reduces the body's production of pregnenolone (PN), the mother of all hormones.

■ PN Produces DHEA in Your Body, According to Your Needs

Scientists agree that if you want to increase your DHEA naturally, you should be taking pregnenolone because it produces DHEA and all the other hormones—*according to the body's daily needs.* In other words, it keeps all your hormones in balance. The reason your DHEA levels drop as you get older is that the quantity of PN in your body diminishes at the same rate.

PN has some other equally important functions as you get older. It controls the adrenal glands, which affect your ability to handle stress. The stress of traffic, driving, traveling, the demands of a job, usually get more difficult to handle as you get older because your PN levels are reduced. Those taking PN daily report that they adapt to stressful situations with greater ease.

PN is very active in the brain. The discoverer of DHEA, Dr. James Flood of St. Louis University Medical School says, "PH is the most potent memory enhancer ever reported." He says the reason is that PN stimulates the amygdala section of the brain, which plays the most prominent role in memory retention.

While PN and DHEA balance and revitalize your hormonal system, and PN restores your memory, the control center of your body, the brain, still slowly deteriorates with age. The main reason for the deterioration has recently been found in the stomach and digestive system.

As we get older, our ability to digest food and extract vital nutrients declines. This is strongly evidenced by young people, who can eat like hogs, yet not have digestion problems. One of the most critical nutrients for the brain, methionine, is deficient in most diets, according to research by Dr. Ted Bottiglieri of the Baylor University Research Center.

Methionine is converted in the body to S-adenosyl-L-methionine (SAM). SAM increases the production of the three major neurotransmitters in the brain: serotonin, norepinephrine and dopamine.

Serotonin is the daytime equivalent of melatonin, the highly publicized anti-aging substance that controls the hourly cycles of body functions at night. At dusk, serotonin is converted into melatonin, according to Dr. J. Axelrod, reporting in the journal, *Science*. Serotonin is also part of our appetite control system. When your serotonin levels drop, you get hungry—even if your body doesn't need food. Keeping your serotonin up will help you keep your weight down.

SAM is the precursor to the body's second most powerful antioxidant and brain food—glutathione. In addition, SAM is the precursor to the body's own pain relievers, enkephalin and endorphins. A lack of those painkillers is what makes us more sensitive to aches and pains as we get older.

The producer of SAM, methionine, can't begin its production unless three nutrients are present—pyridoxine, folate and cobalamin. Those nutrients do a lot more than help metabolize methionine. They help deter cholesterol from clogging your arteries. Biochemists have recently found that the bad cholesterol (LDL) doesn't attach itself to the artery walls until it has been oxidized into foam cells by a process called homocysteinia.

Several years ago, Dr. Kilmer McCully was studying

children with an unknown genetic flaw that caused them to be mentally retarded and have severe artery damage. These children *looked like they were seventy to ninety years old!* He eventually discovered they had a malformed gene that caused their bodies to flood with homocysteine. This strongly illustrates how important it is to eliminate homocysteine, if you want to slow down the aging process, avoid clogged arteries and live a long life.

Dr. Meir Stampfer monitored the homocysteine levels of over 2,000 older physicians for ten years. The doctors with high homocysteine levels had 3.4 times more heart attacks than those with low levels.

SAM has gotten a lot of publicity lately, so you can expect the drug companies to start promoting synthetic SAMe as a cure-all. (The synthetic version has a small "e" on the end.) It won't work. Clinical tests have shown that if SAMe is taken orally, only about 1 percent gets into the bloodstream, according to Dr. Ross J. Baldessarim of Harvard Medical School in a study published in the *American Journal of Medicine.*

SAMe can be injected into the blood vessels with a needle, but realistically, the best way to increase SAM in your body is by taking natural methionine.

Dr. Kilmer added TMG to the children's formula for three reasons. First, it converts homocysteine into beneficial methionine. Second, the children's muscles were sagging like ninety-year-olds, and part of the TMG converts to dimethylglycine (DMG) which is known to rebuild and strengthen muscle and control fat. TMG is commonly used by weight lifters, Olympic and professional athletes to build muscle strength.

Third, homocysteine also causes free radicals, which damage the DNA in our cells. Damaged DNA can cause malformed or tumor cells to be produced instead of normal ones. Malformed cells in organs, such as the liver, stomach and brain reduce the organs' ability to function properly. TMG has the unique ability, through methylation, to protect the DNA from damage.

- **Sagging Muscles May Not Be Due to Lack of Exercise**

By the age of sixty, most people's muscles are beginning to sag. Exercise is important for everyone, but the lack of exercise is not always the major cause of muscle sagging in older people. Glucose and insulin are required to build and maintain your muscles. Normally, whatever glucose isn't consumed by the body in the course of the day is converted to fat. An enzyme from the mineral chromium is the major controller of this process.

Chromium is a powerful antioxidant mineral and is active in heart tissue, controls glucose tolerance and affects muscle and fatty tissue. As was mentioned earlier, when we age, our digestive system doesn't extract nutrients from food as well as it did when we were younger. Chromium is difficult to extract from foods, and in many cases, there is little in the food to begin with. Consequently, without the chromium controller, the muscles don't get adequate glucose and insulin, and most of the glucose is converted to fat. This is why most diabetics are overweight.

Some of you might think that sagging muscles are no big deal but consider this: the most used muscle in your body is your heart. You certainly don't want weak heart muscles.

A study at the government's Human Nutrition Research Center of 216 apparently healthy, affluent individuals showed that over 90 percent were deficient in chromium, and their blood glucose levels were almost double the norm. Dr. Richard Anderson, who led the research team, reported that supplementation of chromium reduced blood glucose levels by 67 percent within a few hours.

A deficiency of chromium is most prevalent in people with clogged arteries, when compared with those not suffering that affliction, according to a test by Dr. H. A. Newman, which was published in the *Journal of Clinical Chemistry*.

Chromium plays an important part in controlling your blood sugar and the insulin sensitivity of heart tissue. Dr. S. Yoneda at the University Medical School in Japan reported that chromium also decreases blood viscosity (thins the blood), making it flow easily to all extremities of the body and reduces the risk of blood clots.

Practically everyone who dies of heart problems is deficient in chromium. The same applies to otherwise healthy people who get late-onset diabetes. The usual symptoms of this type of diabetes are any one or more of the following: drowsiness, shaking, blurred vision or sweating. Dr. Anderson also reported that a patient who had symptoms of late-onset diabetes and was taking insulin, was given chromium to see if it would reverse the condition. Within a few weeks, all signs of the diabetes disappeared.

Two controlled studies were conducted at Bemidji State University in Minnesota on a group of athletes. Half were given chromium and the other half, a placebo. Those taking chromium lost 23 percent of the thickness of their fatty tissue and gained 8 percent in thickness of their muscle tissue. The placebo group gained a little muscle and lost a very small amount of fatty tissue, even though they were exercising regularly.

Along with losing fat, you can expect a drop in bad cholesterol (LDL), when you take chromium. Dr. Raymond Press conducted another double-blind, placebo-controlled trial on a group of average, healthy adults using chromium and a placebo. Those taking chromium had a 16 percent drop in bad cholesterol in six weeks, compared to the placebo group, which showed little change.

Dr. V. M. Dilman reported in the journal *Gerontology* that chromium increased the life span of laboratory animals by an awesome 26 percent. Many scientists believe the reason is that chromium stimulates the production of PN. The chromium we have been referring to is chromium picolinate. Plain chromium is not easily absorbed by the body.

If you know any expectant or new mothers, let them know that government studies show pregnancy severely depletes the chromium stores in the body. Without supplementation, it may take up to three years to replenish it. Also, people who take antacids usually have low chromium levels because antacids flush chromium from the body.

- Sources of Substances Mentioned in this Chapter

The following are available in many health food or vitamin stores. (If you don't find some of these on the shelves, the proprietor can order them for you):

Arginine
Chromium picolinate
Cobalamin (B_{12} vitamin)
Copper (chelated)
DMAE
E vitamin
Folate (folic acid)
Ginger
Ginseng
Lysine
Manganese (chelated)
Melatonin
Methionine
N-acetyl cysteineand glutamic acid (to make
    glutathione)
PABA
Pregnenolone (from which the body manufactures
    DHEA)
Pycnogenol
Pyridoxine (B_6 vitamin)
Selenium
Trimetylglycine (TMG)
Zinc (chelated)

The Human Growth Hormone (GH) and Procaine are available by prescription only.

Gerovital H3 is only available in Europe. However, the American version, Gero Vita GH3 is available from Gero Vita International.

A multiantioxidant called Oxyspectro, which contains Adoxynol (ADN), N-acetyl cysteine, beta-carotene, selenomethionine, zinc, vitamin C and natural vitamin E is available from Gero Vita.

Write or call Gero Vita International
2255-B Queen Street East #820, Dept. Z101
Toronto, Ontario M4E 1G3, Canada
(800) 825-8482, Ext. Z101

24

Healthiest Doctors Take Six Times the RDA of Vitamins and Minerals—and So Should You

THESE DAYS, IT seems almost everywhere you look—from the side of your box of breakfast cereal to television advertising for foods and patent medicines—you'll see boasts about nutritional content. All these claims are designed to prey on our interest in maintaining good health and well-being through proper nutrition. But what do they mean in terms of the nutrients our bodies actually require for optimum health?

According to federal law, the nutritional content of food is given as a percentage of the Recommended Daily Allowance, or RDA. This is the government's estimate of the *minimum* amount of each nutrient the average person in good health requires each day to stay healthy. But as a guideline to our true nutritional needs, many nutritionists and researchers have concluded the RDA is a very poor yardstick for measuring how much of each nutrient you really need. If you get just the minimum RDA, you are on the borderline between sick and healthy.

Before the 1750s, sailors on long sea voyages frequently developed bleeding gums, wounds that refused to heal, rough skin, and muscles wasted, all symptoms that characterize the disease called scurvy. Back then, before refrigeration, sailors subsisted primarily on a diet of biscuits and dried meat, with very few fruits or vegetables. Thus, the stage was set for one of the first scientific experiments in nutrition.

A British Navy doctor divided the sailors aboard the fleet's ships into two groups. Both groups got the usual rations, but one group was also given limes to eat at sea. As expected, the group on the standard rations alone continued to develop scurvy. But the group that got the limes—and in them the key nutrients we now know as vitamin C and bioflavonoids—avoided sickness.

The results of this experiment were too dramatic to ignore, and soon the order went out that all hands were to be given limes or other citrus fruits to eat on long voyages, which is why British sailors are known as "limeys" to this day. In fact, the notion of a disease caused by something lacking in the diet—a deficiency disease—was born.

For years the United States government has sponsored testing to determine how much of a nutrient we need to avoid developing vitamin deficiency diseases. Using rats or mice on a controlled diet, a particular nutrient is eliminated until the animals become sick. Then the researchers gradually add small carefully measured amounts of the nutrient being tested to the diet until obvious signs of deficiency disease disappear and the rats are able to reproduce.

Calculating the weight ratio between the average rat and the average human, and tacking on a small percentage to account for variation in adult human body size and the needs of pregnant women and lactating mothers, the government arrives at its Recommended Daily Allowance—that is, the absolute minimum amount your body requires to avoid vitamin deficiency disease.

But is staying one step ahead of the ravages of deficiency disease the same thing as optimum health? These were the questions that fascinated one of America's most brilliant scientific minds over thirty years ago as he set out to discover what level of nutrition is required to be truly healthy.

Dr. Emanuel Cheraskin, professor emeritus at the University of Alabama Medical School, is both a medical doctor (M.D.) and a dentist (D.M.D.). His curriculum vitae runs to well over forty pages because he has written or co-written twenty-three books and has published over seven hundred scientific papers in prominent medical journals. Dr. Cheraskin has been honored worldwide for his significant medical research and has received two hundred and ten citations in the National Library of Medicine.

Dr. Cheraskin wrote, "America is seventeenth (of the countries of the world) in life expectancy at birth . . . (and) Medicare costs for the oldest (of our citizens) may increase sixfold by the year 2040." "It is unlikely," Dr. Cheraskin continued, "that these projected increases . . . will be restrained solely by cost containment strategies."

Instead of basing his work on calculating the level of malnutrition where rats would develop deficiency diseases in order to deduce human nutritional needs, Dr. Cheraskin took a completely different tack.

Dr. Cheraskin reasoned that if a person was free of any symptoms of illness, such as aches, pains, colds, allergies, and abnormal functions such as high blood pressure, then they must be healthy. He decided to study a group of these very healthy people to see what level of nutrition was contributing to keeping them that way. Being a doctor and a dentist, he didn't have to look far for his experimental group. Medical professionals became Cheraskin's subjects because they knew the importance of good nutrition and a healthy lifestyle. And, they could afford the best food and medical care.

For over twenty years Dr. Cheraskin surveyed, interviewed, and monitored 1,405 dentists and their spouses. To assemble this group, Cheraskin sent thousands of dentists across the country both the Cornell Medical Index Questionnaire and the Standard Food Frequency Questionnaire. The Medical Index asks for the mildest symptoms of ill health, even though actual sickness may not be present. The

Food Questionnaire requests an inventory of what you eat, how much you eat, what supplements you take, and how much of each supplement you take.

The initial survey of dentists revealed what Cheraskin suspected all along—that healthy people kept themselves well nourished, both through diets and by taking supplemental vitamins and minerals. What he didn't expect to see was the dramatic correlation between nutrition and health: The lower the level of nutrition, the higher the incidence of symptoms of poor health—and, conversely, the higher the level of nutrition reported, the less frequent and less severe the symptoms.

For the next twenty years, Dr. Cheraskin conducted hundreds of double-blind studies to scientifically confirm his survey findings of the direct relationship between good nutrition and good health. In these studies, half the subjects were given vitamin supplements and half were given placebos. No one except Dr. Cheraskin knew which participants got the real vitamins and which got the fakes.

Dr. Cheraskin methodically tested every vitamin, every dietary mineral, and every trace nutrient believed necessary to sustain human life—and he tested some that remain controversial to this day. His goal: to establish, based on human testing, the ideal amount of each nutrient required daily for the "most healthy" life.

He proved that the optimally nourished body repairs itself more effectively, fights off germs better and delays cell damage longer. In all his studies, Dr. Cheraskin and his research team consistently found optimum nutrient levels to be *five to nine times greater than the government's RDA*.

During all these years, the government did not significantly change its RDA levels, but Dr. Cheraskin's findings were gaining notice in the scientific community, and other scientists were conducting research of their own.

A study conducted for the Eli Lilly Company by Dr. Judy Z. Miller, for example, examined the effects of vitamin C on child development. Dr. Miller studied identical twins six to eleven years old. One twin ate a normal diet, and the other ate the same diet but *also* took a supplement of vitamin C five times the RDA amount. After only five months, amazing results were already obvious.

While the children on the normal diet grew at the expected rate, all but one of the children receiving the supplementary vitamin C grew faster, outstripping their identical siblings by one-quarter inch to more than a full inch!

In another experiment, Dr. W. A. Harris tested the effects of megadoses of vitamin C on infertile men. Forty men were enrolled in the test. Half were given a gram of vitamin C every day for two months. The other half were given a placebo. In a truly sensational result, *all* of the wives of the men given the vitamin C became pregnant during the experiment, and *none* of the wives of the men taking the placebo conceived.

Perhaps our modern diet is seriously deficient in the level of nutrients needed for optimum health. But don't we eat better now than ever before? Dr. S. B. Eaton reported in the *New England Journal of Medicine* on his team's research into the nutrition of Paleolithic people. They found that the plant and fruit diet of our early ancestors gave them an average daily vitamin C intake of 392 milligrams (very similar to Dr. Cheraskin's ideal level of 349 milligrams)—and way above the RDA.

Dr. Cheraskin's three decades of research revealed that there are some thirty vitamins, minerals, bioflavonoids and enzymes essential to good health—and most of them are needed in amounts far greater than specified by the government's RDA. For example, the healthy, symptom-free people he studied had intakes of vitamin A five times greater than the RDA, intakes of vitamin B_1 nine time greater than the RDA, and consumed more than five times the RDA of vitamin C. And bioflavonoids and enzymes are not on the government list at all, even though research has demonstrated they are essential for good health!

Based on his studies, Dr. Cheraskin estimates that only about 5 percent of the adults in the United States would be rated very healthy, or, as he puts it, "clinically well" after answering the Cornell and Food Frequency questionnaires.

Our most obvious experience with disease is the sudden

onset of an illness such as a cold or the flu. Few of us realize most illnesses are progressive in nature, beginning as a relatively slight imbalance or infection and progressing in severity over time unless the underlying cause is identified and treated.

Dr. Cheraskin theorized that diabetics for example, gradually progress from being just slightly diabetic—say, 5 percent—until they are completely diabetic years later. In many cases, recognizing the symptoms early can be the first step in reversing the progress of the disease before it is too late.

Even relatively minor health problems, according to Dr. Cheraskin's reasoning, can be an indication of a potentially serious health crisis down the road. With this in mind, he looked at his most "symptomless" subjects to help determine his model for what constitutes the nutrition you need for optimum health.

Along with proper nutrition, good health habits are essential for a long and healthy life. One of the best guidelines for developing a healthier lifestyle is a federally funded study conducted in Alameda County, California.

This fourteen-year-plus study of hundreds of Alameda residents revealed that people who practice at least six of seven good health habits live an average of eleven years longer than those who practice fewer than two good health habits.

The good health recommendations studied were:

1. Get eight hours or more of sleep each night.
2. Maintain proper weight for height and bone structure.
3. Refrain from smoking.
4. Drink no more than two glasses of wine or one drink of hard liquor per day.
5. Exercise moderately three times a week.
6. Eat a healthy breakfast daily.
7. Eat meals during regular hours.

These results were confirmed by the nation's largest ever health research program, the decades-long Framingham study of residents of the Boston suburb. In all, hundreds of well-researched, well-reported studies point to the conclusion that it is possible to live longer and healthier by following simple good health habits, including eating a careful diet and taking nutritional supplements.

For years, we've been admonished to eat a sensible balanced diet. But just what constitutes a diet optimized to keep us as healthy as possible? The outline of Dr. Cheraskin's optimal nutrition program is fairly simple, but it is quite different from the typical diet of most Americans. Included in his plan are elements designed to provide the nutrition needed to keep our bodies operating at peak efficiency while helping to ward off infections, to minimize progressive conditions brought about by deficiencies and imbalances and to slow aging.

In the foods we eat, the Cheraskin plan considers our need for organic nutrients, including carbohydrates, proteins, lipids (fats, fatty acids, cholesterols) and vitamins. Organic nutrients are all compounds containing the element carbon. His plan also accounts for our requirements for inorganic compounds—those not bound to carbon—usually referred to as dietary minerals and trace elements. Inorganic compounds we require in amounts greater than 100 milligrams per day are called minerals; those we need in amounts less than 100 milligrams per day are called trace elements.

Proteins, the building blocks of life, should come from a variety of sources to ensure the availability of all the key amino acids. About 125 grams of protein should be eaten per day, about twice the RDA level.

Minerals, inorganic compounds essential to good health, are often overlooked. For example, a survey by Dr. J. Matsovinovic, published in the *Journal of the American Medical Association*, shows that 3 percent of American males and 11 percent of American females display obvious signs of clinical hyperthyroidism as a result of a deficiency of iodine, even though this type of deficiency was thought to be virtually wiped out in the early days of this century. An iodine intake of at least 50 micrograms per day is essential to maintain the body's production of thyroxine, an enzyme that controls metabolism. In contrast with the Matsovinovic study,

Cheraskin's healthy dentists and their families consumed an average of 0.5 milligrams of iodine daily—*five times the RDA level!*

Most minerals we consume are stored in our body tissues, so it's important to guard against becoming too enthusiastic and raising intake to dangerous levels. Even so, Cheraskin found an increasing intake of essential minerals—such as calcium, copper, iron, magnesium, manganese, selenium and zinc—paralleled an increase in overall health and a decrease in reported symptoms.

Vitamins, as we have seen, are not completely understood, even by many so-called experts. The government's RDAs are merely estimates of the amounts needed to prevent full-blown deficiency diseases. Much exciting research on vitamins is being conducted today, but much has already been learned.

In just one example, it is estimated that less than 20 percent of the U.S. population eats enough fresh fruits and vegetables to reach the RDA of 5000 IU (international units) of vitamin A. Cheraskin's studies have demonstrated that the maximum health benefit from vitamin A is reached not at the 5000 IU RDA level, but at 33,000 IU—*nearly seven times as much*. This is truly a tragedy for our national health, especially when you consider that the National Cancer Institute has shown that beta-carotene—another form of vitamin A—can arrest development of certain forms of cancer.

Dr. Cheraskin's results continue to show that RDA vitamin levels are inadequate to maintain optimum health. His healthy subjects took in 9 milligrams of thiamine (vitamin B_1), or *eight times the RDA*—and 115 milligrams of niacin, between *six and seven times the RDA!* Since the B vitamins are critical to brain function, what toll is our national deficiency of these essential vitamins taking on our mental abilities?

Bioflavonoids are a less well-known group of nutrients that appear essential for optimal health.

Scientists have long recognized that vitamins and minerals acting alone do not always have the effects that the same nutrients appear to have when consumed as part of the diet.

For example, vitamin C in its pure state does not cure bleeding gums, but vitamin C consumed as lemon juice has that effect. Clearly, something *else* must be at work that unlocks the power of vitamin C, and scientists have been trying to track down this link for decades.

In 1980, French scientists made a breakthrough when they discovered a compound that appears to protect cell walls in plants. It is found in the rind of citrus fruits, in the bark of most trees and in woody shrubs. This class of substances, known as PAC or pycnogenols, are most commonly called bioflavonoids and act like a "vitamin's vitamin" to help unlock the ability of vitamins to increase our health.

Dr. Cheraskin has clearly demonstrated that adequate nutrition can affect mental attitude and disposition as well as physical health. He describes a fifty-year-old male patient with a "rotten" disposition. The man told the doctor he was "shy and sensitive" but complained of a "violent temper" and of being "nervous under pressure." His sour disposition was destroying his personal and professional relationships.

A few months after beginning Dr. Cheraskin's optimum nutrition plan, the patient reported his mood swings and temper tantrums were gone. And he could perform better in pressure-filled situations, such as discussing sensitive issues with his boss.

Dr. Cheraskin's research established the vital importance of diet in maintaining optimum health, but it also showed that diet alone can't ensure we get all the nutrients we need and get them in the right balance—and that some elements of our diet can be bad for our overall health. Refined carbohydrates—sugar, for example—were shown to influence health. Those who reported eating the most sugar also reported the most symptoms, while those who reported eating the least sugar also reported the fewest symptoms of ill health.

But perhaps even more important, Dr. Cheraskin found that some people in his survey were getting too much of one nutrient and at the same time not enough of another as a result of their eating habits. Rarely did he discover, even among his sophisticated sampling of highly trained medical professionals and their families, people who chose a diet optimized for their health. And, he realized, even if you eat the proper foods and eat them in the right combinations, you would need more food than you could eat to get the proper nutrition.

One reason is that processing, packaging, freezing, and cooking destroy many of the biologically available nutrients in the foods we eat. Our lifestyle often doesn't allow us to prepare foods in the manner that preserves their maximum nutritional value. Yet the stresses and pressures of modern life—such as exposure to pollutants and our ever faster pace—actually can *increase* our requirements for certain nutrients.

Dr. Cheraskin concluded that to ensure the best health, top energy and performance, better mental functions, and your best possible appearance, you should take supplemental nutrients. Because it is nearly impossible to determine how much nutrition we receive from the foods we eat, Dr. Cheraskin advocates taking supplements that provide all of the vitamins, minerals and trace nutrients his research demonstrates we need daily.

Other researchers concur. A study by a team at the University of California of over eleven thousand people demonstrates that supplementing the diet with vitamin C alone can add more than six healthy years to the life expectancy of men and a smaller number of "bonus" years for women.

Dr. Ranjit Chandra of the Memorial University of Newfoundland in St. John's found that senior citizens receiving vitamin and mineral supplements reported 40 to 50 percent fewer days of illness than seniors who received placebos.

Some of the vitamins on Cheraskin's optimum list are antioxidants that combat free radicals that can accelerate aging. Many scientists around the world believe these nutrients are not enough by themselves to counteract the effect of free radicals. In addition to the nutrients on this optimum list, you should also take all the antioxidants listed below.

Here, then, are the daily vitamin and mineral supplements that Dr. Cheraskin's work suggests you need to maintain your peak health.

OPTIMUM DAILY VITAMIN AND MINERAL SUPPLEMENTATION

■ VITAMINS

		(handwritten)
Vitamin A (retinol palmitate)	5,000 IU	
Vitamin A (beta-carotene)	15,000 IU	5,000
Vitamin C	2,000 IU	1,000
Vitamin E (d-alpha tocopherol)	400 IU	800
Vitamin D (cholecalciferol)	1,000 IU	400
Pantothenic acid	70 mg	10
Vitamin B_1 (thiamine)	50 mg	15
Vitamin B_2 (riboflavin)	10 mg	17
Vitamin B_3 (niacinamide)	45 mg	40
Vitamin B_6 (pyridoxine HCL)	50 mg	20
Vitamin B_{12} (cyanocobalamin)	50 mcg	12
Folic acid	400 mcg	400
Biotin	300 mcg	30
Choline	250 mg	
Inositol	30 mg	

■ MINERALS

		(handwritten)
Calcium (carbonate, hydrolyzed protein chelate)	1,000 mg	1200
Magnesium (oxide-chelate and gluconate)	500 mg	100
Potassium (amino acid complex)	50 mg	
Iron (chelate)	18 mg	2.7
Zinc (picolinate)	30 mg	15
Manganese (chelate)	10 mg	5
Copper (chelate)	3 mg	2
Iodine (kelp)	75 mcg	150
Silicon (chelate)	20 mg	
Selenium (chelate)	100 mcg	25
Chromium (picolinate)	300 mcg	200
Molybdenum (chelate)	150 mcg	25

■ BIOFLAVONOIDS

Lemon bioflavonoids	60 mg
Quercetin (saphora japonica)	30 mg
Rutin (saphora japonica)	25 mg
Heseperidin (citrus)	10 mg

Let's take a closer look at these vital nutrients and see just how each is important for your good health.

■ Vitamin A—the Infection Fighter

At one time hailed as the "anti-infective vitamin," later cheered as a cancer fighter, today vitamin A's immune system–stimulating properties are again grabbing headlines. It is recognized as a curative and restorative for the skin and is the basis of the highly publicized drug Retin-A, used to fight acne, wrinkles and balding.

Long recognized as essential for human health, vitamin A is available in meats, carrots, cantaloupes, sweet potatoes and many other fruits and vegetables, especially those with a yellow orange color. Vitamin A is needed for night vision, regulation of cell development and reproduction. Deficiencies can cause changes in the skin and mucous membranes, and possibly lead to precancerous conditions.

In laboratory tests with animals, vitamin A supplements have been shown to increase immunity with increased antibody activity, improve acceptance of skin grafts and lead to faster production of a variety of disease-fighting cells. Giving vitamin A to children in Third World countries where measles is still common has been shown to cut the death rate from the disease by 35 percent.

Very high doses of preformed vitamin A—given for a short time—are prescribed by doctors for cancer patients undergoing radiation and chemotherapy treatments. Vitamin A reduces the destructive consequences of these immuno-suppressive therapies.

Preformed vitamin A can be toxic in large doses, but the precursor, beta-carotene, does not appear to be toxic even in substantial, sustained dosages of as much as 500,000 IU daily. Because of the well-known toxicity of preformed vitamin A supplementation, many doctors warn their patients away from vitamin A, completely ignoring the far safer beta-carotene form.

Beta-carotene used in the same circumstances in animal experiments has much the same beneficial effect with few of the unwanted toxic side effects of preformed vitamin A.

Large population studies suggest beta-carotene has protective effects working directly against various forms of cancer, including those of the bladder, larynx, esophagus, stomach, colon/rectum and prostate.

In healthy males with normal immune functions, research has shown that supplemental beta-carotene increases the number of T-lymphocytes, or "helper" cells, in the immune system. And in the laboratory, the addition of beta-carotene stimulated neutrophiles immune cells to more effectively fight off the yeast infection Candida albicans, commonly known as thrush, which attacks AIDS patients and others with weakened immune systems.

■ Vitamin C—an Anti-Cancer Miracle

So many claims have been made for vitamin C (also known as ascorbic acid) that it's sometimes hard to know what to believe. One thing seems certain: there are more people taking vitamin C supplements today than any other nutrient—with some surveys showing that as much as *half* the U.S. population takes vitamin C daily. No doubt much of the popularity of vitamin C can be attributed to the efforts and visibility of its most famous champion, the Nobel Prize winner Dr. Linus Pauling. For decades, Dr. Pauling has touted the abilities of vitamin C to prevent and alleviate colds and cancer.

Like the sailors of the old British Navy, we can get vitamin C from many fresh fruits and vegetables. Citrus fruits in particular are recognized as a rich source of vitamin C. No studies, however, have demonstrated that the vitamin C we get from our diet or from supplements made from natural sources is any better for us than synthetic ascorbic acid. The key seems to be in the amount that passes through our digestive systems, rather than what is retained in our tissues.

Vitamin C has been clinically demonstrated to significantly reduce the severity of colds and also to help prevent cancer. There is still no hard evidence to show it can *cure* colds or prevent the growth of advanced cancers. An analysis of twelve clinical studies of vitamin C's effectiveness against colds showed that those treated with vitamin C enjoyed an average 37 percent reduction in the duration of their colds.

But colds and cancers are only the beginning of the vitamin C story. It's used in the management of asthma, to protect against cardiovascular disease, to hasten healing, to prevent gum disease, and to protect us from the harmful effects of environmental pollution, including cigarette smoke. Research is on-going to establish whether or not vitamin C is effective in the treatment of some mental disorders, another claim popularized by Dr. Pauling.

Many scientists believe vitamin C's effectiveness against cancers, such as those of the stomach and esophagus, is a result of its antioxidant properties. Chemically, this may have the effect of blocking the formation of cancer-causing nitrosamines within the body.

Vitamin C has also been shown to protect against cervical dysplasia, a condition that predisposes women to cervical cancer. Research has established that women whose daily intake of vitamin C is below 90 milligrams—already 150 percent of the RDA—have a 2.5 times greater chance of developing cervical dysplasia than women consuming more than 90 milligrams.

In warding off infections such as the common cold, vitamin C is thought to work because it is essential to the normal functioning of infection-fighting white blood cells. Levels of vitamin C drop in white blood cells whenever the body is under unusual stress, whether from infection, poisons and pollutants, drugs, radiation, emotional duress or indulgence in alcohol or tobacco. By getting these cells' vitamin C level back up to normal, supplemenation can make our white blood cells more effective when we need them most.

People with coronary artery disease have been observed to have a lower level of vitamin C in their cells than healthy people. Hospital studies of people undergoing surgery demonstrate that those getting a supplement of 1 gram of vitamin C a day were less subject to hazardous blood clots than those who did not get supplements.

Vitamin C also plays a key role in the production of collagen, a protein the body makes that helps to hold together bone and connective tissue. This is thought to be one mechanism by which vitamin C helps speed healing. Studies show, for example, that supplementary doses of vitamin C significantly accelerate healing of corneal burns. It may also be useful in preventing the formation of cataracts and in treating glaucoma.

■ Vitamin E—Guardian of the Nerves

As in the case of vitamin C, many claims have been made for vitamin E over the years, so it's sometimes hard to tell fact from fiction. Recent research, however, shows that vitamin E is essential to all oxygen breathing life, including humans. Vitamin E is the oldest recognized biological antioxidant. It is intricately involved in the production of energy on the biological level. These two functions make vitamin E one of the most important nutrients in Dr. Cheraskin's pantheon. In the diet, vitamin E is available from sources that include whole-grain cereals, eggs, vegetable oils and vegetables, especially leafy greens.

Vitamin E has been shown to be crucial to normal neurological functioning. Vitamin E supplements have been effective in treating various disorders of the nervous system. Deficiencies commonly experienced by those with chronic fat absorption disorders, liver disease, or cystic fibrosis, often lead to nerve damage. Neurological symptoms of these disorders that have been relieved by vitamin E (taken under a doctor's supervision) include muscle weakness, abnormal eye movements, loss of reflexes, restriction of field of vision, unsteady gait and loss of muscle mass. Certain forms of diarrhea can also be symptomatic of a vitamin E deficiency.

Recently, several studies have revealed that children with epilepsy have low vitamin E levels. Supplements of vitamin E help to control seizures among these patients.

One side effect of the long-term use of major tranquilizers used to reduce psychotic behavior is the neurological condition known as tardive dyskinesia, which is characterized by involuntary movements. A double-blind study demonstrated that vitamin E reduced their frequency by as much as 43 percent.

Research concentrating on the immune system demonstrated a correlation between the level of vitamin E and optimum immunity in mice. A human study linked low blood levels of vitamin E to an increased risk of lung cancer.

There are a number of theories on just how vitamin E works to stimulate the immune system. One school of thought continues to investigate the nutrient's antioxidant properties, while an alternative approach suggests vitamin E can block prostaglandins, chemicals that reduce immune responses. Still another beneficial action of vitamin E is its ability to protect cell membranes, reducing their susceptibility to attack by viruses and other pathogens.

Long-term vitamin E therapy has also been shown to be effective against narrowing of the arteries, such as the painful condition of the calves called intermittent claudication. In one study, relief from persistent cramping of the legs and feet was reported by 82 percent of one hundred twenty-five patients given less than 300 IU of vitamin E daily. Five hundred IU of vitamin E per day has also been shown to elevate blood levels of HDL cholesterol—the so-called good cholesterol—by 14 percent. Other studies have indicated vitamin E supplementation can be helpful against conditions ranging from precancerous breast lesions to life-threatening blood clots.

Vitamin E protects us from ozone and nitrogen dioxide, both components of smog, cancer-causing nitrosamines, radiation and chemotherapies and even the toxins in cigarette smoke. There is also experimental evidence that vitamin E can increase the ability of the mineral selenium to inhibit breast cancer and to ward off the formation of other types of tumors. Low blood levels of vitamin E have been linked to a greater risk of lung cancer.

Some doctors use vitamin E, separately or in combination with other therapies, to treat fibrocystic diseases of the breast, such as mammary dysplasia, a precancerous condition. Some 70 percent of women treated with 600 milligrams of vitamin E daily reported relief. And Vitamin E is also used to treat the symptoms of PMS (premenstrual syndrome), with a 400 IU daily dosage being effective in one double-blind study.

■ Vitamin D—the Sunshine Vitamin

Unique among vitamins, vitamin D is the only nutrient whose active form is actually a hormone produced in the skin following exposure to ultraviolet (UV) rays of the sun. Vitamin D can also be taken as a supplement. Vitamin D is available in trace amounts in some foods, principally fatty fish, liver, egg yolks and milk fat. Because these foods are often avoided by people seeking optimum health, and because it is minimal even in these dietary sources, vitamin D is commonly supplemented.

In the years before most milk commercially available in the United States was fortified with vitamin D_2 (one of the nutrient's two major forms), children with vitamin D deficiencies often were afflicted with rickets, a disease characterized by defective mineralization of growing bones. Luckily, this disease is now rare, but it does demonstrate the importance of vitamin D in the regulation of calcium metabolism and its promotion of calcium absorption from the gut.

Just because rickets seems a disease of the past doesn't mean that we can forget about vitamin D. Exciting new studies have shown it to have remarkable powers to optimize our health. For example, much work is being conducted on the role of vitamin D in the proliferation and differentiation of cells. This research is already having an impact on the understanding and treatment of cancer. It also appears vitamin D is crucial to the process of immunomodulation, with effects in the prevention and treatment of infectious diseases. And vitamin D's influence on the fluidity of cell membranes is related to nearly all biological processes, including aging.

Some of the latest research suggests vitamin D protects against colorectal and breast cancer and is beneficial in the treatment of other forms of cancer. Some researchers even speculate that chronic vitamin D deficiency can ultimately lead to breast or colon cancer late in life.

The elderly are at special risk for a deficiency of vitamin D. They may have too little exposure to sunlight, consume inadequate amounts of foods containing vitamin D, or take drugs that interfere with metabolism of the vitamin. Alcoholics, people with malabsorption problems, and those who live in regions with little sunlight can also be vulnerable to vitamin D deficiency.

Since 1985, the evidence has been mounting that vitamin D protects against cancer. Scientists who compared a map of the United States with rates of death from colon and breast cancer discovered that these deaths are most common in areas with the least sunshine.

Also in 1985, a team at the University of California, San Diego, published startling findings based on the nineteen-year-long Western Electric Health Study. This study, begun in 1957, followed two thousand men who worked at Western Electric's Hawthorne Works in Chicago. The data revealed the only significant way in which men who later develop colorectal cancer differed from those who didn't, was that those who came down with cancer consumed much lower amounts of foods containing vitamin D and calcium.

Confirming these findings, scientists have found that vitamin D inhibits the growth of human colon cancer cells, breast cancer cells, leukemia cells, malignant melanoma cells and lymphoma cells in test tubes. It also prevents known carcinogens from causing tumors on mouse skin and inhibits the growth of a common form of eye cancer both when it is applied to tumors and *when included in the diet*.

As if all this weren't enough, vitamin D has also been shown to be effective in treating the skin disorder psoriasis. A Boston University scientist tried vitamin D on the reddish, scaly patches caused by the abnormal growth of skin cells characteristic of this condition. All the patients in the study had normal levels of vitamin D, but when its active form was used as a supplement, many reported sympton relief. Sunlight is also known to help the condition.

Long before the age of wonder drugs, victims of tuberculosis went to the mountains for a rest cure. There, the fresh air and sunshine helped many. Today, we understand that some of these patients were probably suffering from a deficiency of vitamin D and that the sunlight was instrumental in their cure. Two groups of researchers, working independently, have found that the active form of vitamin D stimulates human macrophages—a type of white blood cell—to attack the bacterium that causes tuberculosis and to slow down and even stop its growth.

■ Pantothenic Acid—a New Fountain of Youth

Parts of the B vitamin complex, pantothenic acid and its cousin pantetheine are vital to human metabolism. We depend on them for the proper production of adrenal hormones and for the production of energy. All manner of claims have been made for these nutrients, from protection against cardiovascular disease and elevated cholesterol, to reduction of the negative effects of aging. Organ meats and whole grain cereals are known to be dietary sources of pantothenic acid.

There is inconclusive scientific evidence to support the claim that pantothenic acid heightens energy and athletic ability, but many people enthusiastically claim it does. A number of studies do point to the benefits of pantothenic acid supplementation for arthritis patients. Interestingly, in one study rheumatoid arthritis sufferers were found to have below normal levels of pantothenic acid in their blood. When they received supplements, they reported a marked reduction in the discomfort caused by their arthritic conditions, but the symptoms soon returned when supplements were stopped. In 1980, the General Practitioner Researcher ran a study that revealed "highly significant effects" of oral pantothenic acid in reducing stiffness, pain and overall disability among rheumatoid arthritis patients.

The vitamin also seems to stimulate cell growth in the healing process. In studies with animals, surgical wounds healed faster in those treated with pantothenic acid supplements. Recent experimental evidence suggests that pantotheine can help detoxify alcohol in the bloodstream. It

appears to have an effect against the component acetalde-
hyde, a major factor in the ravages of long-term alcohol
abuse.

In experiments with rats, pantothenic acid deficiencies
have led to graying hair and hair loss. This has encouraged
a claim that the vitamin can cure hair loss in humans and
reverse the graying of hair. While there is some evidence
that pantothenic acid may be effective in these uses, there is
no current scientific evidence to prove it.

Similarly, laboratory studies with mice suggest that pantothenic acid may help re-energize old cells and extend their
life span, as well as diminish the "age spots" that can appear
on the skin. In one experiment, mice given supplements of
pantothenic acid lived 20 percent longer than mice who
didn't receive the supplement.

■ Vitamin B_1—the Drinking Man's Vitamin

Serious vitamin deficiencies are not a widespread problem in most developed countries—with the exception of vitamin B_1. More adults are deficient in this vitamin than in
any other. The reason: the high rate of alcoholism. Alcohol
is especially destructive to thiamine—vitamin B_1—in the
body.

Among alcoholics, vitamin B_1 deficiency is common.
Not only does the alcohol prevent the vitamin stored in the
tissue from being converted to its active form, but alcoholics
often also eat a diet low in vitamin B_1 to begin with. Large
supplemental doses can usually help alcoholics with B_1 deficiencies.

All foods contain some vitamin B_1. Whole grains, brown
rice, seafood and beef are rich sources. Highly refined and
milled foods, such as polished white rice, are robbed of their
vitamin B_1. In the body, vitamin B_1 is an integral part of the
process of converting blood sugar into energy. It is involved
in essential metabolic reactions in nervous tissue, the heart,
new cell formation and is vital in the maintenance of both
smooth and skeletal muscles. If a vitamin B_1 deficiency persists, the deficiency disease beriberi is likely to be the result,
with its symptoms of confusion, visual disturbances, partial

paralysis and balance problems. Another form of the disease affects the heart and circulatory system and can lead to death.

Other signs of a deficiency of vitamin B_1 are uneven heartbeat, shortness of breath, low blood pressure, chest and abdominal pain, kidney failure and heart failure. Except for the last, of course, all these symptoms can be effectively treated and reversed with vitamin B_1 supplements.

In experiments using dogs, vitamin B_1 has been beneficial in treating heart attacks, with injections stimulating contractions and decreasing the heart's demand for oxygen. Russian researchers have reported similar results with humans.

One type of anemia responds to large doses of vitamin B_1. Although most people with this condition have what appear to be normal levels of the vitamin, their conditions improve when treated with relatively high doses of up to 100 milligrams per day.

Lead is one of the most common—and most damaging— pollutants in our environment. Vitamin B_1 has been shown to be effective against the high lead toxicity in the tissues of experimental animals.

■ Vitamin B_2–the Athletic Vitamin

Vitamin B_2, also known as riboflavin, acts together with an enzyme to help produce energy and also to protect against free radical damage. It is a powerful antioxidant. Water soluble, vitamin B_2 cannot be stored in the body and must be replaced continuously to avert a deficiency. Active people, athletes, and women particularly, often need extra vitamin B_2.

Some of the best dietary sources of vitamin B_2 are milk, cheese, and yogurt. Deficiencies are found in people who eat an unbalanced diet, especially the elderly and alcoholics. Vitamin B_2 can also be destroyed by certain drugs, including tranquilizers.

Cracks around the mouth and lips, a reddening of the tongue, and eczema of the face and genitals can all be symptomatic of a deficiency of vitamin B_2. Riboflavin is thought to be important in the absorption of iron, so many people deficient in B_2 are also anemic. Deficiencies of riboflavin have been linked with cancer of the esophagus. The growth of precancerous cells in the esophagus has been reduced with B_2 supplements.

■ Vitamin B_3—the Cholesterol Buster

Vitamin B_3 is a hot topic in medical circles these days because one of its forms is rapidly being accepted as a preferred treatment for lowering blood cholesterol levels. Safer and apparently more effective than multimillion dollar anticholesterol drugs, vitamin B_3 has fewer side effects and *costs forty times less than the designer drugs*.

This miracle nutrient is acknowledged to significantly reduce the risk of death among people who have had heart attacks. And many claim it can treat and even cure schizophrenia. What's more, it is recognized as a detoxifying agent able to rid the body of many poisons, including narcotics.

A true vitamin powerhouse, B_3 is available in lean meats and poultry. Various forms of supplements are also commonly available. As niacin, vitamin B_3 can cause a flushing of the face and neck, itching and dizziness. In the form of niacinamide, these unpleasant side effects will be avoided.

■ Cuts Heart Attacks by 30 percent

As little as two grams a day are now known to reduce blood levels of cholesterol and triglycerides, which can form deposits inside blood vessels and lead to heart attacks and strokes. The Coronary Project Research Group's major 1975 study found that B_3 not only reduces cholesterol, but cuts back the likelihood of subsequent heart attacks by almost 30 percent.

As if this weren't amazing enough, follow-up work to the famous Coronary Drug Project study showed that heart attack patients who took vitamin B_3 instead of a placebo lived longer and had fewer later medical problems in every category: second heart attacks, other cardiovascular diseases, cancer and "all others." The patients who got the vitamin treatment were also less likely to die than those treated with major anti-cholesterol pharmaceuticals. In fact, the expensive drugs were demonstrated to be no more effective than the placebo in preventing death—in other words, they were as good as nothing (but a lot more expensive)!

Vitamin B_3 in moderate doses has also been shown to increase blood levels of HDL (the so-called "good cholesterol") by 33 percent. Many have claimed remarkable success using vitamin B_3 to remove toxins from the system, often in a regimen that includes sauna baths and running. The Foundation for Advancement in Science and Education, based in Los Angeles, confirmed the results of this process as practiced by the drug rehabilitation program Narconon, as well as a simultaneous reduction in cholesterol levels.There have been claims that vitamin B_3 reduces addicts' craving for alcohol and drugs, but they have not been proven. Similarly, vitamin B_3 has also been reported to reduce high blood pressure.

The assertions that mental illness such as schizophrenia can be cured with vitamin B_3 probably originated with its use to treat the deficiency disease pellagra, caused by a lack of B vitamins and typified by symptoms including dementia. No adequate proof of niacin's effectiveness against mental illnesses not caused by a B vitamin deficiency has been reported, but some mental health professionals claim success with this treatment.

■ Vitamin B_6–the Super Immunity Builder

Without vitamin B_6, more than sixty essential enzymes could not function properly. Normal nucleic acid and protein synthesis would grind to a halt. And the multiplication of cells—especially red blood cells and cells of the immune system—would become impossible. The nervous system and brain would cease to function properly as production of neurotransmitters broke down. Deficiency of vitamin B_6 leads to anemia, nervous disorders and skin problems. Women are in particular need of B_6 if they're on the pill, if they're pregnant, or when they're dealing with the effects of PMS. But most important of all is the function of vitamin

B_6 in maintaining our immunity. Of all the B vitamins, B_6 may be most crucial for maintaining a vigorous immune system. B_6 is found in meats, whole grains and brewer's yeast.

Elderly people, alcoholics, lab animals and human volunteers have all demonstrated that a lack of adequate vitamin B_6 leads to a severe compromise of the immune system. Both AIDS victims and cancer patients show low levels of B_6. Supplements of B_6 have boosted immunity among elderly patients and reduced cancerous tumor growth. Vitamin B_6 applied in a cream to melanomas—skin cancers that are highly resistant to treatment—caused reduction and even disappearance of cancerous nodules.

In one study, women treated with vitamin B_6 for the symptoms of premenstrual tensions (headaches, weight gain and irritability) not only enjoyed relief from their symptoms, but many with fertility problems also were able to conceive. In another study of B_6's affect on PMS, women reported it reduced nausea, depression and anxiety.

For decades it's been well-established that a deficiency of B_6 can lead to convulsions and problems with peripheral nerves. And it's been used for forty years to treat convulsions in newborns with metabolic disorders.

More recently, vitamin B_6 has been used successfully to treat carpal tunnel syndrome, a painful compression of the nerves in the wrist that can cause pain and a pins-and-needles sensation extending into the hand as well. While most other treatments are ineffective, 100 to 200 milligrams of B_6 daily usually clears up the condition within about three months.

Diabetics with abnormal metabolism of the amino acid triptophan and the related intolerance of glucose, one of the basic sugars, have been helped with B_6. For some diabetics, B_6 supplements can even reduce the need for insulin. Many women who use oral contraceptives experience the same type of abnormal triptophan metabolism as diabetics. About 5 milligrams of vitamin B_6 taken daily can usually reverse this situation and return glucose tolerance to normal.

■ Vitamin B_{12}—the Super Energy Secret

Because so many claims have been made about B_{12} over the years, many in the medical establishment have dismissed it as a modern day snake oil. They do agree that it is essential in humans for healthy nerve tissues, and they acknowledge deficiency of B_{12} can cause problems ranging from nerve disorders and brain damage to anemia. But only in recent years have its more remarkable properties been gaining credence within the medical establishment.

In the diet, vitamin B_{12} is available in fish, dairy products, organ meats such as liver and kidney, eggs, beef, and pork. Until fairly recently, it was difficult to accurately diagnose a vitamin B_{12} deficiency. If one of the most common symptoms—anemia—was not present, doctors did not believe there could be an inadequate supply of B_{12}. But with today's more sensitive tests, it is possible to discover that people can be suffering from too little vitamin B_{12} even if they are not anemic.

As a treatment for stress, fatigue and recovery from trauma, vitamin B_{12} certainly benefits people with pernicious anemia, but more medical doctors today are admitting that injections of B_{12} appear to have equally dramatic positive effects on patients who do not show signs of B_{12} deficiency. One doctor wrote in *Medical World* that, like " . . . thousands of other physicians . . . " he was convinced B_{12} can help speed recovery from viral and bacterial infections as well as surgery. Like others, he reports it helps restore appetite and a higher energy level.

B_{12} is used to treat various neuropsychiatric problems and to prevent mental deterioration, especially in the elderly who are likely to have B_{12} deficiencies. Of thirty-nine patients treated with vitamin B_{12} for neurologic problems such as abnormal gait, memory loss, poor reflexes, weakness, fatigue and psychiatric disorders, all showed improvement—and some showed dramatic improvement. It is effective in treating neurologic damage.

Vitamin B_{12} has also been demonstrated to help counteract the consequences of cigarette smoking. It has long been recognized that components in cigarette smoke reduce the levels of B_{12} and folic acid in the cells of the lungs and bronchioles. In one experiment, seventy-three longtime heavy smokers were studied. They all had developed precancerous tissue, but none had cancer. They were split into two groups, one being given B_{12} and folic acid, and the other a placebo. Four months later, the treated smokers had significantly fewer precancerous cells than the control group.

Recently, a new study demonstrated that B_{12} blocks allergic reactions to the sulfites used as additives in some foods and wines. These reactions include headache, congestion, runny nose and bronchial spasms. Sulfite sensitive subjects were given 2,000 micrograms of B_{12}, then exposed to sulfites. All except one avoided any allergic reaction. This test, repeated successfully with a second group, suggests B_{12} can help those who suffer from allergies.

- Folic Acid—Can It Help Smokers?

A key player in some of the most basic metabolic processes in our bodies, folic acid is essential in the synthesis of DNA (the blueprint for cell growth and reproduction). It has also recently been promoted as being able to prevent certain cancers and birth defects.

Folic acid is available in fresh leafy green vegetables, yeasts and liver, among other dietary sources. A deficiency of folic acid can show up as a type of anemia termed megaloblastic anemia whose symptoms include a feeling of overall weakness, tiring easily, irritability and cramps. Deficiencies can be caused by poor diet (common among the elderly) and malabsorption problems. Pregnant women are at risk of folic acid deficiency, as are those who are deficient in vitamin B_{12}. Some drugs and blood conditions can also cause folic acid deficiencies.

Studies dating back to the 1970s demonstrated that precancerous cervical cells could be eliminated with large doses of folic acid. National Cancer Institute researchers in 1986 found that smokers showing abnormal bronchial cells (cells recognized as precancerous) had depressed levels of folic acid in their blood. Scientists at the University of Alabama reported in 1988 that they were able to reduce this type of precancerous growth in smokers with a combination of folic acid and vitamin B_{12}.

Too little folic acid increases smokers' susceptibility to cancerous changes in the lung tissue. It can also increase the malignancy potential of cancers in other parts of the body. A University of Vermont researcher reported not long ago that mouse melanoma (skin cancer) cells low in folic acid were much more likely to spread when injected into mice than similar cells with normal folic acid levels. The same study demonstrated that the cancer cells low in folic acid were more likely to spread than those with normal amounts of folic acid even after their folic acid deficiency was brought up to normal levels. This suggests that something irreversible happens to the cells during the time they were deficient in folic acid. Knowing the part folic acid plays in DNA formation, it is suspected this lethal change is breakage of the chromosomes due to folic acid starvation.

More and more is learned about human chromosomes every day. So far, at least fifty-one sites have been identified along the chromosome where breakage is likely to occur— and twenty of these places, when damaged, are associated with the formation of cancer. Test tube studies have shown cells are far more likely to have breaks in the DNA chain— including at these known cancer-stimulating sites—when they are grown with too little folic acid. Based on what is now understood, some scientists believe that oral supplementation of folic acid may lower the risk of developing cancer.

Folic acid is also given to pregnant women to help prevent neural tube defects that can cause mental retardation in their babies. Like Down's syndrome, Fragile X syndrome is an inherited disorder of males that is an identified cause of mental retardation. French scientists reported in 1981 that oral supplements of folic acid were effective at improving some of the behavior abnormalities characteristic of retarded boys with Fragile X syndrome.

A 1986 study of a similar group of boys showed that 10 milligrams a day of folic acid resulted in some improvement in their behavior. Prepubertal boys also showed some increase in IQ, but older boys did not. Studies continue with this population, but evidence so far shows the benefits are most likely to been seen among younger children.

Dr. Kurt Oster and others use folic acid to treat arteriosclerosis. His treatment for patients with arteriosclerotic heart disease is folic acid dosage twice the RDA, which he reports prevents recurrent heart attacks and also reduces angina (pain in the heart) and the need for the common anti-angina drug, nitroglycerine.

Limited tests have also shown folic acid to be beneficial among the elderly in alleviating the symptoms of peripheral nerve diseases. Intravenous folic acid leads to improved vision in less than an hour, but the effects are short-lived. Elderly diabetic patients given folic acid orally also noticed improved vision and skin temperature. These tests suggest that folic acid may help by opening up blood vessels and allowing increased collateral circulation.

▪ Biotin—the Hair Salon Molecule

A water-soluble B vitamin, biotin, is just now beginning to be studied. Nuts, whole grains, milk, vegetables, organ meats and brewer's yeast are all good dietary sources of biotin. Biotin deficiency is rare, but when it is seen its primary symptoms are baldness, dry flaky skin and rashes in the nose or mouth.

Raw egg whites contain a substance that acts as an anti-vitamin and appears to destroy biotin. People who consume a lot of raw eggs are at risk of having this substance bind to biotin and thus prevent its absorption by the body. People on long-term oral antibiotic therapy are also at risk for biotin deficiency.

Luckily, the baldness that can come from biotin deficiency—even when caused by strict dieting—can be reversed with supplementation. Many people believe that biotin can promote healthy hair and help prevent graying and baldness. Numerous hair products contain biotin. It remains to be seen whether these theories will stand up to scientific study, but at least one claim about biotin's effects on the hair is well supported. Children with unruly, "uncombable" hair that insists on sticking out in all directions in a profusion of cowlicks have been helped with biotin. The mechanism by which biotin tames the uncontrollable hair is not understood—but it works.

Because biotin is required for the metabolism of the branched chain amino acids valine, isoleucine and leucine, which some believe can enhance athletic performance, biotin supplementation has been recommended for those wishing to improve their strength and stamina.

■ Choline

For years one of the most popular—and controversial—dietary supplements was lecithin. Many claims have been made about this nutrient's ability to fight cardiovascular disease and boost energy. But as scientific knowledge of nutritional chemistry grows, the mystery surrounding lecithin and its molecular brethren, which include the nutrient choline, has begun to clear up.

New evidence shows that choline can be important in treating major nerve, psychiatric and infectious diseases—and may be beneficial for victims of cardiovascular disease. Choline (from the chemical compound, phosphatidylcholine) is readily available in the diet, because it's found in all plants and meats. Egg yolks, soybeans, cauliflower and cabbage are good sources. It also is one of the very few substances used as a food additive that actually has nutritional value.

The most recent findings suggest that choline elevates the HDL cholesterol (good cholesterol) level. In addition, injections of choline lower blood pressure; choline taken orally doesn't.

Choline also seems to affect memory loss and other diseases of the nervous system. In 1980, *Science* magazine reported that choline improved memory in mice. Choline-rich diets also improved memory in animal experiments, but choline-deficient diets appeared to lead to memory loss. People who take drugs that destroy choline (including antihistamines and some anti-depressants) develop short-term memory loss. Some experiments on humans indicate that choline can improve short-term memory. Early tests suggest it may help the memory—and mood—of some Alzheimer's patients as well.

Diseases that result in abnormal muscular movements and those caused by abnormalities of the neurotransmitter system—including Parkinson's disease and Huntington's disease—can be treated effectively with choline. Mood disorders, such as manic depression, have also been treated with choline. This therapy is much safer—as well as much cheaper—than lithium, which is a standard treatment for depression and other manic symptoms (and which often doesn't work).

There have been a number of recent reports in medical literature, including an article in the *Journal of Czech Medicine*, suggesting that choline can be effective against viral hepatitis A and B. It helped provide a quicker end to symptoms and a shorter time for a return to normal liver cell functioning together with fewer relapses. It is believed that choline works by repairing the membranes of liver cells.

Research at King's College Hospital and Medical School in Great Britain confirms the effectiveness of choline-containing substances against active hepatitis of the type caused by the virus once known as non-A non-B (also known as hepatitis C). Similar results were reported in studies in Italy and Nigeria.

Another choline-containing substance—AL 721—has been proven to inhibit the replication of the AIDS virus in the laboratory. It is being used clinically in an experimental treatment for AIDS. AL 721 has been shown to lessen withdrawal symptoms of morphine-addicted mice in laboratory studies conducted in Israel in 1982 and may be helpful for human drug addicts.

■ Inositol—a Nutritional Nerve Tonic

Another of the little understood nutrients is a complex form of fatty acid called inositol (or its nutritionally active form, myo-inositol). It is known to be linked to messenger molecules within the nervous system, and plays a key role in controlling various cells within the system. Fruits, nuts, beans, grains and vegetables are good sources of inositol. Fresh fruits and vegetables usually contain more inositol than processed or frozen ones.

Many people report that inositol is a natural tranquilizer that relieves anxiety and promotes sleep. It is known that the level of inositol can influence the levels of certain key compounds within brain cells. In any event, inositol is much safer than chemical tranquilizers or sleeping pills.

Diabetics suffer from the disintegration of peripheral nerves as a result of chronic high blood sugar. An investigation of the effects of inositol on this condition showed improved nerve functioning after inositol was taken, compared with those who took a placebo.

■ Calcium—What's Good for the Goose . . .

It's been ten years since a National Institute of Health medical panel dropped a bombshell on the American public: Most American women, it reported, aren't getting enough calcium in their diets. Just one consequence of this deficiency is the degenerative disease osteoporosis, which primarily affects elderly women. In all, there are more than twenty million Americans suffering from osteoporosis today.

But the link between calcium and osteoporosis has turned out to be just the tip of the iceberg. Research next suggested calcium is beneficial in preventing cancer and high blood pressure and in lowering cholesterol. And, perhaps most startling of all, scientists estimate that most Americans are getting as little as one-third of the calcium they need to maintain optimum health.

Children have long been admonished to drink their milk, and it's good advice, because dairy products, including milk, cheese, ice cream, yogurt and buttermilk, are excellent dietary sources of calcium. It's also plentiful in salmon, green leafy vegetables and tofu.

Most of us remember learning back in grade school that calcium is a major part of our bones and teeth. It is also vital for nerve conduction, heartbeat and other types of muscle contractions, coagulation (clotting) of the blood, the production of biological energy and maintenance of our immune systems. Besides the well-recognized problems of osteoporosis and cavities, severe calcium deficiency can cause abnormal heartbeat, convulsions and dementia. Antacids containing aluminum, alcohol, cortisone and some special diets (such as high protein or fiber), can all lead to a calcium deficiency.

The calcium ion is the most sensitive chemical regulator of human cellular activity known. Even the slightest difference in the concentration of calcium can influence our cells and our organs. And if the concentration of calcium ions becomes too high within a cell, toxic oxygen forms will be created and destroy the cell. Magnesium and calcium work together to maintain the proper delicate balance, which suggests that for optimum nutrition, we must have both calcium and magnesium in the proper ratio.

As we grow older, we can have increasing difficulty absorbing calcium. Sometimes, the elderly don't eat a well-balanced diet or supplement their nutrition intake. In the case of calcium, this is playing with fire! Because the body requires calcium so absolutely for the regulation of its biochemical processes, if there is insufficient calcium in the diet, the body will look for calcium anywhere it can be found—and too often this means that we literally begin digesting our own bones and teeth for the calcium our cells crave! This is the genesis of osteoporosis, as well as other degenerative diseases.

Alas, once bone has been lost this way, it cannot be replaced, so the secret to avoiding osteoporosis is prevention—which means including enough calcium in the diet, before the damage has a chance to occur. The National Institute of Health recommend premenopausal women get 1 gram of calcium a day before reaching menopause, and 1,500 milligrams a day after that.

In a nineteen-year study of men in Chicago, the incidence of colorectal cancer was linked to the amount of vitamin D and calcium in the diet. These findings have been corroborated by statistical studies in four Scandinavian countries. Following up on this work, men from families known to be prone to developing colorectal cancers were given 1,250 milligrams of calcium daily. Within two or three months, the abnormal rates of cell division in their colons had slowed to normal. Other experiments suggest this result may be due to calcium's ability to detoxify carcinogenic bile acids.

A recent double-blind study of calcium's effect on high blood pressure confirmed the findings of doctors who noticed that individuals with hypertension have lower levels of calcium in their bodies than do people with normal blood pressure. The experiment showed calcium to be effective at lowering blood pressure, but the extent of the effect varies according to the individual. A daily supplement of 1,500 milligrams of calcium produced a significant lowering of blood pressure in most of those tested.

Calcium can protect against cardiovascular disease in two ways. By lowering blood pressure, it lessens the likelihood of heart attacks and strokes. There has been mounting evidence over the last several decades that calcium also acts directly to lower serum cholesterol levels.

■ Magnesium—the Heart Mineral

Magnesium is a major component of our bodies. It is concentrated in our bones and in the liquid filling our cells with life itself. It is indispensable in every major biological process such as glucose metabolism, the production of cellular energy and synthesizing nucleic acids and proteins.

Magnesium takes part in maintaining the electrical stability of our cells, membrane integrity, muscle contraction, nerve conduction and the health of our veins. It is part of a delicate balance with calcium in producing energy.

Magnesium is found in meats, seafoods, green vegetables and dairy products. A deficiency of magnesium causes loss of appetite, nausea, vomiting, diarrhea, confusion, tremors, loss of coordination and convulsions. Marginal magnesium deficiency is thought to be fairly common. The elderly, those on weight loss diets, diabetics, pregnant women, people who exercise hard and people who take certain drugs are all at risk.

Medical doctors now recognize that even a slight lack of magnesium can cause life-threatening interruptions in the heart's rhythm. And it is thought by some that magnesium supplements can help protect the heart against the oxygen starvation caused by clogged arteries.

Studies have correlated the death rate from heart disease caused by blocked arteries with geographical areas of hard and soft water. They've discovered that locations with high concentrations of minerals—including magnesium—in the water are also areas where the death rate from this type of heart disease are low. Evidence has also been presented that the typical American diet is insufficient in magnesium, which may contribute to our very high rate of cardiovascular disease.

Further studies have shown that in some people, the cellular level of magnesium can be inadequate, even when blood magnesium levels are normal. This situation can also contribute to cardiovascular diseases, including high blood pressure. People who have a recurring problem of calcium-oxalate kidney stones have been helped with supplements of magnesium.

For many years, pregnant women experiencing the life-threatening conditions known as pre-eclampsia and eclampsia have been successfully treated with magnesium. Pre-eclampsia's symptoms include protein in the urine, high blood pressure and swelling of the body. It can lead to the much more serious eclampsia, which can involve convulsions, coma and ultimately death. No one knows precisely how magnesium helps women experiencing this condition, but it is now a standard therapy.

■ Potassium—for High Blood Pressure

Potassium is one of the most studied nutrients, partly because of its well-known influence on blood pressure. It is also vital in muscle contraction, nerve conduction, the beating of the heart, the production of biological energy and the synthesis of nucleic acids and proteins, which are the building blocks of life.

Potassium is widely available in an average diet. Some of the best sources are fresh vegetables and fruits. Bananas in particular are known to be a rich source of potassium. Cantaloupes, oranges, avocadoes, raw spinach, raw celery and raw cabbage are also good sources. A deficiency of potassium shows up as symptoms throughout the body: Fatigue, weakness and muscle pains are often noted. Even death can occur if a lack of potassium goes uncorrected.

Much has been written about the harmful effects on our bodies of too much salt. Potassium helps to counteract the effects of salt, and it is also helpful in reducing the effects of hypertension that too much salt can produce. Some have suggested that high blood pressure is not caused (or worsened) by too much salt, but by a lack of sufficient potassium.

This idea is supported by a number of studies. In one, researchers assessed vegetarians and non-vegetarians in Tel Aviv, Israel, in 1983. Vegetarians are known to have a higher intake of potassium in their diets than meat eaters. Not only was the average blood pressure level lower in the vegetarian group, but among the vegetarians, only 2 percent had what could be considered high blood pressure, while 26 percent of the meat eaters were hypertensive. Of all the factors measured in this study—family history, coffee drinking, smoking and even sodium intake—the only real difference was the level of potassium consumed by the vegetarians.

One of the best pieces of news about the connection between potassium and blood pressure is that, while potassium does not appear to have any effect on *normal* blood pressure, it appears to lower the blood pressure of many people suffering from *high* blood pressure. Evidence shows that there are considerable individual differences in the way people react to both potassium and salt and to how they affect blood pressure.

A high level of potassium consumption has also been shown to protect against death from strokes. A twelve-year study of older Southern Californians revealed that those with the highest levels of potassium in their diets had fewer deaths from strokes, while those who did experience fatal strokes all consumed lower levels of potassium. It is interesting that those conducting this study excluded blood pressure, weight, smoking, blood sugar level and other known risk factors for stroke. The *only* factor that appeared to be different between those who died of strokes and those who avoided strokes was potassium intake.

Vigorous exercise—such as the efforts of an athlete in training—can lead to the loss of potassium through sweat. To counter the consequent symptoms of muscle weakness and fatigue, a supplement of potassium can contribute to improved athletic performance. The best news of all is that a single banana or serving of vegetables is usually enough to make up for the loss and return the athlete's potassium balance to its optimum level.

■ Iron—the Body's Alchemist

Alchemists searched for a way to turn base metals into precious gold. If they had been able to peek inside their own bodies' chemistry, they would have understood that even the simplest "base" metals—such as iron—are more valuable than gold on the cellular level. In fact, without a reliable supply of iron, we would not be able to sustain life at all!

A number of foods provide a good source of iron, but Popeye notwithstanding, spinach is not one of them. Iron is found in meat (especially organ meat such as liver), poultry, fish, and ground soybean hulls. Iron is essential to the process of burning the food we eat on the cellular level and creating the biological energy that keeps us alive. Iron is also vital to hemoglobin, the part of the blood that carries oxygen to the cells. It's also a part of the process of forming carnitine, which is needed to oxidize fatty acids. And collagen and elastin—two components vital to the integrity of our connective tissue—both require iron in their composition. The immune system likewise needs iron as it fights infections and oxidation damage.

One of the most obvious consequences of a lack of iron is iron deficiency anemia, a condition that was recognized as long ago as the days of the Pharaohs, even though the cause wasn't understood. By the seventeenth century, Thomas Sydenham was prescribing iron supplements for chlorosis (green sickness), which today we call iron deficiency anemia.

Iron deficiency is fairly common in infants, adolescents and pregnant women. Even without the telltale anemia, iron deficiency can produce symptoms including behavioral problems, fatigue, muscle weakness and an increased susceptibility to infection. Iron deficiency anemia is the most common deficiency disease in the world, affecting at least a billion people. Iron occurs in two forms: ferrous and ferric. Free (ferrous) iron generates destructive oxygen radicals and is very toxic. Its harmful effects are rare, though, because most dietary iron is tightly bound in biological structures.

An interesting (though fairly unusual) consequence of iron deficiency is a condition called Plummer-Vinson syndrome, in which a membrane grows across the top of the esophagus and prevents swallowing. People with Plummer-Vinson are at increased risk of cancer in the esophagus or stomach. Supplemental iron can eliminate the condition, as well as the cancer risk.

Iron's effect on the immune system is related to its role in the function of the white blood cells. Candida (a yeast infection) and herpes are more likely to strike people who have iron deficiencies. A key enzyme essential to the synthesis of DNA requires iron.

Oxygen free radicals are generally something the body tries to avoid. But, using iron in the process, some types of white blood cells actually create these toxins and aim them as weapons at invading bacteria. The immune system uses iron in another way—by stimulating an enzyme to create iodine to kill bacteria. This same enzyme is found in human breast milk and is believed to be one way a nursing mother passes resistance to infection along to her baby.

A slight iron deficiency, and even when there is no obvious anemia, can cause significant muscle weakness. And since the heart is a muscle, a lack of iron can affect its performance and lead to symptoms of heart failure. Active people such as runners, and women more than men, are subject to these debilitating symptoms that result from even small iron deficiencies.

■ Zinc—the Immunity Tonic

Zinc is widely recognized as a protector of the immune system and a disease fighter in its own right. It has recently also been found to combat a common eye disorder called macular degeneration, which leads to blindness in the elderly. There is increasing evidence that we all may develop a deficiency of zinc as we grow older.

Many foods contain zinc. Some of the best sources are whole grains, brewer's yeast, wheat bran and wheat germ. Some people believe that seafood and meat supply more easily absorbed forms of zinc than do vegetables. There are more than two hundred human enzymes known to require zinc in order to function. They include the enzymes we need to produce DNA and RNA. Zinc also allows proteins to bind with nucleic acids and is a building block of cell membranes.

Severe zinc deficiencies in developed countries are rare; however, marginally low levels of zinc are thought to be common. Deficiency can lead to growth retardation, poor appetite, malfunctioning sex glands, lethargy, slow healing and abnormalities of sense and perception. Low levels of zinc are also linked to increased susceptibility to infection.

Animals and people with zinc absorption difficulties are prey to a variety of infections, proving zinc's usefulness in protecting the immune system. Low levels of zinc have also been discovered in AIDS patients. Many elderly people whose diets are deficient in zinc, needlessly fall victim to infections. In addition, there is new evidence that a lack of zinc leads to the gradual breakdown of aging immune systems and the increase in various autoimmune disorders of the elderly, such as arthritis. Because it is known to boost the immune system and is an anti-viral agent, zinc is now known as an excellent cold preventive.

Much faster healing of surgical wounds and ulcers has been reported when patients receive zinc supplements. So far, it is unclear if the remarkable increases in the speed of healing and recovery that have been observed are related to a pre-existing deficiency of zinc among the patients tested.

Zinc is closely related to testosterone, the male sex hormone. It has helped to increase male potency and sex drive in men with suboptimal zinc levels. A topical application of zinc, together with an antibiotic, helps to improve acne even in people who are not obviously deficient in zinc. Because of their special diets and abnormal metabolisms, diabetics often show symptoms of zinc deficiency. Zinc is also important to the normal production and regulation of insulin. Many people believe zinc supplements can therefore reduce some of the complications of diabetes.

Until recent times, there has been strong resistance in the medical and pharmaceutical communities to treatments using nutrients. Perhaps the example of zinc in the treatment of a rare condition called Wilson's disease argues the case best. Wilson's disease is a fatal disease of copper accumulation. Oral zinc has been shown to be effective against the disease with no side effects. The conventional drug therapy, peninillamine, is toxic to many patients, as well as much more expensive than zinc. Here is another instance in which treatment with nutrition is at least as effective, safer and cheaper than treatment with drugs.

■ Manganese—the Mystery Mineral

Scientists know that manganese makes some of the most basic biological functions possible, including the production of energy. As an antioxidant, manganese may also help to protect us from the toxic effects of some forms of oxygen. But little else is well understood about this enigmatic mineral.

Manganese is available to us in whole grains and nuts, as well as in some fruits and green vegetables, but the amount depends heavily on the level of manganese in the soil where they were grown. Alkaline soils produce vegetables with little manganese content. In grains, manganese tends to be concentrated in the bran, which unfortunately is often removed by milling. It is also present in organ meats, shellfish and milk.

Animals are known to develop manganese deficiency, but its role in human nutrition is still shrouded in mystery. Lowering of serum cholesterol levels, impaired blood clotting, dermatitis and changes in hair color occur in humans lacking in manganese, but deficiencies are not commonly seen.

Dietary manganese is low in toxicity, but people exposed

to a great deal of it develop a syndrome known as manganese intoxication, or manganese madness. Chilean manganese miners with this condition have the following symptoms: impulsiveness, heightened sexuality, unaccountable laughter and hallucinations. These early-stage symptoms progress to a state of deep depression and ultimately to symptoms similar to Parkinson's disease. Like Parkinson's, manganese poisoning is treated with the drug L-dopa.

Manganese has the unusual property of being able to substitute for magnesium in many biochemical processes. When analyzed, tumors typically show decreased levels of manganese, which suggests to some that manganese may play a role—still not understood—in the human degenerative process.

Other possible needs for this mysterious mineral include proper brain function and the synthesis of the neurotransmitter dopamine. Going along with this, there is a school of thought that believes manganese can be useful in the treatment of schizophrenia and other neurological disorders.

Animals deficient in manganese sometimes have reproductive failure. This may be because manganese is involved in the synthesis of sex hormones. Other animal studies suggest that manganese is needed for the development of normal bone structure, particularly the growth of the matrix of cartilage at the ends of the bones where the formation of new bone tissue takes place. This has suggested manganese as a treatment for osteoarthritis, a theory encouraged by studies showing a significantly lowered level of manganese in women with osteoarthritis. A large number of unsubstantiated claims have been made about manganese in humans, and investigation continues.

▪ Copper—the Molecular Fire Department

There is now no question that copper is an essential trace mineral needed for good human health. It is vital to normal respiration. Copper is required (along with iron) for the synthesis of hemoglobin, the substance that carries oxygen in the blood. It is also part of the formation of the protein collagen, which holds together bones, tendon, skin and cartilage. Copper is needed in the production of elastin, which makes our blood vessels, lungs and skin flexible. The neurotransmitter norepinephrine, a key messenger in the nervous system, is produced using copper, as is melanin, which gives pigment to our hair and skin and helps protect us from the ultraviolet (UV) rays of the sun.

Copper also combines to form enzymes that protect the body from oxidation damage. It is one of the most important blood antioxidants. As if all this isn't enough, copper also prevents polyunsaturated fatty acids in our bodies from turning rancid and contributes to the integrity of cell membranes, essential to limiting the production of free radicals.

Dietary copper is available in animal livers, crustaceans, shellfish, nuts, fruits, oysters, kidney and dried legumes. The body chemical ceruloplasmin, dependent on copper, is what is known as an acute-phase reactant. The body produces as much as needed to help combat toxic and infectious agents. Ceruloplasmin acts like the body's fire department—an emergency antioxidant squad rushed to the scene of disaster to quench the cellular fire.

Copper deficiencies are thought to be responsible for lung damage from emphysema. Other symptoms include anemia, low white blood cell count and loss of bone density. High levels of zinc supplementation can cause copper deficiency over time.

As an anti-cancer agent, copper has been tested in a number of experiments. In one, copper protected rats against chemically induced cancers. In another, chicks were protected against a form of cancer caused by a virus. And in still another, a copper salt protected mice against cancerous tumor formation.

Copper deficiency in young men leads to a significant lowering of the level of HDL in the blood. A supporting experiment in mice shows that a copper/zinc imbalance can increase the risk of heart disease by lowering HDL levels. These and other studies suggest that zinc and copper should be balanced at about a ten-to-one ratio.

Copper also appears to have an effect on the immune system. Laboratory rats with copper deficiencies showed a higher mortality rate from salmonella infection than properly nourished rats. Copper deficiencies in mice result in decreased antibody response. More research into this fascinating nutrient mineral is progressing. As the body's volunteer fire department, we depend on copper for long and healthy lives.

■ Iodine—Radiation Protector

Iodine is rare on land, but plentiful in the sea. It is vital for the production of thyroid hormones, which control the production of energy. Deficiency of iodine results in hypothyroidism—an overall slowing down of the bodily functions.

Iodine is available in seafoods, including sea animals and kelp. Years ago, iodine deficiency in the United States was rather common, and led to an enlargement of the thyroid (goiter) and the symptoms of chronic fatigue, apathy, dry skin, sensitivity to cold and weight gain. Luckily, iodine deficiency is relatively rare today because it is now added to table salt.

Unfortunately, we are also now more subject to exposure to unsafe levels of radiation. Here iodine can be protective. Iodine can block the uptake of radioactive iodides by the thyroid. This is effective in preventing the highly toxic effects of radiation on the thyroid, which is particularly vulnerable to attack by radioactive pollutants.

In 1988, a Canadian physician reported that a majority of the women he treated for a painful condition called fibrocystic breasts were completely relieved of their symptoms after being treated with elemental iodine. When the iodine supplement was discontinued, the pain came back, suggesting that this condition is a result of an iodine deficiency.

An iodine-containing compound is also used by physicians to help break up mucus in persistently congested breathing tubes when the congestion causes a cough that never quite goes away. Most familiar is iodine the antiseptic, good for cuts, scrapes and purifying backcountry water.

■ Silicon—for Arteriosclerosis?

Silicon is one of the most common elements on earth and is found in the world around us in forms as varied as sand, glass and computer chips. Recently, some have speculated that it may also be a key to reversing arteriosclerosis—hardening of the arteries—in humans.

In the diet, silicon is available in vegetables, whole grains and seafood. Studies have revealed that, as we age, the levels of silicon in our arteries and skin decline. French researchers report finding a correlation between the level of silicon in the walls of the human aorta and the development of arteriosclerosis.

■ Selenium—a Secret Weapon Against Cancer

In very, very small amounts, selenium can have a major impact on our health. For many years, selenium was ignored as a nutrient because it is highly toxic and because it was thought to be carcinogenic. But recent findings show that not only is it essential for optimum health, but that selenium actually protects against cancer.

Selenium is available in many vegetables, including broccoli, cucumbers, onions, garlic and radishes. The selenium content of foods, however, is extremely dependent on the selenium content of the soils where they are grown, and there are considerable regional differences. Selenium deficiencies are now known to occur in most warm-blooded animals and can cause cataracts, muscular dystrophy, liver disease, infertility, heart problems, cancer and can affect growth. It has been found to protect against a variety of serious, if common, conditions, including arteriosclerosis, cancer, arthritis, cirrhosis and emphysema.

Selenium is incorporated by the body into one of its major defenses against attack, an antioxidant enzyme that places the mineral strategically at each of its active molecular sites. The "micronutrient" selenium is also active against excessive blood clotting, and in this way protects against coronary artery disease, heart attacks and stroke.

There are various theories about why and how we age. It is fascinating to note that no matter which of these theories we consider, selenium plays an essential part in countering the effects of aging. It certainly reduces the likelihood of developing many of the diseases associated with aging.

Scientists have studied the relationship between the level of selenium in the soil and the development of a variety of cancers. Their nearly incontestable conclusion: A high concentration of selenium corresponds to a low rate of these cancers, and a low rate of selenium corresponds to a high rate of cancers.

Venezuela, which has a high selenium content in its soils, has less than one-fourth of the United States' mortality rate from cancer of the large intestine. In Japan, where selenium levels are high, the incidence of breast cancer is low. But when Japanese women move to the United States, their chances of developing breast cancer are just as high as women born here.

Studies from around the world confirm the relationship between adequate levels of serum selenium in the blood and resistance to many cancers. Other experiments suggest that selenium may also be effective against certain types of cancer tumors once they have developed.

On another front, increases in immune responses have been measured in test subjects given large doses of selenium. In experiments, this boost in immunity has been shown to be effective against malaria and, in animals, against eptospirosis. In a study of AIDS patients, selenium levels were found to be subnormal, although it is not yet understood whether a deficiency of selenium contributes to the disease or if AIDS reduces selenium levels.

A swath of the southern United States crossing through Georgia and the Carolinas is known as the stroke belt. Not only does this region have the nation's highest stroke rate, it is also known for a very high incidence of heart disease. Not surprisingly, soils in this area are very low in selenium. This supports the observation that cardiovascular disease increases as selenium absorption decreases. A similar correlation has been found in Finland.

Toxic heavy metals such as mercury and cadmium, as well as alcohol, various drugs and cigarette smoke, can all be detoxified by selenium. It is thought the mineral combines with the toxins to yield inert compounds. Selenium may also be able to detoxify some types of carcinogenic fats.

Selenium has also been shown to contribute to the production of sperm and to sperm motility. As an anti-inflammatory, selenium is an effective treatment for arthritis and other autoimmune diseases. It is used to treat a condition called Kashin-Beck disease, which affects the joints of millions of people in a region of China where the soil is known to be deficient in selenium. In this use, it can be effective against growth retardation, joint enlargement, deformity of the spinal column and muscular atrophy, if diagnosed and treated quickly.

■ Chromium—Dietary Insulin

Prior to the 1950s, chromium was thought to be nothing more than a toxic trace metal. Then, in an experiment with rats, it was discovered that feeding them brewer's yeast corrected glucose intolerance—an inability to remove sugar from the blood to nourish the cells—which is one of the characteristics of diabetes. Much work was conducted to isolate the specific component of the yeast responsible for this remarkable cure. It was finally recognized as a chromium-containing compound now called glucose tolerance factor (GTF).

Chromium is available in whole grain cereals, black pepper, meat products and cheese—as well as in brewer's yeast. A deficiency of chromium, besides leading to glucose intolerance, is now known to cause impaired growth, elevated blood cholesterol, fatty deposits in the arteries, decreased sperm count, and infertility, plus an overall decrease in lifespan.

Marginal chromium deficiency is thought to be fairly common in the United States due to a diet of highly refined foods. Studies have also revealed a dramatic lifelong slide in the level of chromium present in body tissues, accompanied by a slow rise in glucose intolerance. It is theorized that this process may contribute to aging.

We cannot live without glucose, but it must be very precisely regulated in the body. Too much can react adversely with many different biological molecules, including hemoglobin, proteins in membranes and possibly even DNA and RNA. Chromium is vital to the body's sensitivity to insulin, which in turn allows us to regulate the use of glucose. Aging, pregnancy, consumption of refined foods, and even strenuous exercise can all contribute to the depletion of chromium in the body. Hypoglycemic patients—those with dangerously low blood sugar levels—have experienced an increase in blood sugars after taking 200 micrograms of chromium daily.

Chromium may also be a part of the cardiovascular disease puzzle. Some researchers found that patients with coronary artery disease have significantly lower levels of chromium than healthy people. Others have reported supplements of chromium can decrease the overall level of cholesterol in the blood, while increasing the level of high density lipoproteins (HDLs).

■ Molybdenum–Poison Control

Molybdenum is as rare in the crust of the earth we call home as it is in the human body. As a trace mineral, it is found in all tissues of the human body. Molybdenum is required for several key enzymes to function properly.

Recently, scientists have come to understand more about molybdenum's role in the human body and have identified the deficiency symptoms. For example, a high rate of cancer of the esophagus in one area of China has been attributed to a lack of molybdenum.

Perhaps most fascinating of all, the extreme scarcity of molybdenum as a geologically occurring mineral and its widespread presence in living things has been used to support the theory that life was planted on earth by extraterrestrial sources.

Organ meats, grains, legumes, leafy vegetables, milk and

beans are all good dietary sources of molybdenum. In the body, molybdenum activates the enzyme sulfite oxidase, which acts to counteract the toxic effects of some of the hazardous substances we encounter daily. For example, this process is used to counter the poisonous effects of the sulfites that are used extensively as food preservatives.

Without the molybdenum-stimulated response to these poisons, we would experience nausea, diarrhea, acute asthma attacks, loss of consciousness and even death. Additionally, the bisulfate form of this pollutant destroys vitamin B_1 unless it is preserved by molybdenum.

Uric acid—one of the body's most important scavengers of dangerous free radicals—is produced by another molybdenum-activated enzyme. These toxic oxygen radicals are believed to be a major cause of degenerative disease and aging.

▪ Bioflavonoids—the Hidden Protectors

Widely available in the plants we eat, bioflavonoids are found in the leaves, flowers, and stems of plants where they provide protection and color to plant tissues. Good sources for bioflavonoids include fruits (especially citrus fruits such as lemons), vegetables, nuts, seeds and buckwheat. Leaves, flowers and bark can also provide the substances when brewed as tea.

First popularized in human nutritional use decades ago as protectors of capillaries, the tiniest of our blood vessels, the bioflavonoids don't completely fit the definition of a vitamin, and no clear-cut deficiency symptoms have been recognized.

In 1968, spurred by an inconclusive study by the National Academy of Sciences and the National Research Council, the United States Food and Drug Administration (FDA) declared bioflavonoids to be "ineffective for treating any human conditions whatsoever" and ordered them removed from the market as drugs. They have continued to be available to consumers as food supplements sold in health food stores.

But the government's bioflavonoid prohibition, perhaps encouraged by the pharmaceutical industry's interest in pushing nutrition *out* to the margins of accepted health care, did little to reduce the public's interest in alternative—and vastly cheaper—forms of prevention and treatment. Now in demand because of the belief that vitamin C cannot work properly without them, bioflavonoid compounds are often found as part of well-balanced multivitamin formulas.

And, in an interesting example of biological checks and balances, not only do we now believe that bioflavonoids are necessary for vitamin C to work in the body, it has been discovered that vitamin C itself protects the bioflavonoid quercetin from oxidation, enabling it to work!

There is also convincing evidence that bioflavonoids themselves have antioxidant actions. By the 1980s, new studies were being published that suggested bioflavonoids had all sorts of previously unknown beneficial properties.

A 1984 paper published in *Trends in Pharmacological Sciences* stated that bioflavonoids have " . . . potent anti-allergy, anti-inflammatory, and anti-viral activity."

During the Second International Conference on Antiviral Research, a number of researchers reported on anti-viral properties of the bioflavonoids. Derivatives of quercetin were found to be effective against a variety of viruses, including polio, ECHO, coxsackie virus and the rhinoviruses responsible for the common cold. It should come as no surprise that the researchers also discovered quercetin had no anti-viral properties by itself—it had to be used in conjunction with vitamin C!

Hesteperidin and quercetin have also been found to be active against herpes type 1, respiratory viruses and influenza viruses in the laboratory. Tests also suggest they have an effect on cells that cause allergic reactions, slowing the release of the histamines that cause sneezing, running noses and itchy, watering eyes.

Several classes of bioflavonoids have also been found to be anti-inflammatories and anti-spasmodic agents. In recent years, there has been an increased interest in the medicinal properties of herbs. A number of investigators have pointed out that bioflavonoids appear to be the active ingredients in many herbs that have been in use as medicines since the dawn of time.

■ Sources of Subtances Mentioned in this Chapter

All of the vitamins, minerals, bioflavonoids and other nutrients mentioned in this chapter are commonly available in health food and vitamin stores.

■ Conclusion

The information in this book will not be worth anything unless you do something about it. Only you are responsible for your health. Don't wait until you get sick. That's like worrying about tooth decay after all your teeth have fallen out!

References

Abe, N., Ebina, T., and Ishida, N. 1982. Interferon induction by glycyrrhizin and glycyrrhetinic acid in mice. *Microbial Immunol.* 26:535–539.

Abonyi, M., Kisfaludy, S., and Szalay, F. 1984. Therapeutic effect of (+)- cyanidanol-3 in toxic alcoholic liver disease and in chronic active hepatitis. *Acta. Phsiol. Hung.* 64: 455–460.

Adachi, K., and Sadai, M. 1985. "The hair-growing product no. 82447." Japanese patent application.

Adachi, K., 1987. Mechanism on hair-growing effect of PDG. Proceedings of the 17th World Congress of Dermatology.

Ala El Din Barradah, M., Shoukry, I., and Hegazy, M. 1967. Difrarel 100 in the treatment of retinal vascular disorders and high myopia. Bulletin of the Opthamological Society of Egypt. 60:251.

Albert-Puleo, M. 1980. Fennel and anise as estrogenic agents. *J. Ethnopharmacology.* 2:337–344.

Alfieri, R., and Sole, P. 1964. Influences des anthocyanosides admistres par voie parenterale sur l'adaptoelectro-retinogramme du lapin. *C. R. Soc. Biol.* 158:2338.

Altman, L. 1992. "Prostrate drug's effects cited." *New York Times*, June 23.

AMA Laboratories. 1988. Independent unpublished cross-over, double-blind study conducted by AMA Laboratories, of Tri-Genesis Hair Growth Formula.

Annin, P., and Underwood, A. 1993. "A Week of Woes Raises More Questions About Saint Merck", *Newsweek*, Aug. 2.

Ask-Upmark. 1967. Prostatitis and its treatment. *Acta Med. Scand.* 181:355–357.

Aslan, A. 1985. Specifications Regarding the Technique and Action of Gerovital H3 Treatment After 34 Years of Usage. Bucharest, Romania: Natl. Inst. of Ger.

Baetgen, D. 1961. "Results of the treatment of epidemic hepatitis in children with high doses of ascorbic acid." *Medizinische Monatschrift.* 15:30–36.

Bailliart, J. P. 1969. "Tentative d' amelioration de la vision nocturne." *Le Medicine de Reserve.* 121.

Baraona, E., and Lieber, C. 1979. Effects of ethanol on lipid metabolism. *J. Lipid Res.* 20:289–315.

Barker, H., Frank, O., Thind, I. C., et al. 1979. Vitamin profiles in elderly persons living at home or in nursing homes versus profile in healthy young subjects. *J. Am. Geriatrics Society.* 10:444–450.

Barry, M. 1990. Epidemiology and natural history of benign prostatic hyperplasia. *Urologic Clinics of N. Am.* 17 (3) 495–507.

Baur, H., and Staub, H. 1954. Treatment of hepatitis with infusions of ascorbic acid: Comparison with other therapies. *Journal of the AMA.* 156:565.

Beattie, A., Campbell, B., Goldberg, A., and Moore, M. 1976. Blood-lead and hypertension. *Lancet.* ii, 1–3.

Beck, M. 1992. Menopause. *Newsweek*, May 25.

Beisel, W. R. 1990. Future role of micronutrients on immune functions. Annal of the New York Acad. of Sciences. 587:267–274.

Berengo, A., and Esposito, R. 1975 *A double-blind trail of (+)-cyanidanol-3 in viral hepatitis" New Trends in the Therapy of Liver Diseases.* 1177–1181, Springer-Verlang, Basel.

Bever, B., and Zahnd, G. R. 1979. Plants with oral hypoglycemic action. *Quarterly J. Crude Drug Research.* 17: 139–196.

Birchall, J. D., and Espie, A. W. 1986. Biological implications of the interaction of silicon with metal ions. Ciba Foundation Symposium. 121:140.

Blondell, J. M. 1980. The anticarcinogenic effect of magnesium. *Med. Hypotheses.* 6:863–871.

Blum, A., Doelle, W., Kortum, K., et al. 1977. Treatment of acute viral hepatitis with (+)- cyanidanol-3. *Lancet.* ii, 1153–1155.

Boari, C., Montanari, M., Galleti, G. P., et al. 1975. Occupational toxic liver diseases. Therapeutic effects of silymarin. *Min. Med.* 72:2679–2688.

Boeryd, B., and Hallbgren, B. 1980. The influence of the lipid composition of the feed given to mice on the immunocompetence and tumor resistance of the progeny. *Intl. J. Cancer.* 26:241–246.

Bombardierei, G., Minalini, A., Bernardi, L., and Rossi, L. 1985. Effects of s-adenosyl-l-methionine in the treatment of Gilbert's syndrome. *Curr. Ther. Res.* 37:580–585.

Boosalis, M. G., Evans, G. W., and McClain, C. J. 1983. Impaired handling of orally administered zinc in pancreatic insufficiency. *Am. J. Clin. Nutrition.* 37: 268–271.

Bordia, A., and Bansal, H. C. 1973. Essential oil of garlic in prevention of atheroslcerosis. *Lancet.* ii: 1491.

Boyd, E. M., and Berry, N. E. 1939. Prostatic hypertrophy as part of a generalized metabolic disease. Evidence of the presence of a lipopenia. *J. Urol.* 41:406–411.

Brattstrom, L. E., Hultberg, B. L., and Hardebo, J. E. 1985. Folic acid responsive postmenopausal homocysteinemia. *Metabolism.* 34:1073–1077.

Bricklin, M. 1990. "The prostatic cancer group has switched to a low-risk one." pp. 438–439, New York: Penguin Books.

Brohult, A., Brohult, J., Brohult, S., and Joelsson, I. 1977. Effect of alkyglycerols on the frequency of injuries following radiation therapy for carcinoma of the uterine cervix. *Acta Obstet. Gynecol. Scane.* 56 (4) 441.

Canini, F., Bartolucci, A., Cristallini, E., et al. 1985. Use of Silymarin in the treatment of alcoholic hepatic stenosis. *Clin. Ther.* 114:307–314.

Carlisle, E. M. 1986. Silicon as an essential trace element in animal nutrition. Ciba Foundation Symposium. 121:123.

Catheart, R. F. 1981. The method of determining proper doses of vitamin C for the treatment of disease titrating to bowel tolerance. *J. Orthmol. Psychiat.* 10:125–132.

Cavalieri, S. 1974. A controlled clinical trial of Legalon in 40 patients. *Gazz. Med. Ital.* 133:628–635.

Champault, G., Patel, J. C., and Bonard, A. M. 1984. A double-blind trial of an extract of the plant Sereno repens in benign prostatic hyperplasia. *Brit. J. Clin. Pharmacol.* 18:461–462.

Chandra, R. K. 1987. Nutrition and immunity: I. basic considerations. II. practical applications. *J. Dent. Child.* 54 (3) 193–197.

Chang, H. M., and But, P. [eds.] 1986. Pharmacology and applications of Chinese Materia Medica. Teaneck, NJ: World Scientific Publishing Co.

Cohen, L., and Litzes, R. 1981. Infrared spectroscopy and magnesium content of bone mineral in osteoporotic women. *Isr. J. Med. Sci.* 17:1123–1125.

Conn, H. [ed.] 1981. "International Workshop on (+)-Cyanidanol-3 in Diseases of the Liver" Royal Society of Medicine Symposia Series no. 47, Academic Press, London.

Cookson, F. B., Altshcul, R., and Federoff, S. 1967. The effects of alfalfa on serum cholesterol and in modifying or preventing cholesterol induced atherosclerosis in rabbits. *J. Atherosclerosis Res.* 7:69–81.

Costello, C. H., and Lynn, E. V. 1950. Estrogenic substances from plants: glycyrrhiza glabra. *J. Am. Pharm. Assc.* 39:177–180.

Daly, J. M., Dudrick, S. J., and Copeland, E. M. 1978. Effects of protein depletion and repletion on cell-mediated immunity in experimental animals. *Ann. Surg.* 188 (6) 791–796.

De Froment, P. 1974. "Unsaponifiable substance from alfalfa for pharmaceuticals and cosmetic uses." French Patent 2,187,328.

Doheny, K. 1992. "New laser approach to prostate surgery." *Los Angeles Times*, Aug. 12.

Donsbach, K. W. 1989. The Prostate. Rosarito Beach, Mexico: Wholistic Publications.

Dreisbach, R. H. *Handbook of Poisoning*, 11th ed. pp. 80–83. Los Altos, CA: Lange Medical Publication.

Duke, J. A. 1985. *Handbook of Medicinal Herbs*. Boca Raton, FL: CRC Press.

Ehrenpreis, S., Balagot, R. C., Comaty, J. E., and Myles, S. B. 1978. "Naloxone reversible analgesia in mice produced by D-phenylalanine and hydrocinamic acid, inhibitors of carboxypep-tidase A." Advances in Pain Research and Therapy, vol. 3.

Ellis, F., Holesch, S., and Ellis, J. 1972. Incidence of osteoporosis in vegetarians and omnivores. *Am. J. Clin. Nutrition*. 25:555–558.

Evans, G. W. 1980. Normal and abnormal zinc absorption in man and animals: the tryptophan connection. *Nutrition Reviews*. 38:137–141.

Evans, G. W., and Johnson, E. C. 1981. Effect of iron, vitamin B-6 and picolinic acid on zinc absorption in the rat. *J. Nutrition*. 111:68–75.

Evans, Wm., Rosenberg, I. H. 1991. *Biomarkers*. New York: Simon & Shuster.

Faber, K. 1958. The dandelion—Taraxacum officinale Weber. *Pharmazie*. 13:423–435.

Fahim, W. S., Harman, J. M. Clevenger, T. H., et. al. 1982. Effect of panax ginseng on testosterone level and prostate in male rats. *Arch. Androl*.

Feinblatt, H. M., and Gant, J. C. 1958. Palliative treatment of benign prostatic hypertrophy: value of glycine, alanine, glutamic acid combination. *J. Maine Med. Assoc.* 49:99.

Felter, H. W. 1983. *The Eclectic Materia Medica, Pharmacology and Therapeutics*. Portland, OR: Eclectic Medical Publication.

Fisher, J. A. 1990. The Chromium Program. New York: Harper and Row.

Folkers, K. Watanabe, T., and Kaji, M. 1977. Critique of coenzyme Q10 in biochemical research on cardiovascular disease. *J. Mol. Med.* 2:461.

Folkers, K., and Yamamura, Y. eds. 1984. Biomedical and Clinical Aspects of Coenzyme Q, vol. 4. Amsterdam: Elsevier Science Publishers.

Formann, S., Hashell, W. Vranizan, K., et al. 1983. The association of blood pressure and dietary alcohol: difference by age, sex and estrogen use. *Am. J. Epid.* 118:497–507.

Francis, R. M., and Beaumont, D. M. 1987. Involutional osteoporosis. Letter to the Editor. *New Eng. J. Med.* 316: 216.

Freudenheim, M. 1992. Prostate treatment could be bonanza. *New York Times*, June 22.

Frezza, M., Possato, G., Chiesa, L., et al. 1984. Reversal of intrahepatic cholestasis of pregnancy in women after high dose s-adenosyl-l-methionine (SAMe) administration. *Hepatology.* 4:274–278.

Fujimoto, I., Hanai, A., and Oshima, A. 1979. Descriptive epidemiology of cancer in Japan: current cancer incidence and survival data. *Natl. Cancer Ins. Monographs.* 53:5–15.

Gestetner, B., Assa, Y. Henis, Y., Birk, Y., and Bondi, A. 1971. Lucerne saponins. IV. Relation between their chemical constitution and hemolytic and anti-fungal activities. *J. Science, Food and Agriculture.* 22 (4) 168–172.

Gibbs, O. S. 1947. On the curious pharmacology of hydrastis. *Fed. Am. Soc. Exp. Biol. Fed. Proc.* 6 (1) 332.

Gilbert, A., and Carnot, P. 1896. Note prelinair sur l'opotherapie hepatique. *Compt. Rend. Soc. Biol.* 48: 934–937.

Gil Del Rio, E. 1968. Los antocianosidos del Vaccinum myrtillus en optalmologia. *Gaz. Med de France.* vol. 18, June 25.

Gladwell, Malcolm. 1990. "Serious Side Effects Linked

To Many Approved Drugs," The *Washington Post*, May 28.

Glauser, S., Bello, S., and Gauser, E. 1976. Blood-cadmium levels in untreated hypertensive humans. *Lancet*. i:717–718.

Goldin, B. R., and Gorbach, S. L. 1984. The effect of milk and lactobacillus feeding on human intestinal bacterial enzyme activity. *Am. J. Clin. Nutrition*. 39:756–761.

Goldstein, A. 1992. "Overmedication Poses Significant Health Risk." The *Washington Post*. February 8.

Gorman, C. 1992. "Can Drug Firms Be Trusted," *Time* magazine, Feb. 10.

Graber, C. D., Goust, M. M., Glassman, A. D., Kendall, R., and Loadholt, C. B. 1981. Immunomodulating properties of dimethylglycine in humans. *J. Infectious Diseases*. 143 (1) 101–105.

Greenberg, J. 1993. "Your Money Or Your Life," *Playboy*. August.

Grossman, M., Kirsner, J., and Gillespie, I. 1963. Basal and histalog-stimulated gastric secretion in control subjects and in patients with peptic ulcer or gastric cancer. *Gastroenterol.*, 45:14–26

Gruchow, H. W., Sobocinski, M. S., and Barboriak, J. J. 1985. Alcohol, nutrient intake, and hypertension in U.S. adults. *J. AMA* 253:1567–1570.

Gutfeld, R. 1993. "F.D.A. Attacks Drug Makers' Ads To Doctors," The *Wall Street Journal*. August 3.

Habib, F. K., et al. 1976. Metal-androgen interrelationships in carcinoma and hyperplasia of the human prostate. *J. Endocrinol*. 71 (1) 133–141.

Harman, D. 1981. "The aging process." Proceedings of the Nat. Acad. of Sciences, vol. 78, no. 11. pp. 7124–7128, November.

Hartroft, W. S., Porta, E. A., and Suzuki, M. 1964. Effects of choline chloride on hepatic lipids after acute ethanol intoxication. *Q.J. Stuc. Alcohol*. 25:427–434.

Hasegaw, T. [ed.] 1975. Proc. First Intersectional Cong. Int. Assoc. Microbiol. Soc. 3:432–442. Tokyo University Press.

Havsteen, B. 1983. Flavonoids, a class of natural products of high pharmacological potency. *Biochem. Pharm.* 32 (7) 1141–1148.

Hikino, H., Kiso, Y., Wagner, H., and Fiebig, M. 1984. Antihepatotoxic actions of flavonolignans from Silybum marianum fruits. *Planta Medica.* 50:248–250.

Hirayama, S., Kishikawa, H., Kume, T., & Tada, H. 1978. Therapeutic effect of liver hydrolysate on experimental liver cirrhosis. *Nisshin Igaku.* 45:528–533.

Hochschild, R. 1973. Effect of dimethylaminoethanol on the life span of senile male A/J mice. *Exp. Ger.* 8:185–191.

Hodges, R., and Rebello, T. 1983. Carbohydrates and blood pressure. *Ann. Int. Med.* 98:814–838.

Hoffmann, D. 1991. *The New Holistic Herbal.* pp. 69–70. Rockport, MA: Element, Inc.

Holl, M. G., and Allen, L. H. 1988. Comparative effects of meals high in protein, sucrose, or starch on human mineral metabolism and insulin secretion. *Am. J. Clin. Nutrition.* 48:1219.

Honegger, C., and Honegger, R. 1959. Occurrence and quantitative determination of 2–dimethylaminoethanol in animal tissue extracts. *Nature.* 184:550–552.

Horton, R. 1984. Benign prostatic hyperplasia: a disorder of androgen metabolism in the male. *J. Am. Ger. Soc.* 32:380–385.

Hosein, E. A., and Bexton, B. Protective action of carnitine on liver lipid metabolism after ethanol administration to rats. *Biochem. Pharm.* 24:1859–1863.

Hunt, G. L. 1987. "Coenzyme Q10: Miracle Nutrient?" *Omni.* p. 24, Feb.

Hvalik, R., Hubert, H., Fabsitz, R., and Feinleib, M. 1983. Weight and hypertension. *Ann. Int. Med.* 98:855–859.

Hypertension Detection and Follow-Up Program Cooperative Group. 1977. Race, education and prevalence of hypertension. *Am. J. Epidemiol.* 106:351–361.

Infante-Rivard, C., Krieger, M., Gascon-Barre, M., and Rivard, G. E. 1986. Folate deficiency among institutionalized elderly, public health impact. *J. Am. Ger. Soc.* 34:311–214.

The Institute for Advanced Study of Human Sexuality Research Department (IASHSRD), 1990, The Avena sativa Project: A Research Report on Sexual Health Care Products with Extract of Avena sativa. San Francisco, CA.

Intelli-Scope. 1992. "Natural Fat-loss," October, vol. 5.

Jameson, P. G. 1988. *The Herbal Handbook*. London: Brighton Press.

Jayle, G. E., Aubry, M., Gavini, M., and Braccini, G. 1965. Etude concernant l' action sur la vision nocturne des anthocyanosides extraits de Vaccinum myrtillus. *Ann. Ocul.* 198:556.

1988 Joint National Committe. A report on detection, evaluation and treatment of high blood pressure. *Arch. Int. Med.* 148:36–39.

Judd, A. M., MacLeod, R. M., and Login , I. S. 1984. Zinc acutely, selectively and reversibly inhibits pituitary prolactin secretion. *Brain Research.* 294:191–192.

Kagawa, T. 1978. Impact of westernization on the Japanese. Changes in physique, cancer and longevity. *Prev. Med.* 7:205–217.

Kamanna, V. S., and Chandrasekhara, N. 1982. Effect of garlic on serum lipoproteins and lipprotein cholesterol levels in albino rats rendered hypercholesteremic by feeding cholesterol. *Lipids.* 17 (7) 483–488.

Kamen, B. 1989. Startling New Facts About Osteoporosis. Novato, CA: Nutrition Encounter, Inc.

Kaplan, N. M. 1985. Non-drug treatment of hypertension. *Ann. Int. Med.* 102:359–373.

Kershbaum, A., Pappajohn, D., Bellet, S. 1968. Effect of smoking and nicotine on adrenocortical secretion. *J. AMA.* 203:113–116.

Khaw, K. T., and Barrett-Connor, S. 1984. Dietary potassium and blood pressure in a population. *Am. J. Clin. Nutr.* 39:963–968.

Kinsella, K. G. 1992. Changes in life expectancy 1900–1990. *Am. J. Clin. Nutr.* 55:1196S–1202S.

Kiso, Y., Suzuki, Y., Watanabe, N., et al. 1983. Antihepatotoxic principles of curcumba longa rhizomes. *Planta Medica.* 49:185–187.

Klenner, F. R. 1971. Observations on the administration of ascorbic acid when employed beyond the range of a vitamin in human pathology. *J. Applied Nutr.* 23:61–88.

Knodell, R. G., et al. 1981. Vitamin C prohylaxis for post-transfusion hepatitis: lack of an effect in a controlled trial. *Am. J. Clin. Nutr.* 34:20.

Kotulak, R., and Gorner, R. 1991. "Science begins to reset the clock: new insights guide research into living younger, longer." The *Chicago Tribune*, Dec. 8.

Krasinski, S. D., Russell, R. M., Furie, B. C., et al. 1985. "The prevalence of vitamin K deficiency in chronic gastrointestinal disorders. *Am. J. Clin. Nutr.* 41:639–643.

Krieger, I., Cash, R., and Evans, G. W. 1984. Picolinic acid in acrodermatitis enteropathica: evidence or a disorder of tryptophan metabolism. *J. Ped. Gastr. Nutr.* 3:62–68.

Kritchevsky, D. 1975. Effect of garlic oil on experimental atherosclerosis in rabbits. *Artery.* 1 (4) 319–323.

Kuagai, A., Nanboshi, M., Asanuma, Y., et al. 1967. Effects of glycyrrhizin on thymolytic and immunosuppressive action of cortisone. *Endocrinol Japan.* 145:39–42.

Kugler, H. 1989. Tyrosine's effect on the depression syndrome. *Prev. Med. Up-Date.* 2 (6).

Kugler, H. 1990a. Procaine versus the DMAE-PABA formula. *Prev. Med. Up-Date.* 4 (11).

Lahtonen, R. 1985. Zinc and cadmium concentrations in whole tissue and in separated epithelium and stroma from human benign prostatic hypertrophic glands. *Prostate.* 6:177–183.

Lancet. 1986. Citrate for calcium nephrolithiasis. p. 955.

Lang, T., Degoulet, P., Aime, F., et al. 1983. Relationship between coffee drinking and blood pressure: analysis of 6,321 subjects in Paris. *Am. J. Card.* 52:1238–1242.

Leake, A., Chisholm, G. D., and Habib, F. K. 1984a. The effect of zinc on the 5-alpha-reduction of testosterone by the hyperplastic human prostate gland. *J. Steroid Biochem.* 20:651–655.

Leake, A., Chisholm, G. D., Busuttil, A., and Habib, F. K. 1984a. Subcellular distribution of zinc in the benign and malignant human prostate: evidence for a direct zinc androgen interaction. *Acta Endocrinol.* 105:281–288.

Leary, Warren E. 1993. "Companies Accused of Overcharging For Drugs Developed With U.S. Aid." The *New York Times*, Jan. 20.

Lesourd, B. M. 1990. Immunologic aging. Effect on denutrition. *Ann. Biol. Clin.* 48 (5) 309–318.

Leung, A. Y. 1980. *Encyclopedia of Common Natural Ingredients Used in Food, Drugs, and Cosmetics.* New York: John Wiley & Sons.

Levenson 1983. Tyrosine: An Energy Enhancer. *J. Parenteral Enteral Nutr.* 7 (2) 181–183.

Lewis, A. 1990. Dimethylaminoethanol (DMAE): An Overview of its Health Effects and Potential Uses. Belmont Chemicals, Inc.

Lewis, H. L., and Memory P. F. *Medical Botany: Plant's Affecting Man's Health*, p. 401. New York: John Wiley & Sons.

Lewis, N. M. 1989. Calcium supplements and milk: effects on acid-base balance and on retention of calcium, magnesium, and phosphorous. *Am. J. Clin. Nutr.* 49:527.

Lippman, R. 1980. Chemiluminescent measurement of free radicals and antioxidant molecular-protection inside living rat mitochondria. *Exp. Ger.* 15:339–351.

Lucas, R. M. 1991. *Miracle Medicinal Herbs.* Paramus, NJ: Prentice Hall, p. 6.

Malinow, M. R., McLaughlin, P., and Papworth, L. 1976. Hypocholesterolemic effect of alfalfa in cholesterol-fed monkeys. *Intl. Symp. on Atherosclerosis.* Tokyo, Japan.

Mandell, M. 1985. *Lifetime Arthritis Relief System.* New York: Berkley Books.

Maros, T., Racz, G., Katonaj, B., and Kovacs, V. 1966. 1968. The effects of cynara scolymus extracts on the regeneration of the rat liver. *Arzneim-Forsch.* 1966. 16:127–129: 1968. 18:884–886.

Marsh, A., Sanchez, T., Chaffee, F., et al. 1983. Bone mineral mass in adult lacto-ovo-vegetarian and omnivorous adults. *Am. J. Clin. Nutr.* 37:453–456.

Martin, D., Mayes, P., and Rodwell, V. 1983. *Harper's Rev. of Biochemistry.* Los Altos, CA: Lange.

Masquelier, J. 1980. Natural Products as Medicinal Agents. *J. Nat. Products*, July.

Masquelier, J. 1987. "U.S. Patent No. 4,698,360," Oct. 6.

Matson, F., Grudy, S., and Crouse, J. 1982. *Am. J. Clin. Nutr.* 35:697–700.

Maugh, T. H., II. 1992. "Scientists draw back veil on the mystery of aging." The *Los Angeles Times*, Feb. 8.

Maynard, G., Franch, J. P., and Dorne, P. A. 1970. "Use of tetrahydroxy flaven diol in opthamology, in particular in diabetic retinopathies (based on 40 cases)." Lyon Medical, no. 4, Jan. 25.

McCaslin, F. E., Jr., and Janes, J. M. 1959. "The effect of strontium lactate in the treatment of osteoporosis." Proc. Staff Meetings Mayo Clinic, v. 34, p. 329.

Meneely, G., and Battarbee, H. 1976. High sodium-low potassium environment and hypertension. *Am. J. Card.* 38:768–781.

Meydani, S. N., Furukawa, T., Meydani M., and Blumberg, J. B. 1990. "Beneficial effect of dietary antioxidants on the aging immune system." Nutr. Immun. and Tox. Lab., USDA Human Nutr. Res. Center of Aging, Tufts University.

Middleton. E. 1984. "The flavonoids." TIPS, August.

Milkie, G. 1972. "Diet and its effect on the visual system," presented at the Annual Meeting of the Am. Acad. of Optometry, New York, Dec. 19.

Miller, E. 1974. Deanol in treatment of levodopa-induced dyskinesias. *Neurology.* 24:116–119.

Miller, J. Z., Nance, W. E., Norton, J. A., Wolen, R. L., Griffith, R. S., Rose, R. J. 1977. Therapeutic effect of vitamin C, a co-twin control study. *J. AMA.* 237:248–251.

Mindell, E. 1991. *Vitamin Bible*, pp. 64–65. New York: Warner Books.

Mitscher, L., Park, Y., and Clark, D. 1980. Antimicrobial agents from higher plants: antimicrobial isoflavonoids from glycyrrhiza glabra L. var. typica. *J. Nat. Products.* 43:259–269.

Montgomery, R., Dryer, R., Conway, T., and Spector, A. 1980. *Biochemistry: a case-oriented approach*. St. Louis, MO: Mosby.

Montini, M., Levoni, P., Angoro, A., and Pagani, G. 1975. Controlled trial of cynarin in the treatment of the hyperlipemic syndrome. *Arzneim-Forsch*. 25:1311–1314.

Morales, A., Condra, M., Owen, J. A., Surridge, D. H., Fenemore, J., and Harris, C. 1987. Is yohimbine effective in the treatment of organic impotence? Results of a controlled trial. *J. Urol.* 137 (6) 1168–1172.

Morris, D. L. 1992. "Squeeze On Pharmaceuticals," *Chem. Wk.*, Aug. 12.

Mowrey, D. 1986. *The Scientific Validation of Herbal Medicine*. New Canaan, CT: Keats Publishing.

Murata, A. 1975. "Viricidal activity of vitamin C: vitamin C for prevention and treatment of viral diseases" in Hasegawa, T. [ed.]. Proc. First Intersectional Cong. Int. Assoc. Microbiol. Soc. 3:432–442. Tokyo University Press.

Murav'ev, I. A., and Kononikhina, N. F. 1972. Estrogenic properties of glycyrrhiza glabra. *Rastitel'nye Resursy*. 8 (4) 490–497.

Murphree, H., Pfeiffer, C., and Backerman, I. 1959. The stimulant effect of 2–dimethylaminoethanol (deanol) in human volunteer subjects. *Clin. Phar. Ther.* 1 (3) 303–310.

Nagai, K. 1970. A study of the excretory mechanism of the liver-effect of liver hydrolysate on BSP excretion. *Jap. J. Gastroenterol.* 67:633–638.

Nandkarni, A. K. 1954. Indian Materia Medica. *Panvel* 1 (3) 189–190.

National Institutes of Health Consensus Conference: Osteoporosis. 1984. *J. AMA*. 252:799.

Nicar, M. J., and Pak, C.Y.C. 1985. Calcium bioavailability from calcium carbonate and calcium citrate. *J. Clin. Endo. Metab*. 61:391–393.

Nielsen, F. H. 1988. "Boron-an overlooked element of potential nutrition importance." *Nutrition Today*, Jan/Feb., pp. 4–7.

Nishinlhon J. Derm. 1986. LKF-a research team, clinical evaluation of LKF-A on male pattern alopecia. 48 (4) 738–748.

Nomura, A., Henderson, B. E., and Lee, J. 1978. Breast cancer and diet among the Japanese in Hawaii. *Am. J. Clin. Nutr.* 31:2020–2025.

Nutrition Rev. 1984. The function of the vitamin K-dependent proteins, bone GLA protein (BGP) and kidney GLA proteins (KGP). *Nutrional Review.* 42:230–233.

Oba, K. 1986. Development of hair growing product especially with a property of PDG. *Fragrance Journal.* 14 (5) 109–114.

Ohbayashi, A., Akoka, T., and Tasaki, H. 1972. A study of effects of liver hydrolysate on hepatic circulation. *J. Therapy.* 54:1582–1585.

Osvaldo, R. 1974. 2–dimethylaminoethanol deanol: a brief review of its clinical efficacy and postulated mechnism of action. *Curr. Ther. Res.* 16 (11) 1238–1242.

Padova, C., Tritapepe, R., Padova, F., et al. 1984. S-adenosyl-L-methionine antagonizes oral contraceptive-induced bile cholesterol supersaturation in healthy women: preliminary report of a controlled randomized trial. *Am. J. Gastroenterol.* 79:941–944.

Paganelli, G. M., Biasco, G., Brandi, G., 1992. Effect of vitamin A, C, and E supplementation on rectal cell proliferation in patients with colorectal adenomas. *J. Nat. Can. Inst.* 84 (1) 4751.

Par A., Horvath, T., Bero, T., et al. 1984. Inhibition of hepatic drug metabolism by (+)-cyanidanol-3 (catergen) in chronic alcoholic liver disease. *Acta Physiol. Hung.* 54:449–454.

Passwater, R. A. 1987. "Coenzyme Q-10: The Nutrient of the 90's" *Whole Foods*, pp. 9–13, April.

————.1991. *The New Supernutrition*. New York: Pocket Books.

Pauling, L. 1986. *How To Live Longer and Feel Better*. New York: Avon Books.

Pautler, E. L., Mega, J. A., and Tengerdy, C. A pharmacologically potent natural product in the bovine retina. *Exp. Eye Res.* March, 42 (3):285–288.

Pelletier, O. 1968. Smoking and vitamin C levels in humans. *Am. J. Clin. Nutri.*, 21:1254–1258.

Pelton, R., and Pelton, T. C. 1989. *Mind Food & Smart Pills*. New York: Doubleday.

Peltz, James F. 1992, "Insurer To Reimburse Cost of Non-Surgical Heart Care.", The *Los Angles Times*.

Penn, N. D., et al. 1990. "The effect of dietary supplementation with vitamins A, C and E on cell-mediated immune function in elderly long-stay patients." *Age and Aging* 20 (20) 169–174.

Peretz, A. M., et al. 1990. Enhancement of the immune response by selenium: clinical trials. *Artzl. Lab.* 36:299–304.

Petersdorf, R. 1983. Harrison's Princ. of Int. Med. New York: McGraw-Hill.

Piazza, M., Guadagnino, V., Picciotto, J., et al. 1983. "Effect of (+)-cyanidanol-3 in acute HAV, HBV, and non-A, non-B viral hepatitius." *Hepatology*. 3:45–49.

Pierkle, J. L., Scwartz, J. Landis, J. R., and Harlan, W. R. 1985. The relationship between blood lead levels and blood pressure and its cardiovascular risk implications. *Am. J. Epid.* 121:246–258.

Pizzorno, J. E., and Murray, M. T. 1988. *A Textbook of Nat. Med.*, ch. 4, "Hepatoprotection." John Bastyr College Publications.

Pointet-Guillot, U. 1958. *Contribution a l'etude chimique et pharmacologique de la reglisse*. These, Paris.

Pompeii, R., Pani, A., Flore, O., Marcialis, M., and Loddo, B. 1980. Antiviral activity of glycyrrhizic acid. *Experientia*. 36:304–305.

Potter, J. F., and Beevers D. G. 1984. Pressor effect of alcohol in hypertension. *Lancet*. January 21:1 (8369). 119–121.

Poydock, M. E., et al. 1979. Inhibiting effect of vitamins C and B_{12} on the mitotic activity of ascites tumors. *Exp. Cell. Biol.* 47 (3) 210–217.

Pristautz, H. 1975. Cynarin in the modern treatment of hyperlipemias. *Wiener Medizinische Wocheschrift*. 1223:705–709.

Ralz, G. 1993. "Drug Companies' Profit Margins Top Most Industries . . ." The *Wall Street Journal*, Feb. 26.

Ramesha A., Rao N., Rao A. R., et al. 1990. Chemoprevention of 7, 12 dimethylbenz[a]anthracene-induced mammary carcinogensis in rat by the combined actions of selenium, magensium, ascorbic acid, and reintylacetate. *Jap. J. Can. Res.* 81:1239–1246.

Rao, C., Rao, V., and Steinman, B. 1981. Influence of bioflavonoids on the metabolism and crosslinking of collagen. *Ital. J. Biochem.* 30:259–270.

Reap, E. A., and Lawson, J. W. 1990. Stimulation of the immune response by dimethylglycine, a nontoxic metabolite. *J. Lab. Clin. Med.* 115:481–486.

Recker, R. R. 1985. The effect of milk supplements on calcium metabolism and calcium balance. *Am. J. Clin. Nutri.* 41:254.

Regenstein, L. 1982. *America the Poisoned*. Washington, DC: Acropolis.

Reid, K., Surridge, D. H. Morales, A., Condra, M. Harris, C., Owen, J., and Fenemore, J. 1987. Double-blind trial of yohimbine in treatment of psychogenic impotence. *Lancet.* 2 (8556) 421–423.

Robbins, S., Cotran, R., and Kuman, V. 1984. *Pathologic Basis of Disease*. Philadelphia, PA: W. B. Saunders.

Robertson, J., Donner, A., and Trevithick, J. 1991. A possible role for vitamins C and E in cataract prevention. *Am. J. Clin. Nutri.* 53:346–351.

Rogers, L. L., and Pelton, R. B. 1957. Effect of glutamate on IQ scores of mentally deficient children. *Tex. Rep. on Bio. and Children.* 15 (1) 84–90.

Rubenstein, E., and Federman, D. D. 1988. Scientific American medicine. *Scien. Am.* 4 (vii) 1–6.

Rubin, R.; Hawkins, D; Poodolsky, D. 1993. "A Double Dose Of Medicine," *U.S. News and World Report*, July 19.

Rundle, R. L., Stevens, A. 1993. "Investigators Intensify

Crackdown On Fraud In The Health Industry," *The Wall Sreet Journal*, Aug. 16.

Sachan, D. A. and Rhew, T. H. 1983. Lipotropic effect of carnitine on alcohol-induced hepatic stenosis. *Nutri. Rep. Int.* 27:1221–1226.

Sachan, D. S., Rhew, T. H., and Ruark, R. A. 1984. Ameliorating effects of carnitine and its precursors on alcohol-induced fatty liver. *Am. J. Clin. Nutr.* 39:738–744.

Sadai, M. 1987. "Effect of PDG on cultured dermal papilla cells, especially with reference to ATP production and DNA synthesis." Presented at the 17th World Congress of Dermatology.

Salmi, H. A., and Sarna, S. 1982. "Effects of silymarin on chemical, functional and morphological alteration of the liver. A double-blind controlled study." *Scand. J. Gastroenterol.* 17:417–421.

Sanbe, K., Murata, T., Fujisawa, K., et al. 1973. Treatment of liver disease—with particular reference to liver hydrolysates. *Jap. J. Clin, Exp. Med.* 50:2665–2676.

Santillo, H. 1991. *Natural Healing with Herbs*. Prescott, AZ: Hohm Press.

Sarre, H. 1971. Experience in the treatment of chronic hepatopathies with silymarin. *Arzeim-Forsch.* 21:1209–1212.

Scheiber, V., and Wohlzogen, F. X. 1978 Analysis of a certain type of 2 X 3 tables, exemplified by biopsy findings in a controlled clinical trial. *Int. Clin. Pharmacol.* 16:533–535.

Schomerus H., Wieman, K., Dolle, W., et al. 1984. (+)-cyanidanol-3 in the treatment of acute viral hepatitis: a randomized controlled trial. *Hepatology.* 4:331–335.

Scott, W. W. 1945. The lipids of the prostatic fluid, seminal plasma and enlarged prostate gland of man. *J. Uro.* 53:712–718.

Sharaf, A., Gomaa, N., El-Camal, M.H.A. 1975. Glycyrrhetic acid as an active estro genic substance separated from glycyrrhiza glabra (licorice). *Egyp. J. of Pharm. Science*, 16 (2) 245–251.

Sinquin, G., Morfin, R. F., Charles, J. F., and Floch, H. H. Testosterone metabolism by homogenates of human prostates with benign hyperplasia: effects of zinc, cadmium, and other bivalent cations. *J. Steroid Biochem.* 20:733–780.

Skrabal, F. Aubock, J., and Hortnagl, H. 1981. Low sodium/high potassium diet for prevention of hypertension: probable mechanisms of action. *Lancet.* ii., 895–900.

Smith-Barbaro, P., Hanson, D., and Reddy, B. S. 1981. Carcinogen binding to various types of dietary fiber. *J. Nat Canc. Inst.* 67 (2) 495–497.

Stanko, R. T., Mendelow, H., Shinozuka, H., and Adibi, S. A. 1978. Prevention of alcohol-induced fatty liver by natural metabolites and riboflavin. *J. Lab. Clin. Med.* 91:228–235.

Stark, P. 1992. "Not All Drug Lords Are Outlaws," The *New York Times*, August 12.

Stolberg, S. 1992. "Rewiring the mind and body." The *Los Angeles Times*, Nov. 30.

Stone, Leonard. 1990. "F.D.A. Seeks Labeling That Would List Side Effects of Drugs on Elderly." *Louisville Courier Journal*, Louisville, KY. November 6.

Surgeon General's Report on Nutrition and Health. 1988. Washington, DC: U.S. Dept. of Health and Human Serv.

Susset, J. G., Tessier, C. D., Wincze, J., Bansal, S., Malhotra, and Schwacha, M. G. 1989. Effect of yohimbine hydrochloride on erectile impotence: a double-blind study. *J. Uro.* 141 (6) 1360–1363.

Suzuki H., et al. 1986 Cianidanol therapy for HBe-antigen-positive chronic hepatitis: a multicenter, double-blind study. *Liver.* 6:35.

Sydenstricker, V. P., et al. 1940. Observations on the "egg white" injury in man. *J. AMA.* 118:1199–1200.

Theodoropoulos, G., Dinos, A., Dimitriou, P., and Archimandritis, A. 1981. "Effect of (+)- cyanidanol-3 in acute hepatitus" in Conn, H. [ed], Int. Workshop on on (+)-cyanidanol-3 in Diseases of the Liver." *Roy. Soc. of Med. Intl. Symp. Series*, no. 47, Academic Press, London.

Thom, J., Morris, J., Bishop, A., and Blacklock, J.J. 1978. The influence of refined carbohydrate on urinary calcium excretion. *Brit. J. Uro.* 50:459–464.

Thompson, J. S., Robbins, J., and Cooper, J. K. 1987. "Nutrition and immune function in the geriatric population." *Clinic. Geriatr. Med.* 3 (2) 309–317.

Thottam, J. 1993. "Generic Drug Makers Prepare For Next Battle," The *Wall Street Journal.* August 9.

Toufexis, A. 1992. "The new scoop on vitamins." *Time* magazine, pp. 54–59, April 6.

Tregarten, S. 1992. "Prescription To Stop Drug Companies' Profiteering," The *Wall Street Journal.* Mar. 5.

Tyihak, E., and Szende, B. 1970. "Basic plant proteins with antitumor activity." Hungarian Patent 798.

Tyroler, H. A., Heyden, S., and Hames, C. G. 1975. "Weight and hypertension: Evans County studies of blacks and whites." Epidem. and Con. of Hypert., ed. O. Paul, pp. 177–205. New York: Stratton.

U.S. Senate hearing, Dec. 11, 1990, before Senate Committee On Labor and Human Resources on promotional practices in the pharmacutical industry.

Vogel, G., Trost, W., Braatz, R., et al. 1975. Studies on pharmacodynamics, site and mechanism of action of silymarin, the antihepatotoxic principle from Silybum marianum (L.) Gaert. *Arzneim-Forsch.* 25:179–185.

Wagner, H. 1981. "Plant constituents with antihepatotoxic activity" in Beal, J. L., and Reinhard, E. [eds.] *Nat. Prod. as Med. Agents.* Stuttgart: Hippokrates-Velag.

Waldholz, M. 1992. "New prostate drug from Merck wins FDA approval." The *Wall Street Journal*, June 23.

Walker, M. 1990. The *Chelation Way.* Garden City Park, NY: Avery Publishing Groups, Inc.

Wallae, A. M., and Grant, J. E. 1975. Effect of zinc on adrogen metabolism in the human hyperplastic prostate. *Biochem. Soc. Trans.* 3:651–655.

Watanabe, Y. 1982a Enzyme activity of hair follicles—especially with regart to glucose-6-phosphate dehydrogenase (G6PDH). *J. Perf. Cos. Soc. Jap.* 6 (1) 9–414.

Watson, R. R., et al. 1991. Effect of b-carotene on lymphocyte subpopulation in the elderly humans: evidence for a dose-response relationship. *Am. J. Clin. Nutr.* 53 (90–4).

Wattenberg, L. 1975. Effects of dietary constituents on the metabolism of chemical carcinogens. *Can. Res.* 35:3326–3331.

Weiss, R. F. 1988. *Herbal Medicine* Ab Arcanum, Gothenburg, Sweden, Beaconsfield, p. 82. Beaconsfield, England: Publishers LTD.

Werbach, M. R. 1987. Nutritional Influences on Illness, pp. 211–212. Tarzana, CA: Third Line Press.

Werbach, M. R. 1988. Nutritional Influences on Illness, pp. 297–298. Tarzana, CA: Third Line Press.

Williams, D. 1993. "Public Service or Just Advertising Hype?" *Alternatives* Newsletter.

Williams, D. M., Lynch, R. E., and Cartwright, G. E. 1975. Superoxide dismutase activity in copper-deficient swine. *Proc. Soc. Exp. Bio. Med.* 149:534–536.

Williams, L. 1992. "F.D.A. Steps Up Effort To Control Vitamin Claims," The *New York Times*, Aug. 2.

Wisniewska-Knypl, J., Sokal, J., Klimczak, J., et al. 1981. Protective effect of methionine against vinyl chloride-mediated depression of non-protein sulfhydryls and cytochrome P-450. *Toxi. Letters*. 8:147–152.

Wolfe, Sidney. Health Letter, April 1993, Public Citizen Health Research Group.

Wynder, E. L. 1979. Dietary habits and Cancer epidemiology. *Cancer*. Supplement, 43 (5) 155–1961.

Index

Schmidt, V., 174–175
Schubert, H., 48
Schulman, Martin, 249
Schwartz, Arthur, 210, 281
Schwartz, Joel, 210
Searle, Alfred, 224
Seasonal Affective Disorder
    (SAD), 61–62, 133–134,
    255–256, 256
Seaweed, 207–208
Selenium
    for aging, 334
    for arthritis and rheumatism,
        333, 335
    for cancer, 209, 333–335, 334
    for cataracts, 333
    dosage, 301
    for heart disease, 179–180, 270,
        333, 334–335
    for immune system, 197, 334
    for liver disease, 333
    Recommended Daily Allowance
        (RDA), 298
    for smoking, 335
Self-destruction process of aging,
    258
Selhub, Jacob, 181
Semord, Albert, 275
Senility and nutrients, 43
Serenoa repens (Saw palmetto
    berry), 77
Serine, 248
Serotonin, 43, 57, 132, 134, 278,
    285
Sex life, healthy, 91–110
    alpha-2-adrenergic receptors
        and, 96–97, 101
    Angelica sinesis for, 108
    aphrodisiacs, 92
    Aspidosperma quebracho for,
        101–102
    beta-blockers and, 167
    beta-sitosterol for, 98
    Bishop's Hat (Epimedium
        grandiflorum) for, 105–106,
        110
    cholesterol and, 96, 98–102
    Damiana (Turnera), 107–108,
        109, 110

dehydroepiandrosterone
    (DHEA) for, 282
Devil's Thorn (Tribulus
    terrestris) for, 103–105, 110
dihydrotestosterone and, 98
diosgenin for, 108
drugs, problems from, 20
Exsativa for sexual health, 110
Gerovital H3 for, 274
horny goat weed for, 102
licorice (Glycyrrhizae radix) for,
    109
for men, 96
nettle (Urtica dioica) for, 92–95,
    110
oats (Avena sativa) for, 92–95,
    110
oysters for, 97–98
Panax ginseng for, 109
Pausinstalia yohimbe for, 100
plant sterols and, 98
Policias fruticosum for, 106, 110
Pthychopetalum ocaloides for,
    99–101
Sexativa for sexual health, 110
Smilax officinalis for, 98
Spanish Fly for, 102–103
stimulants, 102–109
testes (animal) ingestion for,
    98–99
testosterone and, 96, 103,
    108–109
Texterex for sexual health, 110
tyrosine for, 46
vitamin B_3 for, 51
vitamin B_6 for, 47, 173
for women, 107–109
zinc for, 97–98, 328
Sexativa for sexual health, 110
Shafer, O., 207–208
Shannon, James M., 12
Shark cartilage, 205–206
Shark liver oil, 198
Shay, J., 259
Sherwin, Barbara, 109
Shingles (herpes-zoster), 123–125,
    195, 225
Shortness of breath, 311
Shulman, Robert, 16